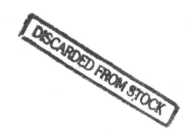

THE PAIN MANAGEMENT HANDBOOK

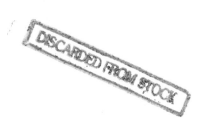

CURRENT ◊ CLINICAL ◊ PRACTICE

THE PAIN MANAGEMENT HANDBOOK

A CONCISE GUIDE TO DIAGNOSIS AND TREATMENT

Edited by

M. ERIC GERSHWIN, MD
and

MAURICE E. HAMILTON, MD
University of California, Davis, CA

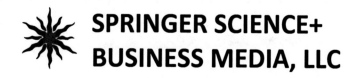

SPRINGER SCIENCE+
BUSINESS MEDIA, LLC

This volume is dedicated by M. Eric Gershwin to his mother, "Gary," for her loving dedication and by Maurice E. Hamilton to the memory of his sister Karen.

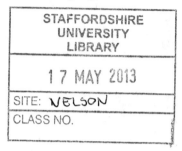
ISBN 978-1-4612-7287-8   ISBN 978-1-4612-1796-1 (eBook)
DOI 10.1007/978-1-4612-1796-1

© 1998 Springer Science+Business Media New York
Originally published by Humana Press Inc. in 1998
Softcover reprint of the hardcover 1st edition 1998

For additional copies, pricing for bulk purchases, and/or information about other Humana titles, contact Humana at the above address or at any of the following numbers: Tel: 973-256-1699; Fax: 973-256-8341; E-mail: humana@humanapr.com

Due diligence has been taken by the publishers, editors, and authors of this book to assure the accuracy of the information published and to describe generally accepted practices. The contributors herein have carefully checked to ensure that the drug selections and dosages set forth in this text are accurate and in accord with the standards accepted at the time of publication. Notwithstanding, as new research, changes in government regulations, and knowledge from clinical experience relating to drug therapy and drug reactions constantly occurs, the reader is advised to check the product information provided by the manufacturer of each drug for any change in dosages or for additional warnings and contraindications. This is of utmost importance when the recommended drug herein is a new or infrequently used drug. It is the responsibility of the treating physician to determine dosages and treatment strategies for individual patients. Further it is the responsibility of the health care provider to ascertain the Food and Drug Administration status of each drug or device used in their clinical practice. The publisher, editors, and authors are not responsible for errors or omissions or for any consequences from the application of the information presented in this book and make no warranty, express or implied, with respect to the contents in this publication.

Cover design by Patricia F. Cleary

This publication is printed on acid-free paper.∞
ANSI Z39.48-1984 (American National Standards Institute) Permanence of Paper for Printed Library Materials.

PREFACE

Those who do not feel pain seldom think that it is felt.

SAMUEL JOHNSON, *The Rambler,* no. 48 (September 1, 1750)

Who among us has not experienced the suffering of a patient with chronic disease, who in addition to the vicissitudes of fatigue, anxiety, and frustration, must also deal with the suffering of pain? Who among us has not considered, and then reconsidered, whether a patient's complaints are worthy of a narcotic and thence worried about the social and legal implications of chronic use? Who among us has not refused pain medications to our patients for fear that use was turning into abuse? Finally, who among us would not have liked a clinical guide to a myriad of syndromes, all of which have pain as their common denominator, in the hopes of developing some strategy to prioritize treatment.

Our purpose in preparing *The Pain Management Handbook* is to provide the information needed by clinicians to develop strategies that optimize pain management. It is the goal of the editors and authors that the present handbook, above all else, will be clinically useful. Its aim is to provide *practical* information regarding the diagnosis and treatment of disorders causing pain, along with tables and graphics to provide the busy practitioner with *rapid* access to *relevant* data. The reader should be able to initiate appropriate diagnostic tests and therapy on the basis of the information in this book without having to consult other references. It is not our intention to be encyclopedic, nor to discuss the pathophysiology of pain. For the latter, there are far more comprehensive texts available. Rather, we aim to provide a comprehensive yet succinct presentation of the causes and treatment of acute and chronic pain across a wide variety of medical conditions, one that is sufficiently detailed to provide all the requisite information, but sufficiently compact to be relatively portable.

We approach *The Pain Management Handbook* as specialists in internal medicine, family practice, rheumatology, neurology, anesthesia, cardiology, gastroenterology, urology, physical medicine and rehabilitation, and oncology—every writer here has had considerable experience in treating patients with pain. We believe that this perspective has helped us create a text that all health care providers will find a highly practical resource for the diagnosis and treatment of patients in clinical practice. Recognizing the diverse and multidisciplinary nature of pain treatment, we have provided multispecialty coverage.

We introduce *The Pain Management Handbook* with a chapter on the medical evaluation of the patient with pain, emphasizing aspects of the history and physical examination that are necessary to correctly diagnose the cause of pain. The following chapters offer a detailed discussion of the differential diagnosis of pain, presented by anatomical region in order to facilitate ready use of this book. Each chapter in this section summarizes diseases that may cause pain in the affected area and describes appropriate laboratory studies that will help confirm the diagnosis. Treatment of these diseases is discussed in practical terms, providing the physician with specific information (including medications and doses) necessary for bedside diagnosis and treatment. These chapters include coverage of pain in the head, neck pain, pain in the shoulders and upper extremities, chest pain, abdominal pain, pelvic, perineal and genital pain, low back pain, and pain in the hips and lower extremities. Where appropriate, reference is made to chapters dealing with specific disorders in more detail.

Causes of more generalized pain, such as systemic rheumatic diseases, are considered in a chapter devoted to musculoskeletal pain. Another chapter describes the treatment of cancer pain. We have also devoted chapters to postoperative pain and other causes of pain, including herpes zoster, postherpetic neuralgia, central pain, and psychogenic pain.

The penultimate chapter describes various general aspects of pain treatment. The pharmacology of analgesic medications is summarized, and adjunctive therapeutic measures, including physical therapy, acupuncture, biofeedback, psychotherapy, and multidisciplinary (pain) clinics, are reviewed. In addition, special considerations related to addiction and legal issues are addressed. Finally, because of the increasing issues of liability, we have included a chapter on key medicolegal aspects of pain management, including a brief discussion of euthanasia.

Many people helped us in the preparation of the book, especially our thoughtful contributors, all from the University of California at Davis. However, we especially want to thank Nikki Phipps, who assembled the manuscripts and typed many of them. Finally, a debt of gratitude is owed Paul Dolgert, our editor at Humana, who encouraged this project and helped in its timely delivery. Whatever flaws, errors, or shortcomings that may yet be found here are ours alone.

M. Eric Gershwin, MD
Maurice E. Hamilton, MD

CONTENTS

CONTRIBUTORS

EZRA A. AMSTERDAM, MD • *Division of Cardiovascular Medicine, University of California at Davis School of Medicine, Davis, CA*

SUSAN L. BALLARD, JD • *Charles Bond & Associates, Berkeley, CA*

CHARLES BOND, JD • *Charles Bond & Associates, Berkeley, CA*

SCOTT CHRISTENSEN, MD • *Division of Hematology and Oncology and the West Coast Center of Palliative Education, University of California at Davis School of Medicine, Davis, CA*

DENNIS L. FUNG, MD • *Department of Anesthesiology, University of California at Davis School of Medicine, Davis, CA*

M. ERIC GERSHWIN, MD • *Division Chief, Rheumatology, Allergy and Clinical Immunology, University of California at Davis, School of Medicine, Davis, CA*

MAURICE E. HAMILTON, MD • *Division of Rheumatology, Allergy and Clinical Immunology, University of California at Davis School of Medicine, Davis, CA*

E. RALPH JOHNSON, MD • *Department of Physical Medicine and Rehabilitation, University of California at Davis School of Medicine, Davis, CA*

JAE H. KIM, MD • *Department of Urology, University of California at Davis School of Medicine, Davis, CA*

JAMES C. LEEK, MD • *Division of Rheumatology, Allergy and Immunology, University of California at Davis School of Medicine, Davis, CA*

WILLIAM R. LEWIS, MD • *Division of Cardiovascular Medicine, Department of Internal Medicine, University of California at Davis School of Medicine, Davis, CA*

JOHN LINDER, LCSW • *Division of Hematology and the West Coast Center of Palliative Education, University of California at Davis School of Medicine, Davis, CA*

FREDERICK J. MEYERS, MD • *Division of Hematology and Oncology and the West Coast Center of Palliative Education, University of California at Davis School of Medicine, Davis, CA*

JOHN MEYERS, PHARM DD • *Pharmaceutical Services, Division of Hematology and Oncology and the West Coast Center of Palliative Education, University of California at Davis School of Medicine, Davis, CA*

STANLEY M. NAGUWA, MD • *Division of Rheumatology, Allergy and Immunology, University of California at Davis School of Medicine, Davis, CA*

R. ERICK PECHA, MD • *Division of Gastroenterology, University of California at Davis School of Medicine, Davis, CA*

THOMAS PRINDIVILLE, MD • *Division of Gastroenterology, University of California at Davis School of Medicine, Davis, CA*

STEVEN RICHEIMER, MD • *Department of Anesthesiology, University of California at Davis School of Medicine, Davis, CA*

ANTHONY R. STONE, MBCHB, FRCS(ED) • *Department of Urology, University of California at Davis School of Medicine, Davis, CA*

VIVIANE UGALDE, MD • *Department of Physical Medicine and Rehabilitation, University of California at Davis School of Medicine, Davis, CA*

N. VIJAYAN, MD • *University of California at Davis Headache Clinic, University of California at Davis School of Medicine, Davis, CA*

RICHARD H. WHITE, MD • *Division of General Medicine, University of California at Davis School of Medicine, Davis, CA*

1 THE ASSESSMENT OF THE PATIENT WITH PAIN

STEVEN H. RICHEIMER, MD

Key Points

- The primary categories of pain are nociceptive and neuropathic.
- The assessment should focus on understanding the category, cause, and additional emotional and environmental factors that relate to the patients's pain.
- Nociceptive pain is usually very responsive to opioids and NSAIDs.
- Neuropathic pain may respond better to antidepressants, anticonvulsants, antiarrhythmics, and sympatholytics.
- Treatment of related emotional and environmental factors will improve outcomes.
- Examining coexisting medical and psychosocial conditions can help to prevent poor outcomes and complications.
- Careful taking of the history and performance of the physical examination should provide the critical diagnostic information.
- Pain medications have considerable potential for side effects and drug interactions. It is important to obtain careful medication histories.
- The evaluation should include a screening assessment of the patient's psychological state, which can uncover signs that more formal psychological assessment is needed.

OVERVIEW

Core Questions to Be Answered as Part of a Pain Assessment

1. What is the type or category of pain?
2. Is there a primary cause of the pain?
3. What additional factors are contributing to the pain?
4. Are treatments available for the primary cause of the pain?
5. Are treatments available for the additional factors which contribute to the pain?
6. Are there other medical or psychosocial conditions that should influence the choice of treatment?

Table 1
Categories of Pain

Nociceptive
 Somatic
  Constant, aching, gnawing, throbbing, well-localized
 Visceral
  Paroxysmal, deep, aching, squeezing, poorly localized
Neuropathic
 Burning, lacinating, electric
 Follows nervous system injury or malfunction
 Central
  May result from chronic pain and persist after healing
 Peripheral

The Methodology of the Pain Assessment

1. History.
2. Past medical history.
3. Current medications.
4. Physical examination.
5. Special tests.
6. Psychological evaluation.
7. Differential diagnosis.

INTRODUCTION

The basics of the assessment of pain are the same as the assessment of other medical complaints. Yet pain is the most common complaint that presents to the primary care practitioner; therefore, it is valuable to give some focused attention to the specifics of the methodology for assessing this problem.

CORE QUESTIONS TO BE ANSWERED AS PART OF A PAIN ASSESSMENT

What Is the Type or Category of Pain? (Table 1) (1)

Nociceptive Pain

This is the typical pain that we have all experienced. It is the signal of tissue irritation, impending injury, or actual injury. Nociceptors in the affected area are activated and then transmit signals via the peripheral nerves and the spinal cord to the brain. Complex spinal reflexes (withdrawal) may be activated, followed by perception, cognitive and affective responses, and possibly voluntary action. The pain is typically perceived as related to the specific stimulus (hot, sharp, and so on) or with an aching or throbbing quality. Visceral pain is a subtype of nociceptive pain. It tends to be paroxysmal and poorly localized, as opposed to somatic pain, which is more constant and well-localized. Nociceptive pain is usually time limited—arthritis is a notable exception—and tends to respond well to treatment with opioids.

Table 2
Neuropathic Pain Problems

Postherpetic neuralgia
Reflex sympathetic dystrophy/causalgia
Cancer pain components
Phantom limb pain
Neuroma
Trigeminal neuralgia
Entrapment neuropathy
Peripheral neuropathy
  Diabetic, alcoholic
Myelopathy—posttraumatic, HIV

Neuropathic Pain (Tables 1 and 2)

Neuropathic pain is the result of a malfunction somewhere in the nervous system. The site of the nervous system injury or malfunction can be either in the peripheral or in the central nervous system. The pain is often triggered by an injury, but this injury may not clearly involve the nervous system, and the pain may persist for months or years beyond the apparent healing of any damaged tissues. In this setting, pain signals no longer represent ongoing or impending injury. The pain frequently has burning, lancinating, or electric shock qualities. Persistent allodynia—pain resulting from a nonpainful stimulus, such as light touch—is also a common characteristic of neuropathic pain. Neuropathic pain is frequently chronic, tending to have a less robust response to treatment with opioids.

Psychogenic Pain

The use of this category should be reserved for those rare situations in which it is clear that no somatic disorder is present. It is universal that psychological factors play a role in the perception and complaint of pain. These psychological factors may lead to an exaggerated or histrionic presentation of the pain problem; but, even in these circumstances, it is rare that the psychological factors represent the exclusive etiology of the patient's pain.

Mixed Category Pain

In some conditions the pain appears to be caused by a complex mixture of nociceptive and neuropathic factors. An initial nervous system dysfunction or injury may trigger the neural release of inflammatory mediators and subsequent neurogenic inflammation. For example, migraine headaches probably represent a mixture of neuropathic and nociceptive pain. Myofascial pain is probably secondary to nociceptive input from the muscles, but the abnormal muscle activity may be the result of neuropathic conditions. Chronic pain, including chronic myofascial pain, may cause the development of ongoing representations of pain within the central nervous system (CNS) which are independent of signals from the periphery. This is called the centralization or encephalization of pain.

Is There a Primary Cause of the Pain?

After determining if the pain is most likely nociceptive or neuropathic, the next step is to determine, as precisely as possible, the cause or specific source of the pain. Frequently, reversible causes can be identified. Nociceptive pain indicates ongoing or impending injury; therefore, identification and removal or treatment of the problem is critical. Is there an underlying sprain, tear, fracture, infection, obstruction, or foreign body? Is there inflammation caused by an underlying arthritic or autoimmune disorder? Myofascial pain may indicate abnormal acute or chronic muscle stresses. Neuropathic pain may also be caused by injury, but the injury in that case is actually to the nervous system. Nerves can be infiltrated or compressed by tumors, strangulated by scar tissue, or inflamed by infection. Some of these, and other neuropathic etiologies, may also be reversible. Usually, neuropathic problems are not fully reversible, but partial improvement is often possible with proper treatment. For example, neuromas may respond to excision or ablation; phantom pain may respond to transcutaneous nerve stimulation (TENS); and peripheral neuropathy may respond to tricyclic antidepressants.

What Additional Factors Are Contributing to the Pain?

For most of the last 300 yr, our understanding of pain has been dominated by the Cartesian model. Viewed from this perspective, the human body is a complex machine separate and distinct from the mind and the process of perception. Therefore, physical pain is a function of the mechanics of the body. In the last 30 yr, we have come to appreciate that pain is an experience rather than a bodily function. Experience is a function of the mind; therefore, the experience of pain cannot be separated from the patient's mental state, including their social–cultural background. We now know that environmental and mental factors can be so critical that they can actually trigger or abolish the experience of pain, independent of what is occurring in the body *(2)*. We now understand some of the mechanisms of how the brain can influence the spinal processing of pain via descending inhibitory and facilitory neural pathways. Furthermore, suffering should not be considered synonymous with pain. The emotional impact and distress caused by pain differs from person to person. Different patients may report very different intensities of pain for similar injuries, but even when they report similar degrees of pain, they may have vastly different amounts of suffering.

When assessing a complaint of pain, it is critical to remember that pain is an experience rather than a bodily function. Therefore it is valuable to investigate the appropriate mental and environmental factors.

Mood Disorder

Depressive disorders are found in approx 50% of chronic pain patients *(3)*. The patient may say, "Cure the pain, and I won't be depressed"; however, it would be a mistake to ignore the depression. Depression can significantly intensify the experience of pain and the associated suffering. In some cases, depression manifests primarily with somatic symptoms and complaints. Therefore, on occasion, depression may even be the primary etiology of the pain.

The Pain Cycle

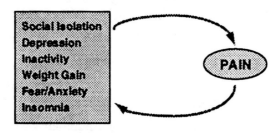

Fig. 1. The pain cycle.

Anxiety Disorder

Again, more than 50% of chronic pain patients suffer with anxiety disorders, which may alter the experience of pain and suffering *(4)*.

Somatization and Hypochondriasis *(5)*

Stress affects the bodily functions and sensations in all people. Emotional distress is often felt and expressed as physical distress. These processes, when predominant, lead to excessive somatic attention and communication in the forms of somatization and hypochondriasis. These can sometimes be primary psychiatric disorders or tendencies, but often they are part of depressive or anxiety disorders. These patients are prone to misinterpreting normal bodily sensations and to exaggerating the symptoms of illness. They are therefore more likely to believe that they are suffering from a catastrophic illness or complication.

Secondary Gain *(5)*

Patients with chronic pain undergo many losses—financial, vocational, recreational, and impaired relationships. They also incur benefits that may be financial or involve emotional support from friends and family. If the secondary gains outweigh the secondary losses, then there may be motivational factors impeding the recovery. These factors are frequently unconscious, and they are not usually the "cause" of the pain. Malingering occurs in those rare situations in which the patient is consciously lying about their condition for reasons of gain. Also rarely, the patient may be consciously lying about symptoms, but without conscious benefit or gain—this represents a factitious disorder.

Other Physical Factors

Other physical factors may also contribute to the experience of pain, including:
- Sleep disturbance.
- Inactivity and poor muscle conditioning.
- Weight gain.
- Other injuries or illnesses.

(*See also* Fig. 1.)

Table 3
Pharmacology
and Neuropathic Pain

Tricyclic antidepressants
Anticonvulsants
Antiarrhythmics
Sympatholytics

Are Treatments Available for the Primary Cause of the Pain? (7,8)

The physician will find it valuable to have some familiarity with the treatments available for various pain syndromes. Subsequent chapters in this handbook will help to find information regarding available therapies.

Nociceptive pain is usually quite responsive to treatment with classical analgesics such as narcotics, nonsteroidal anti-inflammatory drugs (NSAID), or acetaminophen. Frequently, synergistic effects can be achieved by combining these medications. For acute, nociceptive pain, regional or nerve block techniques may also be effective. Clearly, while analgesia is being provided, the clinician must be diligently searching for underlying sources of tissue injury, irritation, or inflammation. TENS (transcutaneous electrical nerve stimulation) units and relaxation training may also benefit the patient suffering with nociceptive pain.

Neuropathic pain (Table 3) also typically responds to treatment with narcotics, but less robustly than does nociceptive pain. Anticonvulsants and tricyclic antidepressants may be particularly beneficial. The allodynia (pain in response to a nonnoxious stimulus) and hyperalgesia present in some neuropathic conditions may, in part, be the result of the production of increased numbers of adrenergic receptors on sensory nerve terminals and on surrounding inflammatory and mast cells. Therefore, sympatholytics such as clonidine, prazosin, and terazosin may be helpful in decreasing allodynia and hyperalgesia. Antiarrhythmics—most notably mexiletine—may alter neuronal sodium channel conduction, thereby decreasing ectopic or abnormal firing within damaged, malfunctioning, pain producing parts of the nervous system. Referral to a pain clinic may be helpful in guiding further treatment or complex pharmacotherapy for the patient with chronic neuropathic pain. Other treatments might include nerve blocks, TENS units, biofeedback, and psychological and physical therapies.

Are Treatments Available
for the Additional Factors that Contribute to the Pain?

For pain treatments to be fully effective it is critical that all factors be treated simultaneously. If depression or anxiety are contributing, these are highly treatable conditions. Appropriate therapy with antidepressants or anxiolytics, together with psychotherapy, should be instituted early in the treatment process.

Somatization and hypochondriasis are more chronic and relatively more refractory conditions. However, here too, psychotherapeutic and possibly psychopharmacologic interventions may be critically helpful components of the treatment for the chronic pain patient. An understanding of these factors will also help to guide all aspects of treatment. For example, the patient who is prone to high levels of somatization is a relatively poor candidate for invasive treatments, since such interventions are likely to exacerbate the patient's somatic concerns and preoccupation *(9)*.

Secondary gain is not an illness, nor is it treated, but we must pay attention to this factor. The physician must be careful not to alter the balance of secondary losses versus secondary gains in such a manner that tips the scales in the direction of greater illness and disability. Psychotherapy may also help the patient to recognize that disability is associated with greater losses and fewer gains than the patient might consciously or unconsciously realize. Factitious disorders, when identified, indicate that treatment must focus on intensive psychotherapy (although it is difficult to get the patient to be compliant with such treatment). Malingering is a moral and legal problem rather than a medical problem, but recognition of malingering can help to avoid unnecessary, costly, and potentially dangerous treatments *(6,9)*.

Other health factors—such as sleep, weight, and overall conditioning—can also contribute to the problem. Like most of the above associated factors, pain can cause these problems and then, in a vicious cycle, be exacerbated by these same problems. Appropriate medical management focused on these problems can be most beneficial.

Are There Other Medical or Psychosocial Conditions that Should Influence the Choice of Treatment? (9)

The previous questions have focused on understanding the nature of the patient's pain and the additional factors contributing to the problem. It is important to consider what other conditions or factors (which are not directly contributory to the pain) might influence the choice of treatment.

Other medical conditions, such cardiac or pulmonary disease, may be relative contraindications for some medications or for various blocks. Examples include arrhythmias (especially bundle branch blocks) as a relative contraindication for tricyclic antidepressants or for right stellate ganglion blocks, bullous emphysema as a contraindication for intercostal nerve blocks, and pulmonary disease in general as a cautionary note regarding the use of narcotics (especially iv narcotics).

Psychiatric conditions may also influence the choice of treatment. A history of mania or bipolar disorder is a relative contraindication for the use of antidepressants; a history of recent drug abuse indicates a need to avoid narcotics or benzodiazepines where possible; and high levels of somatization or anxiety argue against the use of invasive techniques or therapies.

Some of the newer and more invasive pain therapies, such as spinal dorsal column stimulators and intrathecal morphine pumps, require that the patient have a good understanding of the medical condition and be highly compliant with complex treatments.

THE METHODOLOGY OF THE PAIN ASSESSMENT

The previous section reviewed the overall questions that the care provider should keep in mind when assessing a complaint of pain. The next section provides some of the specifics of the data-gathering process.

Table 4
Critical Elements of the Pain History

How the pain developed
The description of the pain
The location of the pain and any spread
The pattern of the pain over time
The patient's level of function and impairment
The previously attempted treatments

History (Table 4) (10,11)

How the Pain Developed

- Was there an injury, illness, or major stress associated with the start of the pain? This may give clues regarding any underlying pathology.
- Did the pain start immediately after the injury or was there a delay of weeks or months? Neuropathic pains such as entrapment neuropathy or complex regional pain syndromes (RSD) frequently develop weeks to months after the injury.
- Is the pain associated with any treatment or medication? Headaches may occur as a rebound phenomena, associated with the use of analgesics. Occasionally, physically manipulative therapies may exacerbate a painful condition.
- Has the condition been stable or deteriorating? Ongoing deterioration mandates a more aggressive search for underlying pathology and possible interventions. Worsening low back pain, especially with deteriorating neurologic signs, may require surgical intervention; this differs from stable, chronic low back pain, for which more conservative measures are usually more appropriate.

Description of the Pain

- What are the adjectives used to describe the pain? The patient's description of the pain can help determine the type of pain. (*See* the previous section on categories of pain.) The patient's choice of adjectives may also provide clues regarding the emotional impact of the pain.
- Are there associated symptoms, such as nausea or sweating, flushing, or sensations of hot or cold in the affected area? These symptoms may indicate a autonomic or sympathetic component of the pain.
- How intense is the pain? There is tremendous individual variation in the perception of the intensity of pain yet obtaining this information is very important to help gage the impact of the pain and to monitor change or progress.
- Standardizing the pain description. The Visual (or Verbal) Analog Scale (VAS) is the most common method for assessing pain intensity, and its change over time.

No pain ——————————————————————— Worst possible pain

The patient is presented with a 10-cm line, labeled as above, and asked to mark an "X" on the line indicating the intensity of their pain. The result is then measured with a metric ruler and scored between 0 and 10. The same scale can be given verbally by asking the

Table 5
Common Examples of Referred Pain

Origin of Pain	Referred to
Pharynx	Ear
Heart	Left shoulder, arm
Esophagus	Substernal
Diaphragm	Shoulder
Pancreas	Mid-back
Bladder, urethra	Perineum, penis

patient, "On a scale of 0–10, with 0 meaning no pain, and 10 meaning the worst pain you can imagine, how much pain are you having now?" These scales can also be used to assess the range of the patient's pain by asking them to indicate their level of pain at its worst, its best, and its average.

Similar scales are available for children. The FACES scale shows cartoon-like pictures of faces in various degrees of distress. The child is asked to choose the one that shows how much pain she is having.

Standardized, multiple choice lists of pain adjectives are also useful, especially in a pain clinic setting. The McGill Pain Inventory is the most commonly used of these. It may also be useful to ask the patient to keep a diary of their pain problem. The downside to this approach is that it asks to the patient to maintain a focus on their pain; this may be counterproductive to their treatment.

The Location of the Pain and Any Spread

- Pain drawings. Ask the patient to draw the distribution of their pain on an outline of the human body.
- Is the pain limited to the distribution of a root or peripheral nerve? Such distributions help to isolate the site and possibly the source of the pathology. Pain that does not have a limited distribution, but instead occurs in multiple sites or has a diffuse distribution, implies a systemic etiology.
- Is the pain in a stocking or glove distribution? A stocking or glove distribution does not indicate a psychogenic etiology. Such a distribution is entirely consistent with a complex regional pain syndrome (RSD or causalgia), or if bilateral with a peripheral neuropathy.
- Could the pain be referred from another site? Possibly because of the convergent structure of the nervous system, it is common for pain to be referred from a separate, possibly quite distant site (Table 5). This is most commonly seen if the site of painful stimulation or irritation is visceral or muscular *(12)*.

How Does the Pain Fluctuate Over Time?

- Is there any daily, monthly, or seasonal pattern associated with the pain? The physician is looking for clues as to the etiology of the pain. Arthritic conditions may be worse in the mornings and during cold seasons. Migraine headaches may occur in patterns associated with a variety of factors, such as stress or menstrual cycling.

- Are there aggravating or alleviating factors that lead to exacerbation or reduction of the pain? Understanding aggravating and alleviating activities can help to pinpoint the diagnosis or refine the treatment. Low back pain, which is worse walking uphill, suggests a diskogenic etiology. If the pain is worse when walking downhill, this points more to facet disease or foraminal stenosis. Some headache syndromes are triggered by specific dietary elements such as alcohol or monosodium glutamate (MSG). Identifying and avoiding these triggers can be most helpful.

What Is the Overall Level of Patient Function?

- Are there changes in the patients weight and sleep pattern? Such changes suggest the need to investigate further regarding possible depression or cancer.
- What is the patient's employment status? Issues of lost productivity and income or workers compensation may affect the patient's emotional and motivational state. It is usually a priority to enable the patient to return to work as soon as possible—vocational rehabilitation may be a crucial part of the treatment.
- What are the patient's daily activities? Understanding the day-to-day activities of the patient and what activities are limited by the pain will help the clinician to focus on the physical and psychological rehabilitation process. If the patient has acquired a totally disabled lifestyle, then it may be important to help the patient understand that he is capable of some productive functioning.
- Is the patient engaging in any exercise and physical activity? Physical activity is critical for preventing further physical deterioration. Exercise is often a crucial part of the treatment process; however, it is important that the patient's physical activities be reviewed, since some activities may exacerbate the problem.
- What is the quality of the family and personal relationships? Chronic pain may lead to irritability and personality changes. Such changes may in turn lead to the deterioration of personal relationships. Such problems should be identified so that interventions can be initiated. Families typically need some education regarding adaptive responses to chronic pain. Overly solicitous responses may reinforce the patient's pain behaviors and undermine the relationship.

What Treatments Have Been Attempted?

- Identifying prior treatment failures will not only prevent unnecessary repetition, but can also help guide the diagnosis. For example, if a variety of sympathetic blocks have not, even briefly, alleviated the pain, then perhaps the pain is not sympathetically mediated.

Past Medical History

In the assessment of the patient with pain, the past medical history should include the following information:

Do Other Medical Problems Relate to the Patient's Complaint of Pain?

For example, a history of diabetes or alcoholism point toward diagnoses of neuropathy. For headaches or abdominal pain, have there been any recent medication changes associated with the onset of the problem.

Table 6
Drugs Associated
with Tolerance

Opioids
Benzodiazepines
Barbituates
Stimulants
Rarely: local anesthetics

Do Other Medical Problems Potentially Affect the Choice of Pain Treatments?

As noted above, the patient's medical condition may present relative contraindications to various medications or procedures.

Does the Patient Have any Prior or Current Substance Abuse History?

Treating chronic pain with narcotics requires special caution with the addiction prone patient. In some patients it may not be possible to use narcotics except in the most dire circumstances.

Current Medications

Dosage and Pattern of Use

Obtain a complete list of the patient's medications and usage. Include over-the-counter medications.

Effectiveness

Note the effectiveness of medications. Analgesics (even if only partially effective) should lead to some increase of function in at least one sphere of the patient's life.

Drug Tolerance

The chronic use of some drugs is associated with tolerance (the gradual need to increase the dose to maintain the same effect) (Table 6). Tolerance does not imply addiction, but the development of physiologic tolerance can be hard to distinguish from inappropriate drug seeking behavior.

Potential for Drug Interactions and Toxicity

Acetaminophen (13). The analgesic ceiling for a single oral dose is reached at 1000 mg. There is the potential for hepatic toxicity; therefore, the daily use should not exceed 4.5 g, and extra caution is warranted if the patient is malnourished or abuses alcohol.

Nonsteroidal Anti-Inflammatory Drugs (NSAIDs) (14,15). Prostaglandins are important factors in the maintenance of renal perfusion in those patients with hypovolemia or reduced renal blood flow. These patients and the elderly are at increased risk for renal damage from NSAIDs. Prostaglandins help maintain gastric mucosal integrity; therefore, NSAIDs may also produce gastroduodenal damage. All NSAIDs may provoke asthmatic reactions in patients with underlying asthma or sensitivity to aspirin or

Table 7
Tricyclic Antidepressant Side Effects

Anticholinergic	Anti-α-adrenergic
Mucosal dryness	Orthostatic hypotension
Constipation	**Antihistaminic**
Urinary retention	Sedation
Confusion	**Quinidine-like**
Blurred vision	Cardiac arrhythmias and block
Aggravation of narrow angle glaucoma	

other NSAIDs. These drugs inhibit platelet function and are associated with increased bruising; they should be discontinued before surgery or other invasive procedures. NSAIDs are relatively contraindicated in patients treated with anticoagulants. There is increased risk of gastrointestinal bleeding, and coumadin levels may be altered secondary to displacement from protein-binding sites.

Tricyclic Antidepressants (16,17). The side effects and toxicity of tricyclics can be exacerbated secondary to drug interactions. Tricyclic levels are increased by the selective serotonin reuptake inhibitors, especially fluoxetine and paroxetine. Neuroleptics, cimetidine, methylphenidate, and estrogens may also increase tricyclic levels. Additive side effects may occur with alcohol, sedatives, or other anticholinergic medications (Table 7). Potentially fatal interactions may occur if tricyclics are given to patients on monoamine oxidase inhibitors (MAOIs). Hypertension and hyperpyrexia may occur secondary to administration with sympathomimetics.

Anticonvulsants (17,18). Carbamazepine has a similar structure to tricyclic antidepressants; it may weakly potentiate tricyclic side effects, and there is a risk of interactions with MAOIs (Table 8). Disulfiram and isoniazid may increase phenytoin levels. Phenytoin may displace coumarin from protein-binding sites and may alter digoxin levels. Propoxyphene may increase carbamazepine levels. Check for altered levels of other antidepressants.

Opioids (9,19). Opioid side effects (Table 9) can vary from one narcotic drug to another in an unpredictable manner for each individual. Meperidine, at doses greater than 1 g/d, is associated with the additional risk of seizures. Meperidine combined with monoamine oxidase inhibitors (MAOIs) can trigger a fatal hyperpyrexic reaction. Opioid side effects may be enhanced by alcohol or sedatives. Propoxyphene may also cause seizures, and overdose may also cause fatal heart block; furthermore, propoxyphene may increase carbamazepine levels.

Sudden discontinuation of opioids is associated with influenza-like symptoms of withdrawal:

- Restlessness & insomnia.
- Nausea & vomiting.
- Diarrhea.
- Backache.
- Leg pain.
- Yawning.
- Lacrimation.
- Rhinorrhea.
- Mydriasis.
- Muscle cramps.

Table 8
Anticonvulsant Side Effects

Carbamazepine	Phenytoin
Sedation	Rash
Headache	Nystagmus, diplopia
Nausea and vomiting	Drowsiness
Leukopnea	Ataxia
Thrombocytopenia	Hepatotoxicity
Agranulocytosis	Gingival hyperplasia
Aplastic anemia	Hirsutism
Hepatotoxicity	Facial coarsening
Stevens-Johnson syndrome	**Valproate**
Clonazepam	Drowsiness
Sedation	Nausea
Cognitive impairment	Weight gain
Ataxia	Tremor
Gabapentin	Menstrual disturbance
Sedation	Thrombocytopenia
Dizziness	Hepatotoxicity
Ataxia	Pancreatitis
Nystagmus	Interstitial nephritis

Table 9
Side Effects of Opioids

Respiratory depression	Sedation[a]
Nausea, vomiting	Cough suppression[a]
Urinary retention	Constipation[a]
Mental clouding	Euphoria[a]
Tolerance and dependence	Pruritis
Ileus	Biliary spasm

[a]These effects are occasionally desirable.

If it is necessary to withdraw a patient from an opioid medication, it is best to decrease the dose by approx 10% every 24–72 h; further individual tailoring may be necessary.

Physical Examination (10,11)

In pain assessments, there are rarely tests available that will "make the diagnosis." Instead, the clinician must rely on the presenting signs and symptoms. The history will often generate a differential diagnosis; the physical exam will often lead to the selection of the primary diagnosis; and occasionally a test will help to confirm this diagnosis. For example, an MRI scan that reveals an L5-S1 disk herniation is only helpful insofar as it confirms or contradicts the findings of the history and physical examination.

When preparing to do a physical examination, it is important to warn the patient as you approach potentially painful areas. It is also good policy to use chaperones whenever examining patients of the opposite sex.

Mental Status Exam

- Cognitive functions: Impairment implies the presence of delirium or dementia.
- Mood and affect: Provide clues regarding the emotional state of the patient and the presence of anxiety or depression.
- Thought process and content: Check if the patient is having suicidal ideation, or if there are signs of thought disorder and possible psychosis.
- Judgment and insight: Many treatments, such as the prescribing of narcotics or the use of relaxation training, require intact judgment and insight.

Vital Signs

- Vital signs are often elevated in acute pain.

Inspection

- Posture, guarding, splinting: If chronic, these behaviors may compound and exacerbate the pain problem, as the patient places abnormal stresses on the body.
- Color and pigmentary changes: These skin changes may indicate sympathetic dysfunction, inflammation, or a prior herpes zoster eruption.
- Sweating: Abnormal or asymmetric sweating indicates sympathetic dysfunction.
- Piloerection, gooseflesh (cutis anserina): Areas involved in neuropathic pain may briefly demonstrate this after disrobing.
- Hair, nail changes: evidence of neuropathic injury or sympathetic dysfunction.
- Swelling, edema: indicate inflammation or sympathetic dysfunction.
- Atrophy: may indicate guarding and lack of use, or denervation.
- Poor healing: indicates poor perfusion possibly associated with ischemic injuries, diabetic neuropathy, or sympathetic dysfunction.

Palpation and Musculoskeletal Exam

- Temperature changes: indicate inflammation or altered perfusion associated with sympathetic dysfunction.
- Edema: Subtle, subcutaneous edema can be appreciated by wrinkling the skin over affected and unaffected areas. Affected areas will not wrinkle into fine lines, but will look more dimpled, like orange peels. This indicates neural injury with denervation or sympathetic dysfunction.
- Muscle tenderness: Examination of muscles may reveal tender areas or actual trigger points. The extent of the tenderness and the amount of pressure required to elicit pain should be observed. Reproduction of the patient's characteristic pain is particularly noteworthy.
- Joints: can be examined for effusions, ROM, and pain with compression or distraction.

Table 10
Upper Extremities[a]

C5	Motor	Raised elbows (axillary n.)
	Reflex	Biceps (musculocutaneous n.)
	Sensory	Upper, lateral arm, near/over deltoid (axillary n.)
	Pain	Upper, lateral arm, never below elbow
C6	Motor	Elbow supination (radial n.) / pronation (median n.)
	Reflex	Brachioradialis (radial n.)
	Sensory	Lateral forearm (musculocutaneous n.)
	Pain	Lower lateral arm, possibly into thumb
C7	Motor	Elbow extension (radial n.)
	Reflex	Triceps (radial n.)
	Sensory	Over triceps, mid-forearm, and middle finger
	Pain	Deep pain in triceps, front and back of forearm and into middle finger
C8	Motor	Thumb index pinch (ant. interosseus n. off median n. at the elbow)
	Reflex	
	Sensory	Medial forearm (antebrachial cutaneous n.)
	Pain	Medial forearm, into the 2 medial fingers
T1	Motor	Finger abduction (ulnar n.)
	Reflex	
	Sensory	Medial arm (brachial cutaneous n.)
	Pain	Deep pain in axilla & shoulder w/ some radiation down inside of arm

[a]Cervical spondylosis or disk protrusion can produce cord compression (upper motor neuron signs) or root compression (lower motor neuron signs). C5-6 disk protrusions are the most common cervical disk problems; they can compress the C6 root and also produce C7 upper motor signs.

Neurologic

- Cranial nerve assessment: especially crucial in the evaluation of head and neck pain.
- Physical examination for radiculopathy (*see* Tables 10–13) *(20,21)*.
- Gait: Observation of gait can help identify weakness or pain (antalgic gait). Distortion of the patient's gait may also lead to improper muscle use and strain, leading to further pain.
- Sensory dysfunction: Neuropathic pain is associated with nerve injury or dysfunction. Frequently, it is possible to demonstrate sensory impairment in one or more modalities, including temperature, light touch, sharp/dull discrimination, position, and vibration. The examiner should test the involved areas for at least one function of large fibers, such as vibration or light touch, and one small fiber function, such as temperature (using an ice cube or alcohol swab) or sharp/dull discrimination. The examination should also make note of the presence and distribution of abnormal pain responses (Table 14).

Peripheral Nerve and Dermatome Map (Fig. 2)

- Motor dysfunction: Assessment of motor strength can help identify neural injury and the roots or peripheral nerves involved (Table 15).

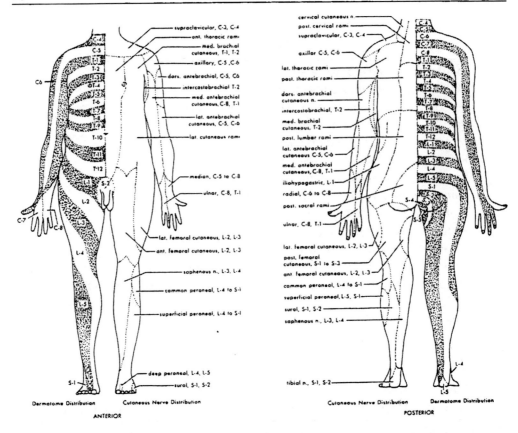

Fig. 2. System dermatomes. (From DeGowin EL, DeGowin RL. Bedside Diagnostic Examination, 3rd ed. New York: Macmillan, 1976; pp. 809,810).

Table 11
Special Tests

Cervical distraction—relieves pain
Cervical compression—provokes radicular pain from the foraminal stenosis
Valsalva—provokes pain, especially from central cervical canal stenosis
Swallowing—provokes pain, especially from anterior cervical spine lesions
Adson—diminished radial pulse with abduction, extension, external rotation
  of arm and head turned toward arm suggests thoracic outlet syndrome

- Abnormal Reflexes *(22): See* Table 16 for a grading of deep reflexes.
    1. Hyporeflexia.
       a. Focal: indicates lower motor neuron pathology at the level of the peripheral nerve or root.
       b. Generalized: peripheral neuropathies—diabetic, alcoholic, inflammatory (Guillain-Barre). Myopathy may also cause hyporeflexia.
    2. Hyperreflexia.
       a. Focal: indicative of upper motor neuron pathology; frequently associated with upgoing toes on testing of the Babinski's sign—this cannot

Table 12
Lower Extremities[a]

L2	Motor	Hip flexion (femoral n.)
	Reflex	
	Sensory	Often no loss, anterior mid-thigh (femoral n. and lat. femoral cut br.)
	Pain	Across thigh
L3	Motor	Knee extension (femoral n.), thigh adduction (obturator n.)
	Reflex	Hip adductors (obturator n.)
	Sensory	Often no loss, anterior thigh just above the knee cap
	Pain	Across thigh
L4	Motor	Inversion of the foot (tibial and peroneal n.)
	Reflex	Knee jerk (femoral n.)
	Sensory	Medial lower leg
	Pain	Across knee and down to medial malleolus
L5	Motor	Dorsiflex great toe (deep peroneal n.)
	Reflex	
	Sensory	Especially dorsum of the foot (peroneal n.)
	Pain	Back of thigh to lateral lower leg, dorsum and sole of foot, especially big toe
S1	Motor	Eversion of the foot (peroneal n.)
	Reflex	Ankle jerk (tibial n.)
	Sensory	Behind the lateral malleolus
	Pain	Back of thigh and calf to lateral foot

[a]It is important to note that lumbar disk lesions can only cause root (lower motor neuron) syndromes. Hyperreflexia is a sign of disease or injury at a higher level, in the spinal cord or brain. Ninety-five percent of lumbar disk lesions involve L5 or S1.

be secondary to lumbar spine disease since there are no UMNs in the lumbar spine.
  b. Generalized: suggestive of increased arousal, hyperthyroidism, drug toxicity.

Diagnostic Testing (24)

Radiographic

- No matter which radiographic technique is used, the results must always be correlated with clinical findings. As Table 17 *(25–36)* of diagnostic tests for low back pain demonstrates, radiographic tests are far from perfect and serve best to confirm a clinically suspected diagnosis.
- Plain films: Value is limited to demonstrating bony pathology; some soft tissue tumors can be seen.
- Myelograms: Involve the injection of contrast into the intrathecal space. For most of the common spinal diagnostic problems, CT or MRI are superior and free of the risk of postdural puncture headaches.

Table 13
Special Tests

Straight let raising—provokes radicular pain, lower slightly and dorsiflex the foot to again reproduce the pain

Crossed leg raising—raising the "good" leg provokes radicular pain in the "bad" leg

Kernig—flex head to stretch the spinal cord and provoke root irritation pain

Milgram—bilateral straight leg raising ×2 in., ×30 s, or Valsalva; provokes root irritation pain

Pelvic compression—provokes SI joint pain

Gaenslen's sign—knee flexed, lower other leg-buttock off edge of table, provokes SI pain

Patrick or Fabere—fully flex, abduct, and externally rotate the hip, provokes hip or SI pain

Homans' sign—dorsiflex foot of extended leg and deeply palpate calf for thrombophlebitic pain

Table 14
Table of Terms (23)

Pain	An unpleasant sensory and emotional experience associated with actual or potential tissue damage.
Allodynia	Pain due to a stimulus that does not normally provoke pain.
Analgesia	Absence of pain in response to stimulation that would normally be painful.
Anesthesia dolorosa	Pain in an area or region that is anesthetic.
Dysesthesia	An unpleasant abnormal sensation, whether spontaneous or evoked.
Hyperalgesia	An increased response to a stimulus that is normally painful.
Hyperesthesia	Increased sensitivity to stimulation, excluding the special senses.
Hyperpathia	A painful syndrome characterized by an abnormally painful reaction to a stimulus, especially a repetitive stimulus, as well as an increased threshold.
Hypoalgesia	Diminished pain in response to a normally painful stimulus.
Hypesthesia = Hypoesthesia	Decreased sensitivity to stimulation, excluding the special senses.
Noxious stimulus	A stimulus that is damaging to normal tissues.
Paresthesia	An abnormal sensation, whether spontaneous or evoked.

Table 15
Grading of Muscle Strength[a]

Grade 0	0%	Zero	No evidence of contractility
Grade 1	10%	Trace	Slight contractility but no joint motion
Grade 2	25%	Poor	Complete motion but with gravity eliminated
Grade 3	50%	Fair	Barely complete motion against gravity
Grade 4	75%	Good	Complete motion against gravity and some resistance
Grade 5	100%	Normal	Complete motion against gravity and full resistance

[a]DeGowin EL, DeGowin RL. Bedside Diagnostic Examination, 3rd ed. Macmillan, New York, 1976, p. 768.

Table 16
Grading Deep Reflexes[a]

Grade 0	0	Absent
Grade 1	+	Diminished but present
Grade 2	++	Normal
Grade 3	+++	Normal
Grade 4	++++	Hyperractive
Grade 5	+++++	Hyperractive with clonus

[a]From DeGowin EL, DeGowin RL. Bedside Diagnostic Examination, 3rd ed. Macmillan, New York, 1976, p. 791.

Table 17
Diagnostic Tests for Low Back Pain

	Accuracy (% agree with surgery)	Sensitivity	Specificity
		(range of estimates)	
Clinical exam	46–76	0.80	0.82
Radiography	34	—	—
Myelography	72–91	0.67–0.95	0.76–0.96
CT or MRI	70–100	0.80–0.95	0.68–0.95
Discography	30	0.83	0.63–0.78
Electromyograph	78	0.66–0.72	—

- Computerized Tomography (CT): more bony detail and superior to MRI for bone or joint disease of the spine, including foraminal bony stenosis.
- Magnetic Resonance Imaging (MRI): superior soft tissue contrast and superior to CT or myelography for diagnosis of spinal disk disease or neural compression secondary to spinal stenosis. Also best for evaluating spinal alignment, infection, or tumor.
- Bone scans: radionuclide bone imaging identifies osteoblastic activity and can help with the diagnosis of bone tumor or metastatic disease, osteomyelitis, fractures, joint disease, avascular necrosis, and Paget's disease.

Diagnostic Blocks (37)

- Nerve blocks with local anesthetics can help to distinguish focal from referred pain, somatic from sympathetically mediated pain, central from peripheral pain, and can help identify which peripheral nerves may be involved. This can help to guide treatment with further blocks or with other medical and surgical interventions.

Electromyography and Nerve-Conduction Studies (EMG/NCS)

- These studies can assist in identifying and localizing functional lesions of peripheral nerves, motor units, and muscle lesions. Such tests of function can be followed over time and complement the anatomic radiology studies.
- NCS generally reflect conduction in the larger, faster, myelinated nerves.

Somatosensory-Evoked Potential Testing (SSEP)

- SSEPs are better than EMG/NCS tests for assessing upper motor neuron diseases such as MS, syringomyelia, or spinal cord ischemia. SSEP testing involves the senses of touch, position, and vibration, rather than pain or temperature.

Other Quantitative Sensory Testing (QST)

- Pain syndromes may represent dysfunction more specific to the small A-delta and C fibers (Table 18). Testing of small fiber function is possible with devices that test thermal or electrical thresholds to perception and pain. Such testing is less invasive and may also be useful to monitor hyperesthetic responses.

Psychological Evaluation

As discussed earlier, the clinician should always assess the patient's psychological state and the emotions surrounding the pain problem. It is particularly valuable to inquire regarding:

- Neurovegetative symptoms.

  1. Sleep disturbance.
  2. Appetite disturbance.
  3. Loss of energy.
  4. Loss of libido.
  5. Anhedonia.
  6. Impaired concentration.
  7. Suicidal ideation.

- Impact of the pain on the patient's:

  1. Day-to-day activities.
  2. Work and finances.
  3. Personal relationships.
  4. Recreational pursuits.

Factors suggesting the need for more formal psychological evaluation include:

- Evidence of mood or anxiety disorders.
- Evidence of substance abuse.
- Evidence of psychotic disorder.
- Evidence of cognitive impairment.
- Evidence of overwhelmed coping capacities or suicidal ideation.
- Evidence of prominent secondary gain.
- Problems with hostility and anger, or a personality disorder.
- Suspicion of malingering or factitious disorder (e.g., inconsistent findings).
- Prolonged and extensive course of treatment failures.
- Need for high-dose opiates for nonmalignant pain.
- Assessment of suitability for aggressive invasive treatments.

Differential Diagnosis

After completing the data-gathering process, it is time to consolidate the findings into a differential diagnosis. During this process the clinician should consider:

Table 18
Nerve Fiber Characteristics

Fiber Type (Group)	Innervation/Function (1,38,39)	Myelin	Mean Diameter, μm	Mean Conduction Velocity, m/s
A-alpha (II)	Primary motor and propioception	+++	15	100
A-beta (II)	Cutaneous touch and pressure (and motor fibers)	++	8	50
A-gamma	Muscle tone (spindle efferents)	++	6	30
A-delta (III)	Mechanoreceptors, nociceptors, and thermoreceptors	++	3	20
B	Sympathetic preganglionics	+	3	7
C (IV)	Nociceptors, mechanoreceptors, thermoreceptors, sympathetic postganglionic	–	1	1

The meaning of inconsistent findings?

- Consider psychogenic or malingering diagnoses, but beware that the emotional turmoil that surrounds chronic pain may falsely suggest these diagnoses.
- Be cautious about reaching a psychogenic diagnosis simply because the pain symptoms cannot be understood physiologically. The clinical and basic sciences of pain are rapidly progressing—what is not understood today may be understood tomorrow.
- Be wary of obvious diagnoses or therapies that were missed by other clinicians. Check with prior physicians about their findings.

Do the signs and symptoms indicate the nature of the pain?

- Nociceptive—suggesting tissue injury or inflammation.
- Neuropathic—indicating central or peripheral dysfunction of the nervous system.
- Pain with mixed features—such as migraine or possibly myogenic or myofascial pain.

Summary

A careful assessment of the patient with pain should include efforts to categorize the pain, to determine its etiology, and to consider associated medical, social, emotional, and psychological factors. If the clinician can answer the six questions listed at the start of this chapter, then the patient will be well on the way toward receiving appropriate and comprehensive treatment.

REFERENCES

1. Cousins MJ. Introduction to acute and chronic pain. In: Cousins MJ, Bridenbaugh PO, eds. Neural Blockade in Clinical Anesthesia and Management of Pain. Philadelphia: JB Lippincott, 1988.
2. Wall PD. Introduction to the edition after this one. In: Wall PD, Melzack R, eds. Textbook of Pain. Edinburgh: Churchill Livingstone, 1994.

3. Smith RG. The epidemiology and treatment of depression when it coexists with somatoform disorders, somatization, or pain. Gen Hosp Psychiat 1992; 14: 265–272.
4. Fishbain DA, et al. Male and female chronic pain patients categorized by DSM-III psychiatric diagnostic criteria. Pain 1986; 26(2): 181–197.
5. Sullivan M, Katon W. Somatization: the path between distress and somatic symptoms. APS J 1993; 2: 141–149.
6. Fishbain DA, Rosomoff HL, Cutler RB. Secondary gain: a review of the scientific evidence. Clin J Pain 1995; 11: 6–21.
7. Moulin DE. Medical management of chronic nonmalignant pain. In: Campbell JN, ed. Pain 1996—An Updated Review. Seattle: IASP, 1996.
8. Tasker RR. Neurostimulation and percutaneous neural destructive techniques. In: Cousins MJ, Bridenbaugh PO, eds. Neural Blockade in Clinical Anesthesia and Management of Pain. Philadelphia: JB Lippincott, 1988.
9. Richeimer SH, Macres SM. Psychological and medical complications of chronic pain management. Seminars in Anesthesiology, 1996; in press.
10. Bonica JJ, Loeser JD: Medical evaluation of the patient with pain. In: Bonica JJ, ed. The Management of Pain, 2nd ed. Philadelphia: Lea & Febiger, 1990.
11. Donohoe CD. Evaluation of the patient in pain—targeted history and physical examination. In: Waldman SD, Winnie AP, eds. Interventional Pain Management. Philadelphia: WB Saunders, 1996.
12. Bonica JJ, Procacci P. General considerations of acute pain. In: Bonica JJ, ed. The Management of Pain, 2nd ed. Philadelphia: Lea & Febiger, 1990.
13. Drug Evaluations, American Medical Association, vol I., Pain Section 1994; 1: 29–30.
14. Kenny GNC. Potential renal, haematological and allergic adverse effects associated with nonsteroidal anti-inflammatory drugs. Drugs 1992; 44 (suppl 5): 31–37.
15. Mather LE. Do the pharmacodynamics of the nonsteroidal anti-inflammatory drugs suggest a role in the management of postoperative pain? Drugs 1992; 44 (suppl 5): 1–13.
16. Csernansky JG, Whiteford HA. Clinically significant psychoactive drug interactions. In: Hales RE, Frances AJ, eds. Psychiatry Update, Annual Review, vol. 6, American Psychiatric, 1987; 802–815.
17. Guze BH, Ferng HK, Szuba MP, Richeimer SH. The Psychiatric Drug Handbook, Mosby Year Book, 1992.
18. Abramowicz M. ed. Drugs for epilepsy. The Medical Letter 1995; 37: 37–40.
19. Sjogren P, Eriksen J. Opioid toxicity. Current Opin Anaesthesiol, 1994; 7: 465–469.
20. Hoppenfeld S. Physical Examination of the Spine and Extremities. New York: Appleton-Century-Crofts, 1976.
21. Patten J. Neurological Differential Diagnosis. New York: Springer-Verlag, 1977.
22. Weiner HL, Levitt LP. Neurology for the House Officer. Baltimore: Williams & Wilkins, 1978.
23. Merskey H, Bogduk N, eds. Classification of Chronic Pain, 2nd ed. Seattle: International Association for the Study of Pain Press, 1994.
24. Waldman HJ. Neurophysiologic testing in the evaluation of the patient in pain. In: Waldman SD, Winnie AP, eds. Interventional Pain Management. Philadelphia: WB Saunders, 1996.
25. Bell GR, Rothman RH, Booth RE, et al. A Study of computer-Assisted Tomography: Comparison of Metrizmide Myelography and Computed Tomography in the Diagnosis of Herniated Lumbar Disc and Spinal Stenosis. Spine, 1984, 9: 552–556.
26. Boden SD, Davis DO, Dina TS, et al. Abnormal magnetic-resonance scans of the lumbar spine in asymptomatic subjects: a prospective investigation. J Bone Joint Surg [Am] 1990; 72: 403–408.
27. Deyo RA, Bigos SJ, Maravilla KR. Diagnostic Imaging Procedures for the Lumbar Spine (editorial). Annals of Internal Medicine, December 1989; 111: 865–867.
28. Hakelius A, Hindmarsh J. The comparative reliability of preoperative diagnostic methods in lumbar fisc surgery. Acta Orthop Scandinav 1972; 43: 234–238.
29. Hakelius A, Hindmarsh J. The significance of neurological signs and myelographic findings in the diagnosis of lumbar root compression. Acta Orthop Scandinav 1972; 43: 239–246.
30. Holt EP. The question of lumbar discography. J Bone Joint Surg 1968; 50A: 720–726.
31. Hudgins WR. Computer-aided diagnosis of lumbar disc herniation. Spine 1983; 8: 604–615.

32. Kent DL, Haynor DR, Larson EB, Deyo RA. Diagnosis of lumbar spinal stenosis in adults: a metaanalysis of the accuracy of CT, MRI, and myelography. AJR May 1992; 158: 1135–1144.
33. Kortelainen P, Puranen J, Koivisto E, et al. Symptoms and signs of sciatica & their relation to the localization of the lumbar disc herniation. Spine 1985; 10: 88–92.
34. Modic MT, Masaryk TJ, Boumphrey F, et al. Lumbar herniated disk disease and canal stenosis: prospective evaluation by surface coil MR, CT and myelography. AJR 1986; 147: 757–765.
35. Tabaraud F, Hugon J, Chazot F, et al. Motor evoked responses after lumbar spinal stimulation in patients with L5 or S1 radicular involvement. Electroencephalography and Clinical Neurophysiology Apr 1989; 72(4): 334–339.
36. Wiesel SW, Tsourmas N, Feffer HL, et al. A study of computer-assisted tomography: I. The incidence of positive CAT scans in an asymptomatic group of patients. Spine 1984, 9: 549–551.
37. Boas RA, Cousins MJ. Diagnostic neural blockade. In: Cousins MJ, Bridenbaugh PO, eds. Neural Blockade in Clinical Anesthesia and Management of Pain. Philadelphia: JB Lippincott, 1988.
38. Bonica JJ. Anatomic and physiologic basis of nociception and pain. In: Bonica JJ, ed. The Management of Pain. Philadelphia: Lea & Febiger, 1990; p. 31.
39. Netter FH. Nervous system—anatomy and physiology. In: The CIBA Collection of Medical Drawings, vol. 1, CIBA, 1991; p. 157.

2 PAIN IN THE HEAD

N. VIJAYAN, MD

Key Points

- Head pain is one of the most common symptoms for which patients consult their physicians.
- Head and face pain can originate from any of the pain-sensitive structures within the intracranial cavity, scalp, face, or neck.
- Primary headache syndromes, which include migraine and tension-type headache, are the most common causes of recurrent or chronic headache.
- Migraine is an inherited disorder, which results in intermittent dysfunction affecting central neurotransmitters, especially serotonin-containing neurons, leading to physiological disturbances of the trigeminovascular pathways causing pain and other associated clinical features.
- Aura occurs in only 20% of migraine headaches and should therefore not be the major criterion for the diagnosis of migraine headache.
- Tension-type of headache may also be caused by a dysfunction of the central pain-modulating systems.
- Combination of tension and migraine headache is seen often in the same patient.
- Specific therapeutic agents appropriate for the type of headache should be used in their management, and analgesics should be used only as "rescue" medications in order to prevent dependency and "analgesic rebound headache."
- Cluster headache appears to have a different pathogenetic mechanism from migraine, even though several migraine medications are effective in controlling cluster headache as well.
- Even though headache is a common symptom in patients with brain tumors, brain tumor is a rare cause of headache.

INTRODUCTION

Head and face are the two most common locations where patients complain of pain. Most sufferers assume that pain in these areas is caused by a serious underlying illness.

Fortunately most of the common causes of pain in the head and face regions are relatively benign. Appropriate management requires accurate diagnosis of the underlying disorder. Clinical features and management of the most commonly encountered head and face pain syndromes will be discussed in this chapter.

HEADACHE

Headache is one of the most common complaints for which patients consult their physicians. It is estimated that at least 80% of the population have experienced headache at one time or other during their lifetime. Approximately 25% of the population suffers from recurrent headache requiring medical consultation or treatment.

Headache problems can be broadly grouped into benign or primary headache syndromes, which include migraine, cluster headache, and tension-type headache, as well as symptomatic headache resulting from identifiable underlying disease processes.

Benign or Primary Headache Syndromes

Introduction and Mechanism of Headache Pain

Primary headache syndromes are currently thought to result from a dysfunction of certain neurobiological functions without any demonstrable structural correlates. Pain is the end result of the changes inflicted on the target organs, primarily the vascular system and musculature of the head, neck, and face regions. Ground-breaking research done by Harold Wolff and his colleagues in the 1940s identified the pain-sensitive structures of the head and the mechanisms by which pain is elicited from these structures (*see* Tables 1 and 2) *(1)*. A knowledge of this is very important in understanding headache mechanisms.

- Pain can be induced in the pain-sensitive structures (Table 1) by the following mechanisms: blood vessels (traction, displacement, dilatation); nerves (pressure, invasion); ventricles (dilatation, collapse); inflammation of all pain-sensitive structures.

Overview of Classification

Most of the research work published in the past was difficult to interpret because there were no clearly defined criteria established for the diagnosis of different types of headache. This problem was addressed by the International Headache Society (IHS) in 1988 when the "Classification and Diagnostic Criteria for Headache Disorders, Cranial Neuralgias and Facial Pain" was published *(2)*. All the publications subsequent to that have relied on these criteria for the diagnosis of various headache syndromes. A familiarity with this classification will be worthwhile. Some aspects of the classification and diagnostic criteria will be detailed in the following sections.

Migraine Headache

Incidence. Current epidemiological studies conclude that approx 16% of females and 7% of males in the United States suffer from migraine headache. Most workers believe that this is a gross underestimation. There is no evidence for any socioeconomic differences in the incidence of migraine.

Table 1
Pain-Sensitive Structures

Scalp (all layers)
Muscles
Periostium
Dura (mostly basal)
Arteries
  Extracranial Dural
  Intracranial (proximal)
Veins
  Extracranial
  Intracranial
  Sinuses

Table 2
Pain-Insensitive Structures

Cranial bone
Diploic veins
Brain Parenchyma
Ependymal lining
Choroid plexus
Pia-arachnoid

Pathogenesis. There is increasing evidence that migraine is a genetically determined disorder.

- Recent studies report that the defective gene is located on chromosome 19 in familial hemiplegic migraine *(3)*. Until the actual gene is identified and its messenger defined, we cannot be certain about the actual pathogenesis.
- There is enough information available to support the hypothesis that the neurotransmitter serotonin is involved in the pathogenesis and that the serotoninergic neurons influence the trigeminovascular system, which in turn leads to dilation and neurogenic inflammation of the blood vessels. This knowledge base is expanding rapidly, especially since the introduction of designer drugs like sumatriptan for the treatment of migraine *(4)*.

Classification. Following is the currently approved classification of migraine *(2)*.

1. Migraine without aura.
2. Migraine with aura.
   a. Migraine with typical aura.
   b. Migraine with prolonged aura.
   c. Familial hemiplegic migraine.
   d. Basilar migraine.
   e. Migraine aura without headache.
   f. Migraine with acute onset aura.

3. Ophthalmoplegic migraine.
4. Retinal migraine.
5. Childhood periodic syndromes that may be precursors to or associated with migraine.
    a. Benign paroxysmal vertigo of childhood.
    b. Alternating hemiplegia of childhood.
6. Complications of migraine.
    a. Status migrainosus.
    b. Migrainous infarction.
7. Migrainous disorder not fulfilling above criteria.

- Migraine without aura is the same as "common migraine," and migraine with aura is the same as "classic migraine," according to the old classification. The former constitutes 75–80% of all migraines. This is an important point to remember because 80% of migraines will be missed if one insists that aura of migraine is essential to make the diagnosis.

Clinical Features and Diagnosis

- Diagnosis of migraine headache is based on the history, absence of any other cause for headache, and a normal neurological examination.

Typically migraine headache is a stereotyped intermittent syndrome characterized by the occurrence of various neurological prodromes or aura in 20% of patients, followed by unilateral or bilateral pain, which steadily increases in intensity and is associated with nausea, vomiting, photophobia, and sonophobia. The exact nature of the pain is variable.

- Even though throbbing pain is the most characteristic, that particular feature need not be present to make the diagnosis, provided other clinical characteristics support such a diagnosis.
- Headache lasts usually 4–72 h. Diagnosis of "status migrainosus" is made if the pain lasts for more than 72 h.

The following sections show the IHS criteria for the diagnosis of migraine.

DIAGNOSTIC CRITERIA—MIGRAINE WITHOUT AURA (2)

1. At least five attacks fulfilling items 2–4.
2. Headache attacks lasting 4–72 h.
3. Headache has at least two of the following characteristics:
    a. Unilateral location.
    b. Pulsating quality.
    c. Moderate to severe intensity (inhibits or prohibits daily activities).
    d. Aggravation by walking up stairs or similar routine physical activities.
4. During headache at least one of the following:
    a. Nausea and/or vomiting.
    b. Photophobia and phonophobia.
5. There is no evidence of an underlying disorder by history, physical, neurological examination, and, if necessary, after appropriate investigations to rule out such underlying disorders that might cause similar headache (summary of the actual wording used by IHS classification).

DIAGNOSTIC CRITERIA—MIGRAINE WITH AURA

1. At least two attacks fulfilling item 2.
2. At least three of the following four characteristics:
    a. One or more fully reversible aura symptoms indicating focal cerebral cortical and/or brainstem dysfunction.
    b. At least one aura symptom developing gradually over more than 4 min, or two or more symptoms occurring in succession.
    c. No aura symptoms lasting more than 60 min. If more than one aura symptom is present, accepted duration is proportionally increased.
    d. Headache following aura with a free interval of less than 60 min. (It may also begin before or simultaneously with the aura.)
3. There is no evidence of an underlying disorder by history, physical, neurological examination, and, if necessary, after appropriate investigations to rule out such underlying disorders that might cause similar headache (summary of the actual wording used by IHS classification).

- Diagnosis of migraine is helped by identifying triggering factors. One should however remember that these factors do not apply universally to all patients and that, in the same patient, these factors may not trigger a headache consistently. The most common triggering factors are:

    a. Alcohol, especially red wine.
    b. Emotional changes, especially "let-down" periods after stress.
    c. Hormonal changes, e.g., menstruation, ovulation, birth control pills.
    d. Too little or excess sleep, exhaustion.
    e. Dietary factors like chocolate, cheese, MSG, cured meats, and so on.
    f. Weather changes, e.g., barometric pressure changes, exposure to sun, and so on.

Management. A small percentage of patients with mild symptoms of migraine may not require any specific treatment. Changes in personal habits of eating and sleeping routines, adequate exercise, and improving general health status often will improve the symptoms.

- Specific therapy can generally be divided into abortive and prophylactic.

ABORTIVE TREATMENT OF MIGRAINE

1. Vasoconstrictors.
    a. Isometheptane mucate (4–6 caps/headache).
    b. Ergotamine tartarate (2–4 mg), DHE-45 (0.5–1.0 mg/headache).
    c. Sumatriptan (6 mg sc or 25–100 mg po).
2. Antiemetics (compazine, promethazine).
3. Sedatives (promethazine 25–50 mg).
4. Nonnarcotic analgesics (NSAIDs).
5. Steroids (short course in intractable cases).

PROPHYLACTIC TREATMENT OF MIGRAINE

- Before placing a patient on a prophylactic agent, one should document the frequency, duration, severity, degree of disability from headache, and response to abortive therapy. The decision should be discussed with the patient in detail, including the implications of daily therapy with drugs that may cause side effects.

The following categories of drugs are available for prophylaxis:

1. Beta-blockers (propranolol) (60–480 mg/d).
2. Calcium channel blockers (verapamil) (120–480 mg/d).
3. Tricyclic antidepressants (amitriptyline, nortriptyline) (10–75 mg/d).
4. Nonsteroidal anti-inflammatory agents.
5. Serotonin antagonists (methysergide 6–8 mg/d).
6. Valproic acid (therapeutic range of 50–100 µg/mL).

- The choice and dosage of these agents have to be individualized.
- The primary goal is to use a single drug and push it to the maximum, provided there are no side effects.
- Coexisting medical conditions will preclude the use of some of these agents. For example, one should not use propranolol in an individual with bronchial asthma or depression. On the other hand, a tricyclic may be a better choice in a person with mood disorders or sleep problems, and valproic acid in someone with depression or bipolar disease.
- If the major, first-line drugs (propranolol, verapamil, and valproic acid) are only partially effective, an ancillary drug like a tricyclic could be added. One should be familiar with the possible side effects and interactions of these drugs and discuss these with the patient.
- Another important point to remember is that many of these drugs do not become effective immediately; therefore the patient should be started on a small standard dose, which is gradually increased as tolerated over a period of 3–4 mo.
- Behavior modification therapy, including biofeedback, may be of additional help in some patients.

Cluster Headache

Incidence. There are no accurate data regarding the incidence of cluster headache. It is estimated, extrapolating from several small studies, that approx 0.4% of men (400,000) and 0.08% of women (90,000) in the United States suffer from cluster headache *(5)*.

Pathogenesis. The exact pathogenesis of this disorder is unknown. The two most common views are: (1) it is due to a functional abnormality in the hypothalamic region (the central theory); (2) it is due to abnormalities in and around the carotid artery, especially in the cavernous sinus (the peripheral theory). An inflammatory process in these areas has been suggested but is not proven *(6)*. Involvement of the trigeminovascular system, similar to migraine pathogenesis as discussed earlier, has also been implicated in the genesis of cluster headache.

Classification. There are two types of cluster headache: episodic and chronic variety. A third category is the "cluster-variants," which are cases that do not fall into the exact criteria satisfying the episodic and chronic varieties. Following is the IHS classification of cluster headache (2) and chronic paroxysmal hemicrania:

1. Cluster headache.
   a. Cluster headache, periodicity undetermined.
   b. Episodic cluster headache.
   c. Chronic cluster headache: unremitting from onset; evolved from episodic.
2. Chronic paroxysmal hemicrania.
3. Cluster headache-like disorder not fulfilling above criteria.

Clinical Features and Diagnostic Criteria

- It is a predominantly male disorder. The most commonly reported ratio is 1:4 (F:M).
- The mean age of onset is 30 yr, later than in migraine. Familial occurrence is rare. Eighty percent of patients have episodic type cluster headache.
- The brief duration of headache with strict lateralization and localization associated with typical autonomic disturbances make the diagnosis fairly easy.

IHS Diagnostic Criteria for Cluster Headache (2)

1. At least five attacks fulfilling items 2–5.
2. Severe unilateral orbital, supraorbital, and/or temporal pain lasting 15–180 min untreated.
3. Headache is associated with at least one of the following signs, which have to be present on the pain-side:
   a. Conjunctival injection.
   b. Lacrimation.
   c. Nasal congestion.
   d. Rhinorrhea.
   e. Forehead and facial sweating.
   f. Miosis.
   g. Ptosis.
   h. Eyelid edema.
4. Frequency of attacks: from 1 every other day to 8 per day.
5. There is no evidence of an underlying disorder by history, physical, neurological examination, and, if necessary, after appropriate investigations to rule out such underlying disorders that might cause similar headache (summary of the actual wording used by IHS classification).

- Episodic cluster headache occurs in periods lasting for 7 d to one yr, separated by pain-free periods lasting at least 14 d. Cluster periods usually last between 2 wk and 3 mo.
- Chronic cluster headache is diagnosed if the attacks occur for more than 1 yr without remission or with remissions lasting less than 14 d.
- The variant form called "chronic paroxysmal hemicrania" (CPH) predominantly occurs in females. Daily frequency is much higher (average cluster headache frequency is 1–2/d, whereas in CPH the average is more than 8/d) and the duration is much shorter. Other characteristics are the same, except that this variety of headache responds dramatically to treatment with indomethacin (7).
- Alcohol appears to be the only consistent triggering factor, if ingested during the headache cycle but not in between.

Management. Unlike migraines, most cluster headache patients require specific therapy because the pain is excruciating.

ABORTIVE TREATMENT OF CLUSTER HEADACHE

1. Oxygen inhalation (100% oxygen at 7–10 L/min for 15 min).
2. Sumatriptan (6 mg sc).
3. Ergotamine preparations (1–2 mg).
4. Analgesics and anti-inflammatory agents (rarely useful).

PROPHYLACTIC TREATMENT OF CLUSTER HEADACHE

Episodic cluster headache:

1. Methysergide (4–6 mg/d, maximum 6 mo).
2. Calcium channel blockers (verapamil 240–480 mg/d).
3. Steroids (short course with rapid taper, 40–60 mg/d for 2 wk).
4. Lithium carbonate (dose to attain usual therapeutic range).
5. Ergotamine tartarate (2–4 mg/d for a short period).
6. Indomethacin (75–150 mg/d for CPH).

Chronic cluster headache:

1. Lithium carbonate (dose to attain usual therapeutic range).
2. Verapamil (240–480 mg/d).
3. Intermittent courses of methysergide or prednisone.
4. Temporary or permanent denervation of trigeminal nerve.

*   A small percentage of chronic cluster headache patients may become resistant to all forms of medical therapy. In this situation, selective lesions made in the trigeminal pain pathways may have to be used for pain relief.

Tension-Type Headache

Incidence. The actual incidence of tension-type headache is not known. Mild and intermittent varieties of tension-type headache are very frequent and most of the sufferers do not seek medical care. This is thought to be the most common form of headache.

*   Chronic variety of tension-type headache can be disabling and require long-term treatment. This occurs at least as frequently as migraine headache.

Pathogenesis. Exact pathogenesis is unknown. It is believed that there is an alteration of central nociceptive system, which leads to the development of this type of headache. However, peripheral mechanisms in the scalp muscles may play a role in generating the symptoms. Some of the recent neurophysiological studies reveal abnormalities in the polysynaptic brainstem pathways, but it is not clear exactly how this leads to the development of tension-type headache.

*   Emotional and psychological problems are assumed to play a significant role in its pathogenesis.

Classification of Tension-Type Headache (2)

1. Episodic tension-type headache.
    a. Episodic tension-type headache associated with disorder of pericranial muscles.

   b. Episodic tension-type headache unassociated with disorder of pericranial
      muscles.
   2. Chronic tension-type headache.
   a. Chronic tension-type headache associated with disorder of pericranial muscles.
   b. Chronic tension-type headache unassociated with disorder of pericranial muscles.
   3. Headache of the tension-type not fulfilling above criteria.

The phrase "disorder of pericranial muscles" denotes the presence of tenderness in
these muscles.

Clinical Features and Diagnosis. Episodic tension-type headache is very common
and is self-limited. However, a certain percentage of patients experience these headaches
more and more frequently and progress to the chronic variety. Following are the diagnostic criteria *(2)*:
Episodic tension-type headache:

   1. At least 10 previous headache episodes fulfilling criteria in items 2–4. Number
      of days with such headache <180/yr (<15/mo).
   2. Headache lasting from 30 min to 7 d.
   3. At least two of the following pain characteristics:
   a. Pressing/tightening (nonpulsating) quality.
   b. Mild or moderate intensity (may inhibit, but does not prohibit activities).
   c. Bilateral location.
   d. No aggravation by walking stairs or similar routine physical activity.
   4. Both of the following:
   a. No nausea or vomiting (anorexia may occur).
   b. Photophobia and phonophobia are absent, or one but not the other is present.
   5. There is no evidence of an underlying disorder by history, physical, neurologi-
      cal examination, and, if necessary, after appropriate investigations to rule out
      such underlying disorders that might cause similar headache (summary of the
      actual wording used by IHS classification).

Chronic tension-type headache:

   1. Average headache frequency 15 d/mo (180/yr) for 6 mo or longer, fulfilling
      criteria in items 2–4.
   2. At least two of the following pain characteristics:
   a. Pressing/tightening (nonpulsating) quality.
   b. Mild or moderate intensity (may inhibit, but does not prohibit activities).
   c. Bilateral location.
   d. No aggravation by walking stairs or similar routine physical activity.
   3. Both of the following:
   a. No vomiting.
   b. No more than one of the following: nausea, photophobia, or phonophobia.
   4. There is no evidence of an underlying disorder by history, physical, neurologi-
      cal examination, and, if necessary, after appropriate investigations to rule out
      such underlying disorders that might cause similar headache (summary of the
      actual wording used by IHS classification).

Treatment of tension-type headache:

1. Muscle relaxants (intermittent use during flare-ups).
2. Anti-inflammatory agents.
3. Analgesics (less than 3 d/wk to avoid rebound and dependency).
4. Ice packs, stretching, and massage.
5. Tricyclic antidepressants (low dose therapy, 10–50 mg).
6. Behavior modification therapy, biofeedback.

Chronic Daily Headache

In the last few years a group of patients have been identified who started out with intermittent migraine headaches and eventually developed daily headache with intermittent exacerbations. This type of transformed migraine has been described as "chronic daily headache." This terminology has not been approved by the IHS as a separate type of headache in their classification. The common characteristics of these headaches evolved from an analysis of 615 patients by Saper *(8)*. These included the following:

- Headache starting out as typical migraines
- Over a period of 7–14 yr, patients developed features of daily tension type of pain involving the head and neck regions with superimposed acute episodes of migraine.
- Many of these patients had significant depression and overused analgesics.
- Eighty-eight percent of these patients had a family history of headache in a close relative.

Many investigators believe that this represents a combination of migraine and chronic tension-type headache rather than a specific entity.

Causes of Chronic Daily Headache

?Central abnormality
Emotional disturbances
Analgesic overuse
Vasoconstrictor overuse

Treatment. Preventing the transformation of migraine to chronic daily headache is the most important part of treatment. Using appropriate abortive medications, controlling the frequency of use of analgesics and ergots (not more than 3 d/wk) and using prophylactic agents when needed will play a significant role in prevention. Once the problem develops, treating the emotional aspects, withdrawing offending agents (especially analgesics and vasoconstrictors), and using prophylactic therapy are the cornerstones of management.

Symptomatic Headache

Tumor, Pseudotumor, Postlumbar Puncture Headache

Brain Tumor. Both physicians and patients worry that headache may be a symptom of brain tumor.

- In fact brain tumor is one of the least common causes of headache. Headache is an initial symptom of tumor only in 10–30% of patients, but rarely is headache the only symptom. As the tumor evolves, eventually up to 80% of patients do experience headache as one of the many other symptoms.
- There are no typical headache features that distinguish brain tumor headache from other causes. Most often it is a nonspecific headache *(9)*.
- Early morning headache with projectile vomiting has been described as typical for brain tumor. This is very uncommon.
- Tumors that obstruct CSF pathways (for example, those in the posterior fossa) tend to cause headache earlier than tumors in other locations.

Generally, headache in brain tumor lateralizes to the side of the tumor. Headache becomes more generalized once the CSF dynamics are altered.

Pseudotumor. Pseudotumor (benign intracranial hypertension) is a term applied to a condition in which there is evidence of increased intracranial pressure as indicated by papilledema, but investigations fail to reveal a cause for the increased intracranial pressure. Headache is the most common symptom of this disorder and is generalized and nonspecific in nature. It occurs most commonly in young, obese females.

- Loss of vision can occur as the intracranial pressure increases.
- Double vision due to paralysis of sixth nerve, which is a "false-localizing sign," may occur in a small number of patients.
- Brain scan reveals no mass lesions but may show small ventricles.
- Elevated CSF pressure establishes the diagnosis and, in many patients, lumbar puncture provides temporary relief of headache.
- The exact etiology is unknown, but there are several predisposing factors: drugs (corticosteroids, birth control pills, antibiotics [tetracyclines, nitrofurantoin, nalidixic acid]), Addison's disease, hypoparathyroidism, lupus, severe anemia, vitamin A intoxication.

Treatment is aimed toward lowering the intracranial pressure by use of large doses of acetazolamide (250–500 mg two to three times a day). Visual acuity and fields have to be monitored regularly. Lumbo-peritoneal shunt can be used to control the pressure if acetazolamide is not effective or visual changes occur.

Postlumbar Puncture Headache. Postlumbar puncture headache occurs in approx 15–30% of patients. This is due to continued leakage of the fluid through the rent in the dura leading to lowered intracranial pressure. Patients complain of orthostatic headache.

- IHS diagnostic criteria are *(2)*:

1. Bilateral headache developing less than 7 d after lumbar puncture.
2. Headache occurs or worsens within 15 min of assuming upright position and disappears or improves less than 30 min after resuming the recumbent position.
3. Headache disappears within 14 d after the lumbar puncture (presence of CSF fistula should be considered if headache persists after 14 d).

- Forced recumbency for 3–4 h after the lumbar puncture is the most effective preventive measure. In most patients, headache subsides with bed rest within 24–48 h, but in some it may last up to 14 d.

- Epidural blood patch is effective in majority of patients if headache persists.

Temporal (Giant Cell) Arteritis

This is a disease of the elderly occurring primarily in patients over 60 yr of age. Headache is of recent onset, persistent and often associated with palpable and tender scalp vessels.

- Headache may be associated with systemic symptoms like malaise, loss of appetite, low-grade fever, arthralgia, and myalgia, which is termed "polymyalgia rheumatica."
- Jaw claudication, if present, is a classical symptom of this disease.
- High sedimentation rate (over 45) strongly supports the diagnosis. Diagnosis is confirmed by temporal artery biopsy, which reveals giant cell arteritis.

Once the diagnosis is suspected and a high sedimentation rate is seen, treatment with prednisone (oral dose of 60 mg/d) is initiated and then biopsy done. Urgent treatment is important to avoid loss of vision, which is the most feared complication. Many patients may require long-term treatment before the steroids can be completely tapered off.

Posttraumatic Headache

Persistent headache following resolution of acute symptoms after head and neck injury is very common. The majority of patients recover spontaneously. In the majority of patients, headache results from injury to soft tissues of the head and neck regions. Headache due to involvement of intracranial structures is very infrequent. There are four types of posttraumatic headache described (1).

- Type I is the most common and is related to scalp and neck muscle injury. This has features of tension-type headache.
- Type II is the so-called "site of injury headache," leading to localized burning and sharp shooting pains of a constant nature overlying an area of direct injury to the scalp. This is thought to be due to entrapment of sensory nerve endings in the scar tissue (10).
- Type III has features of intermittent vasodilatory headache resembling migraine without aura.
- Type IV is a vasodilatory headache associated with prominent autonomic disturbances ("posttraumatic dysautonomic cephalgia") (11).

Often patients have combinations of these varieties of headaches. Treatment is symptomatic depending on the nature of headache.

Cervical Spine Disease and Headache

Patients with cervical spine disease often complain of pain radiating to the occipital region. This can either be due to irritation of the greater occipital nerve with features of neuralgic pain or secondary to paracervical and scalp muscle spasm.

- At times, pain from cervical spine disease can be primarily referred to the anterior portions of the head, most frequently to the temporal, periorbital, or frontal regions.

CNS Infections

Headache is a prominent symptom of meningitis, encephalitis, or brain abscess. There is nothing specific about headache associated with these disorders except that they all have other neurological symptoms and signs characteristic of the underlying disorders.

Stroke, Hypertension, Carotidynia, Pericarotid Syndrome

- Approximately 30–50% of patients experience transient headache in association with an acute stroke.
- Headache is more prevalent in strokes affecting the posterior circulation. Often the symptom of headache is mild and does not require any specific therapy.
- Patients with subarachnoid or intracerebral hemorrhage have severe and often persistent headache in the early stages.
- Elevated blood pressure *per se* is not a cause of headache except in situations of hypertensive encephalopathy (malignant hypertension), in which headache is common. There is evidence of associated increase in intracranial pressure with papilledema in these patients.
- Some patients with migraine headache complain of pain and tenderness over the carotid artery in the neck ipsilaterally; this is often referred to as carotidynia. Occasionally this may outlast the headache or may be more severe than the head pain. Appropriate treatment of migraine usually controls the pain.

A small number of patients have been identified who—following trauma, dissection or inflammation around the cervical carotid artery—complain of head pain over the frontal and temporal regions ("pericarotid syndrome"). Experimental studies in the past have concluded that stimulation of the carotid artery leads to referral pain to these areas. This can often be associated with autonomic disturbances due to stimulation or paralysis of the perivascular sympathetic fibers (12). Investigations to rule out structural abnormalities in the neck will be warranted. This may include soft tissue imaging and carotid angiogram besides physical examination of the pericarotid region. Treatment is symptomatic.

Exertional Headache, Orasmic Headache

- Physical activities that increase intracranial pressure can trigger intense but short-duration headache in some patients described as benign cough or exertional headache.
- This can be triggered by coughing, sneezing, laughing, straining at stools, stooping, lifting, or running. Headache associated with sexual intercourse (orgasmic or coital cephalalgia), especially at the time of climax, has also been described.
- Approximately 10% of these patients have intracranial tumors. Therefore these patients have to be investigated.
- If it turns out to be the benign form of exertional headache, treatment with 75–150 mg of indomethacin is often helpful in controlling these headaches.

Central Pain Syndromes Involving Head and Face

This entity refers to pain caused by an abnormality in the CNS, resulting in pain in the head and face regions. This can result from lesions in the thalamus or the spinothalamic pathways due to strokes, trauma, or demyelinating disease like multiple sclerosis. Upper cervical spinal cord and brain-stem lesions, especially syringobulbia, can lead to facial pain. Treatment modalities include analgesics, tricyclics, anticonvulsants like carbamazepine, GABA-ergic drugs like clonazepam, valproic acid or baclofen, and alpha-2 agonists like clonidine. TENS can sometimes be helpful in the short term.

CRANIAL NEURALGIAS

Trigeminal Neuralgia

This is the most common type of neuralgia and most frequently involves the mandibular and maxillary divisions. It is most commonly seen in 50- to 70-yr-olds. The pain is sharp and brief and can occur in paroxysms or individual episodes with a lancinating quality.

- Constant and continuous pain is not characteristic of trigeminal neuralgia.
- Pain is often triggered by talking, chewing, or a cold blast of air or touching the so-called "trigger points" on the face. There is no neurological abnormality on examination.

Neuralgic pain in the trigeminal distribution may be either symptomatic due to easily identifiable structural changes in the nerve like MS plaques, tumors or irritation due to dilated vessels in the posterior fossa, or a primary variety in which there are no identifiable structural changes. The majority of patients suffer from the primary variety.

- It is, however, believed that the majority of patients with trigeminal neuralgia of the primary variety may have dilated posterior fossa vessels impinging on the nerve. These cannot be easily identified by the usual investigations, but microvascular procedures with relocation of the offending vessel often seem to relieve the pain. This type of abnormality is found in 90% of patients during surgery.
- In glossopharyngeal neuralgia, pain occurs in the vagal-glossopharyngeal distribution involving the tonsillar region, base of the tongue, and larynx. Pain is often precipitated by swallowing.

Management of neuralgic pain can most often be achieved with medications. The most commonly used medications are: Carbamazepine (300–1200 mg), Phenytoin (300–600 mg), Lioresal (10–80 mg), Valproic acid (500–2000 mg).

- Carbamazepine is the most effective drug. In some patients, if it is not effective by itself, lioresal can be added to the regimen.
- Surgical procedures to interrupt the pain pathways and microvascular decompression are available if medical therapy fails.

TEMPOROMANDIBULAR JOINT DYSFUNCTION (TMJ) AND PRIMARY MYOFASCIAL PAIN DYSFUNCTION SYNDROME (MPD)

- The majority of patients with these disorders do not have any identifiable structural changes in the TM joints.

Primary symptom is pain around the joint and radiating pain in the temporal and adjacent facial areas. Pain is increased by chewing, and there is limitation of mouth opening (<40 mm). Clicking of the joint and deviation of the mandible can be seen on examination. Trigger points may be present in the muscles. Pain may be unilateral but bilateral involvement is very common.

- In the majority of patients, the disorder is thought to originate from excessive muscle tension with clenching and grinding and is seen in a setting of anxiety and depression. This is typical of MPD.

Malocclusion may result from or lead to structural changes in TM joints, which may set in over the long term. Primary disease of the joint (for example, owing to trauma, degenerative joint disease, or inflammatory arthritis) can lead to a similar condition in a small number of patients when it can be classified as symptomatic TMJ syndrome.

- MPD is best treated with antianxiety agents, antidepressants, muscle relaxants, anti-inflammatories, physical therapy, and behavior modification. Surgical treatment may become necessary on rare occasions when structural changes warrant this.

OCULAR PAIN

Tolosa Hunt Syndrome

- This is a rare condition associated with ocular pain and cranial nerve palsies causing ophthalmoplegia. This can occur in a recurrent fashion.
- This is associated with nonspecific granulomatous inflammatory change in the cavernous sinus and superior orbital fissure. Structural lesions in these locations may lead to a similar clinical presentation. Such lesions have to be ruled out before the diagnosis of this benign syndrome is considered.
- This syndrome responds to short courses of steroids.

Jabs and Jolts, "Needle-in-the-Eye" Syndrome, Ice-Pick Headache

It is common for patients with migraine headache to report occasional sharp shooting pains in the head or in the eyes. This may herald the onset of migraine or may occur concomitantly. This has also been observed in patients with other kinds of headaches like cluster and post-traumatic headache. In certain patients, these symptoms become very prominent and may be the main complaint. This may occur all through the day, often every few minutes. Even though the pain is brief, it is severe. The exact causation is unknown, but it is believed that this is a manifestation related to vascular headache syndromes of a benign nature.

- Indomethacin in doses of 75–150 mg/d is the most effective therapy in the majority of patients.

Glaucoma

- Chronic open-angle glaucoma rarely causes pain but leads to slowly progressive visual loss, which may go unnoticed for long periods of time. On the other hand, acute angle-closure glaucoma leads to eye pain, injection of the eye, dilated unresponsive pupils, clouding of the cornea, and decreased vision.

- Immediate treatment is required to save vision and prevent recurrence. Laser iridotomy is the preferred treatment in acute angle-closure glaucoma.

Inflammation, Pseudotumor

Inflammation of the ocular structures obviously causes eye pain. Inflammation of the iris, ciliary body, and choroid plexus occurs as a part of several systemic disorders, including ileocolitis, Crohn's disease, Whipple's disease, and systemic rheumatological illness. Direct infection due to various microorganisms can also cause inflammation of these structures.

- Nonspecific granulomatous inflammation of the orbital tissues leads to pain, displacement of the globe, diplopia, and formation of a mass in the orbit (pseudotumor). Ultrasound examination of the orbit helps in the diagnosis. This responds to steroid therapy.

Herpes Zoster and Postherpetic Neuralgia

Herpes zoster infection in the distribution of the ophthalmic division of the trigeminal nerve is common in the elderly or otherwise immunocompromised individuals. Eye involvement often occurs in these patients. Pain occurs both in the acute stage and also as part of the postherpetic neuralgia. Acute pain is related to the infection and involvement of the ocular structures, especially cornea. If there is severe infection, visual loss can result.

- Postherpetic neuralgia is defined as pain persisting beyond a month after the eruptions have healed.

Incidence of this is much higher in the elderly. The pain may occur in the eye and/or in the surrounding areas of the face. There are two types of pain described, one being the constant burning variety and the other is the sharp neuralgic type of pain. This may gradually subside or may persist.

- There is some evidence to suggest that treatment of the infection with an antiviral agent (like acyclovir or a similar drug) in combination with steroids reduces the pain during the acute stage *(13)*.
- The burning type of postherpetic pain best responds to local application of lidocaine cream and tricyclics.
- Sharp neuralgic pain responds best to drugs like carbamazepine or phenytoin.

Optic Neuritis

- Acute optic neuritis is associated with decreased vision and pain in the eye. Pain is usually temporary and is increased by eye movements. Pain subsides within a few days.
- The most common cause in a young, otherwise healthy, person is multiple sclerosis.
- Fundoscopic examination in the acute stages reveals either a normal disk, if it is retrobulbar neuritis, or evidence of papillitis with swelling of the disk.
- Prognosis for improvement of vision is excellent, with over 87% recovering vision to better than 20/40 within 6 mo.

- One of the recent studies concluded that a 3-d course of iv methylprednisolone followed by an 11-d course of oral prednisone results in the best visual outcome and reduces the recurrence rate *(14).*

Anterior ischemic optic neuropathy on the other hand occurs as a result of occlusion of posterior ciliary vessels. Patients present with acute onset of visual loss of an altitudinal type. Pain is not a prominent symptom. This occurs under the setting of generalized arteriosclerotic disease or specific varieties of arteritis. Treatment is aimed toward the underlying disorder.

FACIAL PAIN

Sinus Disease

Acute sinus infection or blockage of the drainage of the sinus cavities leads to pain, which is generally located over the involved sinus. Sphenoid sinus pain radiates to vertex, temples, and (rarely) to the occipital areas. An acute infection will usually have all the systemic effects of infection in addition to the local signs. Under these circumstances, diagnosis is easily made on clinical grounds. This can be confirmed by X-rays or, more efficiently, by CT scanning.

- Conservative therapy with antibiotics and irrigation generally clears the infection.
- Surgical treatment may become necessary in recurrent and chronic situations.
- It is not uncommon to see evidence of sinus mucosal thickening in CT or MRI scan in a patient with past history of infection, and this is rarely an indication for surgical treatment with the hope of helping nonspecific headache symptoms.

Atypical Facial Pain

There are several patients with chronic vague facial pain lacking the features of neuralgia. There are no clinical signs of neurologic impairment and investigations do not reveal any evidence of underlying pathology.

- This is more common in women, and most patients are anxious or depressed.
- Pain is resistant to the usual analgesic and narcotic medications.
- Small amounts of tricyclic antidepressants provide the best results.

Neuritis, Nerve Infiltration

- Facial pain may occur as a result of nonspecific inflammation or neuritis of the trigeminal nerve. This can occur in systemic disorders, including rheumatological illnesses. Usually this is short-lived and self-limited.
- Infiltration of the trigeminal nerves and its branches in the facial tissues (due to local malignancies like squamous-cell carcinoma) or infiltrative lesions at the base of the skull may lead to facial pain. This is associated with loss of sensation, and one may be able to detect the presence of the underlying pathology with clinical examination and appropriate investigations.

Ice Cream Headache

This results from ingestion of cold liquids or solids, which leads to rapid onset of sharp pain in the forehead and temple.

- This occurs more often in migraine patients.
- This is thought to be brought on by stimulation of the pain receptors in the posterior pharyngeal wall.

EAR PAIN

Acute Bacterial Infections

Ear pain with infections in the external ear canal is easy to diagnose and treat. If the pain arises from the middle-ear structures or mastoids, one will have to resort to otoscopy, tympanometry, audiometry, and radiological studies to arrive at the correct diagnosis. The pain also radiates to the surrounding scalp regions and sometimes to the whole half of the head.

Herpes Zoster

- Herpes zoster infection may be confined to the ear canal without facial eruptions.
- This is characterized by ear pain, facial palsy, and often loss of taste over the anterior two-thirds of the tongue (Ramsey Hunt syndrome). Postherpetic neuralgia may follow.
- Prognosis for recovery of facial paralysis is poorer than in Bell's palsy.
- Management is the same as discussed under zoster ophthalmicus.

Bell's Palsy

This is not a common cause of facial pain, but the majority of patients complain of discomfort and pain behind the ear in the early stages of Bell's palsy. No specific therapy is required for the pain itself in the majority of patients.

Relapsing Polychondritis

- This is a rare autoimmune disorder, characterized by recurrent episodes of inflammation and progressive loss of structural integrity of cartilaginous tissues. Ear cartilage is a common target for this.
- As the acute phase subsides, it may leave the patient with a drooping external ear. The episodes of inflammation are painful.
- This is a systemic disorder, and life-threatening complications like tracheobronchial collapse and severe aortic insufficiency may occur.
- Coricosteroid therapy usually controls the symptoms and patients often require long-term maintenance therapy.

DENTAL PAIN

- Dental pathology is not a frequent cause of head pain. However pain from infections or other diseases of teeth can be referred to the face and head. Often the diagnosis is easy because the primary location of the pain is in the gum or tooth.

- Atypical odontalgia is another entity that has been described as a syndrome of pain in a tooth where there is no identifiable pathology. Some investigators have suggested that this is similar to atypical facial pain. Others have suggested this may be a neurovascular disorder, similar to migraine or a sympathetically mediated pain problem. No specific therapy is available.

REFERENCES

1. Dalessio DJ (ed) Wolff's Headache and other Head Pain. Oxford Universiy Press, UK, 1980.
2. Classification and Diagnostic Criteria for Headache Disorders, Cranial Neuralgia and Facial Pain. Cephalalgia 1988; 8: suppl 7.
3. Joutel A, Bousser MG, Biousse V, Labauge P, Chabriat H, Nibbio A, Tournier-Lasserve E, et al. A gene for familial hemiplegic migraine maps to chromosome 19. Nature Genet 1993; 5: 40–45.
4. Moskowitz MA. The neurobiology of vascular head pain. Ann Neurol 1984; 16: 157–168.
5. Kudrow L. Cluster Headache. Mechanism and Management. Oxford, UK, 1980.
6. Hannerz J, Ericson K, Bergstrand G. Orbital phlebography in patients with cluster headache. Cephalalgia 1987; 7: 207–211.
7. Sjaastad O. Chronic paroxysmal hemicrania. Cluster Headache Syndrome. Saunders, 1992.
8. Saper JR. Changing perspectives on chronic headache. Clin J Pain 1986; 2: 19–28.
9. Forsyth PA, Posner JB. Headache in patients with brain tumors: a study of 111 patients. Ann Neurol 1992; 32: 289.
10. Vijayan N, Watson C. Site of injury headache. Headache 1989; 29: 502–506.
11. Vijayan N, Dreyfus, PM. Post-traumatic dysautonomic cephalgia. Arch Neurol 1975; 32: 649–652.
12. Vijayan N, Watson C. Pericarotid syndrome. Headache 1978; 18: 244–254.
13. Wood AJJ. Postherpetic neuralgia—pathogenesis, treatment and prevention. N Engl J Med 1996; 335: 32–42.
14. Beck RW et al, the Optic Neuritis Study Group. A randomized, controlled trial of corticosteroids in the treatment of acute optic neuritis. N Engl J Med 1992; 326: 581–588.

3 NECK PAIN

N. VIJAYAN, MD
STANLEY M. NAGUWA, MD

Key Points

- Carotidynia refers to pain and tenderness over the carotid artery in the neck. The most common cause is pain associated with migraine headache.

- Carotidynia can occur independent of migraine in patients who have a history of migraine.

- Carotidynia also results from local disease of the artery due to dissection, trauma, inflammation, or infiltration.

- Pain originating from the carotid artery is often referred to the same side of the face and head.

- Patients who have migraine history and carotidynia respond to the usual antimigraine medications.

- Compression or distortion of the cervical nerve roots can cause neuralgic symptoms. The most well-known are greater and lesser occipital neuralgia. Typical neuralgic (brief, sharp, shooting) pain is uncommon. More often there is a constant pain with some superimposed sharp pains.

- Degenerative disease in the cervical spine is the most common cause for cervical neuralgia.

- Pain from the cervical region can be referred to the chest, mimicking cardiac pain, or cardiac pain may be referred to the anterior cervical region, confusing the diagnosis.

- In rheumatoid arthritis, loosening of the C1-2 transverse ligament can create a dangerous situation.

- Osteoarthritis X-ray changes may be seen in the absence of symptoms.

- The neck may be involved in 50% of spondyloarthritis.

- Fibromyalgia may be the most commonly diagnosed etiology of neck pain in a primary care setting.

- Isolated osteomyelitis of the spine is uncommon.

- The severity of trauma is prognostic in neck injury, though in older patients comorbidities are a factor.
- Tumors of the cervical spine are usually metastatic.

CAROTIDYNIA

This term refers to a clinical syndrome of episodic pain and tenderness of the carotid artery in the neck *(1)*. The pain is most prominent in the region of the carotid bifurcation. Pain may radiate to the adjacent areas of the neck, face, and head. It was originally demonstrated by Fay, the first to use the term carotidynia, that stimulation of the carotid artery in the neck resulted in referral of pain to the face and head on the same side *(2)*. There are several clinical situations associated with pain in the region of the carotid artery:

Causes of Carotidynia

Migraine
Dissection of carotid artery
Inflammation
Trauma
Infiltrative disease

- Migraine patients often complain of pain in the region of the carotid artery during a headache, which subsides with the headache. Tenderness may be elicited in this location during and shortly after the resolution of headache.

Lovshin *(3)* reported 100 patients with "vascular headache of the neck" who complained of intermittent episodes of pain and tenderness in the carotid region. Sixty-seven percent of these patients had a history of migraine. Besides, there was a high incidence of positive family history of migraine in these patients. It was therefore concluded that this syndrome is a migrainous phenomenon with the same pathophysiologic mechanisms, causing dilation and inflammation of the carotid artery. Evans and Steinberg demonstrated distention of the carotid sinus in an angiogram during migraine, thereby supporting this theory *(4)*.

- Carotid dissection, spontaneous or traumatic, may be accompanied by pain in the carotid region. This can be associated with ipsilateral Homer's syndrome (ptosis and miosis), unilateral face and head pain, and (if there is significant occlusion of the vessel) contralateral neurological manifestations.
- Inflammation, especially of viral etiology, has been suggested in some patients with this syndrome. Roseman *(5)* described a group of patients with carotidynia that developed in association with symptoms of upper respiratory infection.
- Pain in the region of the carotid artery and headache on the same side has been described under the term "pericarotid syndrome," which may follow trauma or other pathologic processes in the region of the carotid artery *(1)*.

Specific inflammatory disorders like vasculitis can also be associated with a similar syndrome. Tumors, in or around the carotid artery, may also lead to pain in this area. Management depends on the underlying cause.

- Patients with a history of migraine respond to the usual abortive medications, especially ergotamines *(6)*. There are no reports so far regarding the use of sumatriptan, but (logically) this drug also should be effective. If the carotidynia is part of the migraine headache, no more specific therapy other than treating the migraine is required.
- In patients with suspected carotid dissection, angiographic studies to document the dissection and appropriate management should be undertaken.
- Specific type of vasculitic disorders can be treated with steroids.

NEURALGIAS

1   The classical trigeminal neuralgia (*see* Chapter 2) does not affect the neck region.
2. In glossopharyngeal neuralgia, the pain is often localized to the lateral aspect of the throat. Details of this disorder are discussed in Chapter 2.
3. Distortion or compression of the cervical nerve roots causes pain in the distribution of these nerves.
    a. The most well-known of these roots that causes pain in the upper neck and occipital regions is the greater occipital nerve, which contains fibers from the C2. This nerve supplies the scalp almost up to the coronal suture. The lesser occipital nerve, with fibers from C2 and C3, overlaps the area of innervation of the greater occipital nerve and also supplies the upper pole of the pinna of the ear. Trauma and degenerative changes of the cervical spine are the most common causes for pain in the distribution of these nerves. Generally the pain is continuous and aching, with some burning quality. Superimposed episodes of sharp shooting pain are also seen in most patients. The typical neuralgic pain by itself is rarely seen in these situations.
        i.   Movements of the neck, compression of the cervical region by pressing down on the head *(7)*, and direct pressure over the nerve as it emerges into the scalp will induce or aggravate the pain.
        ii. It is rare to have sensory loss in this distribution unless there is severe damage to the nerve.
        iii. Occasionally, pain in the distribution of the nerve is caused by compression of the neurovascular structures owing to entrapment.
        iv. Cervical spine X-rays and (if needed) imaging studies will often reveal the cause. Treatment should be directed toward the underlying cause.
        v.   Local anesthetic and steroid injections have been used extensively in the treatment of pain in these areas, but there is no reliable documentation of the effectiveness of these forms of therapy by double blind studies.
        vi. Decompression of the neurovascular structures may relieve the pain if entrapment is present.
        vii. Symptomatic treatment with anti-inflammatories, tricyclics, and muscle relaxants may often be of help. In rare instances, section of the nerve may have to be done to provide relief of intractable pain if medical therapy fails.

Other causes of cervical root compression are:

    b. Compression of the upper cervical nerves owing such developmental anomalies as Arnold-Chiari malformation. Herniation of cerebellar tonsils in this anomaly can often be associated with upper cervical and occipital pain.

    c. Posterior fossa expanding lesions can similarly cause pain in the upper neck owing to compression of these nerves. Lesions in the region of foremen magnum (meningioma, basal invagination, and so on) may also lead to pain in these areas.

    d. Lance and Anthony (1980) described patients who developed upper cervical or occipital pain and paresthesia on the same side of the tongue on turning of the head. This was termed "neck-tongue syndrome" by the authors. Tongue paresthesia is thought to be due to the presence of C2-C3 afferents in the ansa hypoglossi *(8)*.

4. Herpes zoster and postherpetic neuralgia can occur in the cervical region. Refer to Chapter 2 for the clinical features and management of these disorders.

REFERRED PAIN

- Pain originating from the lower cervical roots can be referred to the precordium and may mimic cardiac pain. This type of pain can be reproduced by neck movements, which helps in the differential diagnosis. This is most often seen in patients with degenerative disk disease in the lower cervical spine.
- Pain of cardiac origin can be referred to the anterior part of the neck and jaw. This type of radiation may occur in the absence of the classical precordial or left upper extremity pain, making the diagnosis more difficult. Awareness of this possibility and the circumstances under which the pain occurs will help in suspecting a cardiac origin for the pain. Appropriate cardiac investigations will establish the diagnosis.
- Pain originating from upper cervical spine can sometimes be referred to the frontal and periorbital areas of the ipsilateral forehead. Patients with cervical spondylosis may thus present with frontal headache.

RHEUMATOID ARTHRITIS (RA)

Rheumatoid arthritis (RA) is a relatively common, erosive, inflammatory joint disease affecting approx 1% of the population. As many as 60–70% of rheumatoid arthritis patients have neck symptoms, especially with concomitant severe symmetric polyarticular peripheral joint disease *(9)*.

The hallmark of the pathophysiology of rheumatoid arthritis is a proliferative synovitis with lymphocyte infiltration and rheumatoid factor production. The process also involves the tenosynovium and bursae. In the neck, the synovium-lined apophyseal and uncovertebral joints are involved. The annulus fibrosis and vertebral disks may be affected by adjacent inflamed structures *(10)* (Fig. 1).

An especially dangerous situation can occur with loosening of the transverse ligaments that stabilize C1 (atlas) on C2 (axis). As depicted in Fig. 1, it is easy to see the danger. The loosening is felt to be a result of a bursitis around these ligaments. Perhaps more catastrophic than the posterior movement of the axis is the dorsal migration of the axis into the foramen magnum.

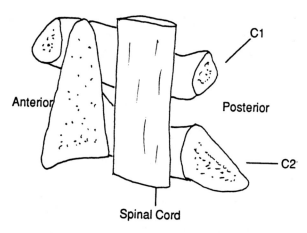

Anterior

Posterior

C1

C2

Spinal Cord

Fig. 1. Sagittal diagram of C1 and C2.

Plain films of flexion and extension of the neck are necessary to demonstrate any C1–2 subluxation, though caution must be exercised if a severe subluxation is suspected. Neck films should be obtained early in the course of RA and even in the absence of symptoms, as there is not a necessary correlation between X-ray changes and symptoms. As in the peripheral joints, the major portion of damage may occur in the first 2 yr of disease *(10)*.

CT scan and MRI are used when a more precise definition of structural damage is needed, especially its impact on neural structures.

Treatment of rheumatoid arthritis of the cervical spine is exactly the same as the treatment of the peripheral joints. NSAIDs and judicious doses of corticosteroids are used to control symptoms and swelling. Disease-modifying agents, such as methotrexate and hydroxychloroquine, must be employed early to affect the course of the disease. A splint (cervical collar) should be prescribed if there is any evidence of C1–C2 subluxation and the patient referred for appropriate rheumatology and neurosurgical consultations. Nonpharmocologic treatment, such as heat/cold or ultrasound, may also provide symptom relief.

OSTEOARTHRITIS

It is not unexpected that osteoarthritis would occur in the neck, with its complex anatomy and frequent motion. The neck moves hundreds of times per hour *(11)* supporting and stabilizing a heavy object (head) at one end while secured to a large base (body) at the other. Such a stressful arrangement would be expected to place the neck at a high risk for micro and macro trauma.

When the age-related changes of cartilage, bone, and vertebral disk are coupled with these stresses and trauma, degenerative changes frequently occur. The affected structures are no longer able to handle day-to-day motions of the neck and respond with structural changes. When imaged, these are seen as joint space loss, bony sclerosis, osteophytes, and abnormal bone alignment involving the vertebral bodies, disks, apophyseal facet joints, and joints of Luschka.

While these structures possess pain fibers, it is unclear as to where neck pain originates in every case, as X-ray changes may be seen in the absence of symptoms. In addition to pain, a patient may complain of neurologic symptoms if the herniating disk or vertebral osteophyte impinges on the spinal cord, or if the facet osteophyte narrows the neural foramen.

Diagnosis is made by careful history-taking and examination with imaging modalities selected to define the structural changes.

The extent of treatment should parallel the severity of symptoms. A patient with mild pain with little effect on the activities of daily living can be managed with analgesics or low-dose nonsteroidal anti-inflammatory drugs (NSAID). If there is secondary muscle spasm, management can include muscle relaxants, cervical collar, and gentle stretch of the muscle, either at home or at a physical therapy facility *(12)*. Heat and cold may also help with muscle relaxation and pain relief.

If the pain is debilitating or the neurologic symptoms are not improved with conservative management, surgical consultation should be obtained.

SPONDYLOARTHROPATHIES

The spondyloarthropathies (including ankylosing spondylitis, Reiter's syndrome, psoriatic arthritis, enteropathic arthritis) are a group of arthritides that share several features:

1. An association with HLA-B27.
2. Sacroiliac joint involvement.
3. Axial skeleton inflammatory involvement with syndesmophytes.
4. Extra-articular involvement of eye, skin, lungs, heart, GI tract, GU tract.
5. Enthesitis, inflammation of the transitional tissue between tendon/ligament and bone.

While the axial skeleton involvement is most commonly of the low back, the neck may be involved in 50% of patients *(13)*.

Clues that would suggest a specific type of spondyloarthropathy in a patient with neck pain include:

1. Ankylosing spondylitis: chronic low back pain, young male, bilateral sacroiliitis on X-rays.
2. Reiter's syndrome: large joint, asymmetric lower extremity arthritis; concomitant genitourinary tract infection.
3. Enteropathic arthritis: unexplained diarrhea, known inflammatory bowel disease.
4. Psoriatic arthritis: psoriasis (may be obscure and miniscule lesions in the umbilicus, gluteal cleft, or postauricular areas).

The neck lesions of the spondyloarthropathies are a result of inflammation of the synovium and entheses. The lesions may result in erosions, such as the "squaring off" of the vertebral body as a result of enthesitis at the annulus and vertebra interface. A later sequela of the inflammatory disease is ossification and the formation of syndesmophytes between vertebrae and ankylosis of the facet joints. Though ankylosis of the cervical spine may ameliorate the neck pain, the rigid spine is more susceptible to fracture with its neurologic sequelae.

Imaging of the SI joints for sacroiliitis and neck for the previously mentioned changes and investigation of extra-articular symptoms should allow the diagnosis of a spondyloarthropathy. There is a subset of patients who have minor sacroiliitis and enthesopathy but no distinguishing extra-articular features; they cannot be further classified. These patients may in the future develop symptoms to permit classification.

HLA-B27 testing is rarely required in the evaluation of a suspected spondyloarthropathy.

Though molecular genetics may in the future provide a cure for the spondyloarthropathies, medications are presently used to provide relief of symptoms, which is important to permit patients to exercise and maintain a near-normal posture.

NSAIDs are the primary treatment and high doses are often required, with serial monitoring for gastropathy, renal, and hepatic effects imperative. As a precaution, NSAIDs may occasionally worsen psoriasis and enteropathic symptoms. If the joint inflammation is not sufficiently controlled by the NSAIDs, then other medications, such as sulfasalazine or methotrexate (MTX), can be used.

FIBROMYALGIA SYNDROME (FMS)

FMS may be the most commonly diagnosed etiology of neck pain, comprising 2–5% of diagnoses in a primary care practice (14). Neck pain is part of the symptom complex that includes characteristic tender points, nonrestorative sleep, and fatigue. Three of the nine pairs of tender points as specified in the 1990 American College of Rheumatology (ACR) criteria for FMS involve the neck: (1) insertion point of muscles into the occiput, (2) upper border of the mid-trapezius, and (3) anterior aspects of C5-7 transverse spaces. FMS is associated with irritable bowel syndrome (IBS), tension headaches, and depression, as well as other nonspecific complaints. FMS may follow or be triggered by infection, injury, stress, or almost any illness (14) (Fig. 2).

The etiology of FMS is unknown. Several lines of investigation have revealed abnormalities in muscle structure, muscle microcirculation, and metabolism (15). Application of the ACR criteria and exclusion of other disorders, such as hypothyroidism, will give one the best opportunity to make the diagnosis of FMS. FMS may be difficult to diagnose, as most of the symptoms are nonspecific and will test the clinical skills of a physician.

Education is paramount in the treatment of FMS, as there is no cure. The approach to FMS management is tripartite: (1) control of pain, (2) promotion of restorative sleep, and (3) aerobic conditioning. Pharmacologic agents for pain control—e.g., acetaminophen and nonsteroidal anti-inflammatory drugs (NSAIDs)—should be selected for the best risk–benefit ratio for the individual patient. Nonpharmacologic treatments such as biofeedback and meditation may work for some patients. Tricyclic antidepressants (TCA) and serotonin reuptake inhibitors in low doses may promote sleep and offer the additional benefit of assisting in pain control.

A gradual aerobic conditioning program may have the best long-term benefit in the treatment of FMS (16). A careful explanation of goals should be undertaken. The patient should select a type of exercise that is enjoyable, as FMS management is a long-term

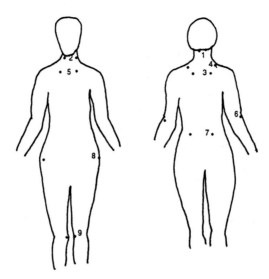

Fig. 2. 1990 ACR criteria for the classification of Fibromyalgia (Wolfe F et al. Arthritis Rheum 90; 33: 160–172). History of widespread pain involving axial skeleton , R & L sides, above and below the waist, greater than 3 mo duration. Pain in 11 of 18 tender points.1, suboccipital muscle insertion; 2, anterior aspects of transverse spaces C 3–7; 3, upper border of the mid-trapezius; 4, supraspinatus near the media border; 5, immediately lateral to 2nd costo-chondral junction; 6, 2 cm distal to the lateral epicondyle; 7, upper outer quadrant of buttocks; 8, posterior to greater trochanter; medial fat pads proximal to joint line.

commitment. The exercise level should be graded, with small increments of duration and intensity, so as to minimize postexertional myalgias/fatigue. A common but not absolute guideline is that postexertional pain/fatigue should not last more than 2 h. Adjustment in the exercise program will need to be made when it is interrupted, such as by illness.

OSTEOMYELITIS

Osteomyelitis is the infection of bone by bacterial or fungal organisms. The organisms enter the bone by the hematogenous route, spread from a contiguous infection, or inoculate directly via trauma. Risk factors for osteomyelitis include infection, diabetes, and intravenous drug abuse *(17)*.

The spine is commonly involved in osteomyelitis that is hematogenously acquired, but cervical spine *(17,18)* involvement is uncommon, occurring in only about 15% of cases.

Clinically, neck pain with localized tenderness on examination is almost invariably present. When accompanied by an elevated erythrocyte sedimentation rate *(17)*, it would strongly suggest the possibility of a cervical osteomyelitis (unless the patient has or is suspected of having a known inflammatory arthritis, e.g., RA [and then one would be more circumspect]). Unless there was spread of the infection beyond the bony borders or vertebral collapse, neurologic symptoms would not be expected. Despite being an infection, fever and an elevated white blood cell count are noted in only a half of cases of osteomyelitis *(17)*.

Diagnostically, X-rays will suffice in most cases and would show bony erosions. However, in early disease or osteomyelitis from low virulence organisms, bone scan, CT scan, or MRI may be required. Identification of an organism is definitely required to best manage the patient. Blood cultures and primary infection cultures may be sufficient in many cases, but if these are negative a specimen from the involved area is required. Organisms expected are *Staphylococcus aureus* for most cases, with Gram-negative organisms in intravenous drug abusers and immunosuppressed patients. Other less common organisms are seen in certain circumstances, such as tuberculosis in immunosuppressed patients or patients from third-world countries.

Management is primarily with parenteral antimicrobials and stabilization of the neck. However, if neurologic sequela has occurred, surgical relief may be required.

Organism	Occurrence
Staphylococcus	Most frequent
Tuberculosis	HIV patients, immigrants from endemic areas
Gram-negative organism	Intravenous drug abusers, immunosuppressed patients
Coccidioidomycosis	Patients who reside in or have traveled into endemic areas
Blastomycosis	Patients who reside in South and North Central United States

TRAUMA

Posttraumatic neck pain is probably best evaluated by separating patients into two age groups: those less than 65 yr old and those older. In the younger group, motor vehicle accidents are the predominant etiology, especially "whiplash" injury. In those greater than 65 yr old, falls are the most common etiology.

The preinjury state and severity of the trauma are important factors in determining the prognosis of the patient. In the younger population, a patient with a history of headaches preinjury would be expected to complain of exacerbation of the headaches and is less likely to recover fully *(19)*. An older patient with osteoarthritis of the cervical spine has a more rigid lower cervical spine, which predisposes to C1–2 injury, in contrast to a younger patient who would more likely injure C3–7 *(20)*.

The severity of trauma, as expected, correlates with the severity of neurologic deficit and (in the younger patient) is prognostic. The older patient usually injures himself in a minor fall; however, his recovery is more prolonged and less assured than a younger patient similarly affected, secondary to a greater number of preexisting health problems and diminished "functional reserve" *(20)*.

While a complete history and neurologic examination of a patient complaining of posttraumatic neck pain is standard, the radiologic evaluation of such a patient is currently being debated because of the low benefit–cost ratio when all patients are imaged. Although routine X-rays are of low sensitivity and specificity, they are the present standard in a patient suffering "major" trauma *(21)*.

Criteria are being developed and studied to improve the benefit–cost ratio in determining who should receive X-rays and the more costly CT-scan, MRI, and bone-scan studies *(21)*. Larger and more definitive studies are being performed to validate the criteria.

Management of neck pain is multimodality and adapted to the individual patient. Pain control may be achieved with acetaminophen, nonsteroidal anti-inflammatory drugs, opiates, and tricyclic antidepressants or a combination thereof. Stabilization of the neck with collar, traction, or halo devices can serve to prevent further neural injury, allow bone healing, decrease inflammation, and ameliorate pain. If there is a muscle spasm, hot and cold cycles, muscle relaxants and benzodiazepines may help. Careful exercises are important to maintain muscle function.

If (despite the conservative treatment) the patient fails to improve or if there is a significant neurologic deficit initially, prompt neurology–neurosurgery consultation should be obtained.

TUMORS

Neck pain owing to tumor is usually due to metastatic disease to the vertebral bodies *(22)* from breast, prostate, lung, renal, and thyroid primaries. Metastatic neoplasms are about 10 times more common than primary cervical spine tumors *(23)*. Pain is the earliest symptom, followed by neurologic impairment with local epidural metastasis (from the vertebral lesion) or bony collapse. Neck involvement occurs much less frequently than thoracolumbar disease, however *(23)*.

Primary tumors of the cervical spine are uncommon and may originate from vertebrae or intradural structures *(22)*. There is a definite age pattern of tumor involvement of the vertebrae. Ewing's sarcoma is a disease of the young, whereas myeloma is the most common primary vertebral tumor in adults *(23)*.

Aside from history and physical examination, looking for evidence of a neoplasm via laboratory testing and radiologic imaging are valuable adjuncts in the evaluation. A complete blood count, urinalysis, chemistry panel, including alkaline phosphatase, prostate specific antigen and serum protein electrophoresis may identify tumor effects. Imaging can start with a plain radiograph, though it is not very sensitive. Bone scans are more sensitive (except for myeloma), but they are not particularly specific *(22)*. CT scan and MRI may be required to more accurately define the tumor effect.

Primary treatment of the tumor is the management modality of choice along with pain control. If there is extensive bony destruction, a cervical collar should be employed. With rapidly expanding tumors, palliative treatment may be necessary.

REFERENCES

1. Vijayan N, Watson C. Raeder's syndrome, pericarotid syndrome and carotidynia. In: Vinken, Bruyn, Klawans, eds. Handbook of Clinical Neurology 1986; 48: 329–341.
2. Fay T. Atypical facial neuralgia, a syndrome of vascular pain. Ann Otol Rhinol Laryngol 1932; 41: 1030–1062.
3. Lovshin LL. Carotidynia. Headache 1977; 17: 192–195.
4. Evans JA, Steinberg I. Evaluation of angiographic techniques of extracranial circulation. J Amer Med Assoc 1962; 181: 678–681.
5. Roseman DM. Carotidynia, a distinct syndrome. Arch Otolaryngol 1967; 85: 81–84.
6. Raskin NH, Prusiner S. Carotidynia. Neurology 1977; 27: 43–46.
7. Dugan MC, Locke S, Gallagher JR. Occipital neuralgia in adolescents and young adults. N Engl J Med 1962; 267: 1166–1172.

8. Lance JW, Anthony M. Neck-tongue syndrome on sudden turning of the head. J Neurol Neurosurg Psychiatry 1980; 43: 97–101.
9. Resnick CS, Resnick D. Radiology. In: Utsinger PD, Zvaifler NJ, Ehrlich GE, eds. Rheumatoid Arthritis. Philadelphia: J. B. Lippincott, 1985; 172–174.
10. McKenna F, Wright V. Clinical manifestations. In: Utsinger PD, Zvaifler NJ, Ehrlich GE, eds. Rheumatoid Arthritis. Philadelphia: J.B. Lippincott, 1985; 291,292.
11. Nakano KK. Neck pain. In: Kelly WN, Harris ED, Ruddy S, Sledge CB, eds. The Textbook of Rheumatology. Philadelphia: W. B. Saunders, 1993; 397–416.
12. Emery SE, Bohiman HH. Osteoarthritis of the cervical spine. In: Moskowitz RW, Howell DS, Goldberg VM, Mankin HJ, eds. Osteoarthritis: Diagnosis and Medical/Surgical Management. Philadelphia: W. B. Saunders, 1992; 651–668.
13. Christian CL. Medical Management of cervical spine disease. In: Camins MB, O'Leary PF, eds. Disorder of the Cervical Spine. Baltimore: William & Wilkins, 1992; 147–155.
14. Bennett RM. The fibromyalgia syndrome: myofascial pain and chronic fatigue syndrome. In: Kelly WM, Harris ED, Ruddy S, Sledge CB, eds. Textbook of Rheumatology. Philadelphia: W. B. Saunders, 1993; 471–481.
15. Geel SE. The fibromyalgia syndrome: musculoskeletal pathophysiology. Semin Arthritis Rheum 1994; 23: 347–353.
16. McCain GA, Bell DA, Mai FM, Halliday PD. A controlled study of the effects of a supervised cardiovascular fitness training program on the manifestations of primary fibromyalgia. Arthritis Rheum 1988; 31: 1135–1141.
17. Sapico FL, Montgomerie JZ. Vertebral osteomyelitis. Infect Dis Clinic N America. 1990; 4: 539–550.
18. Waldvogel FA, Medoff G, Swartz MN. Osteomyelitis: a review of clinical features, therapeutic considerations and unusual aspects. N Engl J Med 1970; 282: 198–206, 260–266, 316–322.
19. Radanov BP, Sturzenegger M, Distefano G. Long-term outcome after whiplash injury. Medicine 1995; 74: 281–297.
20. Spivak JM, Weiss MA, Colter JM, Call M. Cervical spine injuries in patients 65 and older. Spine 1994; 20: 2302–2306.
21. Lindsay RW, Diliberti TC, Doherty BH, Watson AB. Efficacy of radiographic evaluation of the cervical spine in emergency situations. South Med J 1993, 86; 1253–1255.
22. Tsairis P, Jordan B. Neurological evaluation of cervical spine disorders. In: Camins MB, O'Leary PF, eds. Disorders of the Cervical Spine. Baltimore: William & Wilkins, 1992; 11–22.
23. Bruckner JD, Conrad KU, Anderson PA, Montesano PX. Tumors of the spine. In: Chapman MW, Madison M, eds. Operative Orthopedics. Philadelphia: J. B. Lippincott, 1993; 2883–2897.

4 PAIN IN THE SHOULDERS AND UPPER EXTREMITIES

James C. Leek, MD

Key Points

- Musculoskeletal conditions of the upper extremity are among the most common painful conditions seen in office practice. Disorders of the soft tissue (muscles, tendons, ligaments, and entheses) are particularly common.

- Monoarticular arthritis is usually due to infection, crystal induced arthritis such as gout or pseudogout, or trauma.

- Osteoarthritis in the upper extremities is usually limited to the interphalangeal joints of the hands and basilar joint of the thumb.

- Common inflammatory arthritides of the upper extremity include rheumatoid arthritis, Reiter's syndrome, and psoriatic arthritis.

- Polymyalgia rheumatica is a syndrome of synovitis causing proximal myalgias and stiffness of the neck, shoulder, and pelvic girdle in individuals over age 50. Identification of coexisting temporal arteritis, which may occur in 20% of patients, is crucial for appropriate treatment.

- Shoulder pain is most commonly due to periarticular involvement, particularly involvement of the rotator cuff.

- Shoulder pain with nonpainful normal range of motion suggests involvement of adjacent structures or referred pain.

- Lateral epicondylitis is one of the most common causes of elbow pain. Painful and limited range of motion of the elbow suggests involvement of the elbow joint itself.

- Carpal tunnel syndrome is the most common cause of paresthesias of the hand. Splinting, nonsteroidal anti-inflammatory drugs, and activity modifications are the key to conservative management.

- Tendonitis of the hands and wrists are commonly due to repetitive and forceful movements, where the hands and wrists are often formed in nonphysiologic conditions.

Table 1
Common Monoarticular Arthritis

1. Septic arthritis
2. Gout
3. Pseudogout
4. Traumatic arthritis
5. Hemarthrosis
     (anticoagulation, hemophilia, Von Willebrand's disease)
6. Monoarticular presentation of a polyarticular disease
     (juvenile rheumatoid arthritis, Reiter's syndrome, psoriatic arthritis, rheumatoid arthritis)

INTRODUCTION

Musculoskeletal problems of the upper extremity are among the most common painful conditions seen in office practice. A careful history and physical examination are required to distinguish the presence of systemic disease from local structural problems and from referred pain. More than one potentially painful condition often coexists, particularly in older individuals. Upper-extremity pain may be caused by disorders of the soft tissues (which are particularly common), bones, joints, nerves, and vascular structures.

ARTHRITIC DISEASES

• Differential diagnosis of arthritis is simplified by distinguishing monoarticular diseases from polyarticular diseases.

Monoarticular Arthritis

The common causes of monoarticular arthritis in the upper extremity are listed in Table 1.

Septic Arthritis

Septic arthritis may occur in any joints of the upper extremity but is most commonly seen in the wrists, elbows, and the metacarpophalangeal (MCP) joints. Involvement of the acromioclavicular joint is occasionally seen, particularly in intravenous drug abusers. Septic arthritis presents as a single red-hot swollen joint with marked pain and limitation of range of motion. The presence of significant loss of range of motion is helpful in distinguishing an infected joint from an overlying soft tissue infection in which joint range of motion would be much less affected. A large joint effusion is usually present, and the diagnosis is made by aspiration of purulent joint fluid. In pyogenic arthritis, the synovial fluid generally has a white blood count of greater than 100,000/mm^3, and the differential white count is greater than 90% granulocytes. In gonococcal arthritis, the synovial fluid white count may be much lower and is sometimes as low as 10,000–20,000/mm^3, although the differential white count of greater than 90% granulocytes is present. Synovial fluid Gram stain will be positive in the majority of pyogenic septic joints; however the synovial fluid Gram stain is much less frequently positive in gonococcal arthritis (1).

- Treatment of pyogenic arthritis consists of appropriate intravenous antibiotics and daily arthrocentesis to remove purulent synovial fluid.

The joint may be splinted for the first several days for pain relief; however, range of motion exercises should be started as soon as possible.

Gout

Gout is an intermittent, very painful, and highly inflammatory monoarthritis due to uric acid crystals, which more commonly involves the distal joints of the lower extremity, particularly the first metatarsophalangeal joint of the foot. It can involve any distal joint as its course progresses. Gout in the upper extremity commonly involves the interphalangeal joints of the hand, the wrist, or the olecranon bursa. Usually in upper-extremity involvement, there will be a history of previous self- limited episodes of acute arthritis in the foot or ankle; and there may be tophi (deposits of urate) in the feet, the small joints of the hands or the olecranon bursa, and occasionally in the periphery of the ears.

- Acute gout must be differentiated from infectious arthritis by arthrocentesis.

Negatively birefringent uric acid crystals in the joint fluid are diagnostic. The synovial fluid white count is inflammatory with predominantly granulocytes on differential count and may achieve white counts seen in joint infection. Treatment of the acute episodes is by nonsteroidal anti-inflammatory drugs given in doses at the upper end of their therapeutic range, colchicine, or intra-articular steroids (if coexisting infection has been excluded). Urate lowering therapy should be deferred until the acute attack has completely resolved *(2)*.

Pseudogout

Pseudogout is a syndrome of acute joint inflammation caused by the deposition of calcium pyrophosphate dihydrate crystals, usually involving one or several joints at a time with a spontaneous resolution of individual attacks. The wrist is second only to the knee as the most frequent site of acute pseudogout. As with gout, surgery or underlying medical illness may often precipitate an acute episode. Pseudogout is seen in predominantly older individuals with onset of disease usually after age 50, and an increasing prevalence with advancing age. It may be seen in younger individuals in the presence of certain associated metabolic conditions, including hyperparathyroidism, hypothyroidism, and hemochromatosis. Diagnosis is made by demonstrating weakly positively birefringent crystals on synovial fluid analysis and by characteristic chondrocalcinosis (radiographic calcification of joint cartilage). Calcification of fibrocartilage—such as the menisci of the knee, the triangular ligament of the wrists, and the symphysis pubis— is the most frequent; however, calcification of hyaline articular cartilage also occurs. Joint radiographs may also show so-called calcium pyrophosphate arthropathy with findings similar to particularly severe osteoarthritis along with involvement of joints not usually involved by such primary osteoarthritis as the wrist, elbow, and metacarpophalangeal joints, with increased frequency of subchondral cysts. Therapy of the acute attacks is with intra-articular corticosteroid injections or nonsteroidal anti-inflammatory drugs *(3)*.

Polyarthritis

Rheumatoid Arthritis

Rheumatoid arthritis is the prototype of polyarticular inflammatory arthritis and is a symmetrical arthritis that may involve all of the joints of the upper extremity, with the exception of the distal interphalangeal joints. The wrists and the MCP joints are involved symmetrically, and there is fusiform swelling of the proximal interphalangeal joints (PIP). Extensor tendons at the dorsum of the wrist are often involved early. Fatigue and morning stiffness of the joints, which lasts for several hours, are characteristic. Rheumatoid arthritis may involve any peripheral diarthroidal joint, except the DIPs. Spinal involvement is limited to the cervical spine. Laboratory findings show a mild anemia. The erythrocyte sedimentation rate (ESR) is elevated and tends to parallel disease activity. Rheumatoid factor is usually present, and high titers may indicate a more progressive erosive course. The presence of rheumatoid factor in itself is not diagnostic of rheumatoid arthritis.

Radiographically, the earliest finding is periarticular osteopenia, followed by the development of joint space narrowing and characteristic marginal bony erosions. Early erosive changes are commonly found at the MCP joints, the MTP joints of the feet, and the ulnar styloid process. The differential diagnosis of rheumatoid arthritis in its early stages includes a long list of diseases that cause polyarthritis, including systemic lupus erythematosus, scleroderma, psoriatic arthritis, inflammatory bowel disease, sarcoidosis, and hematomacrosis, to name a few. This differential diagnosis and management of rheumatoid arthritis will be further considered in Chapter 10.

Reiter's Syndrome and Psoriatic Arthritis

Reiter's syndrome and psoriatic arthritis are representative of the seronegative spondyloarthropathies, a group of arthritis characterized by the absence of rheumatoid factor and involvement of the sacroiliac joints and spine. These have distinctive arthritic involvement in the upper extremity. The psoriatic arthritis particularly involves the DIP joint and is characterized by asymmetric arthritis, similar to that seen in Reiter's syndrome. A distinctive finding in Reiter's arthritis in the upper extremity is the sausage digit, in which there is diffuse swelling of the entire digit, with particular involvement of the PIP. Similar lesions are also seen in the toes. Typical nail changes of onycholysis and subungual hyperkeratosis are seen in both Reiter's syndrome and psoriatic arthritis; however, nail pitting is seen only in psoriatic arthritis *(4)*.

Osteoarthritis in the Upper Extremity

Osteoarthritis is usually limited to the interphalangeal joints of the hands and the first carpometacarpal joint at the base of the thumb. Joint space narrowing and osteophyte (bony spur) formation occur. Osteophytes in the DIPs are known as Heberden's nodes; in the PIP they are known as Bouchard's nodes. Osteoarthritis also occurs at the acromioclavicular joint and generally spares the other joints of the upper extremity unless there are unusual occupational factors or unless other pre-existing joint disease is present. When osteoarthritic changes are seen in the wrists, elbows, or shoulders, calcium pyrophosphate arthropathy should be considered. In osteoarthritis of the hands, there is little soft tissue swelling, although cysts resembling ganglia may occur at the DIP and PIP joints. There is relatively brief morning stiffness and pain is precipitated by joint use and relieved by rest.

Osteoarthritis of the hands is managed by preventing overuse of the joint and by modifying utensils and activities to protect the joints as much as possible. Local heat administered by warm soaks or paraffin baths may be helpful. Analgesics and nonsteroidal anti-inflammatory drugs (NSAIDs) are useful. Involvement of the first carpometacarpal joint at the base of the thumb may respond to splinting or intra-articular steroid injection. Joint arthroplasty is successful for severe cases that do not respond to these measures *(5)*.

Polymyalgia Rheumatica

Polymyalgia rheumatica is a syndrome of proximal aching and stiffness of the neck, shoulder girdle, and pelvic girdle in older individuals. This syndrome occurs only after age 50. The great majority are over 60 yr old and the typical patient is often in the 70s. Pain is often attributed to muscles but is in fact due to synovitis of the large joints. Onset is often abrupt. Other systemic symptoms—including fatigue, weight loss, and fevers—are frequent. Up to 20% of patients have associated temporal arteritis. Examination generally reveals few abnormalities, although mild synovitis may be present in the wrists, knees, and the sternoclavicular joints. Muscle strength is normal except as limited by pain. Muscle enzymes, EMGs, and muscle biopsies are normal and are not diagnostically useful. The predominant laboratory finding is an elevated sedimentation rate that is nearly always greater than 50 mm/h and is often greater than 100 mm/h. Mild-to-moderate anemia is often present. Mild liver function abnormalities may be present *(6)*.

The diagnosis of polymyalgia rheumatica is clinical and is confirmed by a diagnostic trial of low dose corticosteroids. Ten to twenty milligrams of prednisone daily will result in the prompt improvement in all symptoms within 1–2 wk, with gradual improvement of the sedimentation rate. This dose of prednisone, although effective for the symptoms of polymyalgia, is not adequate to control temporal arteritis. (*Note:* The presence of temporal arteritis symptoms or findings such as a unilateral headache, temporal tenderness, jaw claudication, or visual symptoms demands immediate treatment with 60 mg of prednisone daily followed by temporal artery biopsy.) Patients with polymyalgia rheumatica without symptoms or signs of temporal arteritis do not require temporal artery biopsy. Steroid dosage is gradually tapered to the lowest dose effective in controlling persistent arthralgias and myalgias. Some patients may be controlled satisfactorily on nonsteroidal anti-inflammatory drugs alone. Symptoms of polymyalgia rheumatica often require treatment for several years or longer.

Patients in this age group frequently have additional co-existing problems such as degenerative disease of the cervical and lumbar spine and abnormalities of the shoulders and hip, which may account for similar symptoms so that careful history taking and a high index of suspicion are required to avoid missing this rather common condition.

SHOULDER AND UPPER-ARM PAIN

Periarticular Shoulder Pain (Table 2)

Rotator Cuff Tendonitis (Table 3)

Shoulder pain is a particularly common cause of musculoskeletal pain and is seen most frequently in individuals above the age of 40. The large majority of painful shoulder

Table 2
Causes of Shoulder Pain

Periarticular	Glenohumeral Joint	Adjacent Structures	Reflex Sympathetic Dystrophy	Referred Pain
1. Rotator cuff tendonitis	1. Adhesive capsulitis	1. Acromioclavicular joint		1. Subdiaphragmatic processes
2. Bicipital tendonitis	2. Inflammatory arthritis	a. Osteoarthritis		a. Cholecystitis
3. Rotator cuff tear	3. Cuff tear arthropathy	b. Inflammatory arthritis		b. Splenic process
4. Calcific tendonitis	(Milwaukee shoulder)	c. Infection (Iv drug use)		c. Subphrenic abscess
	4. Infection	2. Cervical radiculopathy		2. Myocardial ischemia
	5. Ischemic necrosis	3. Entrapment neuropathy		
	6. Osteochondritis dessicans	a. Supraclavicular nerve		
	7. Shoulder subluxation	b. Long thoracic nerve		
		4. Myofascial pain		
		5. Pancoast syndrome		

Table 3
Features of Rotator Cuff Tendonitis

1. Lateral shoulder pain is present, most often referred to the deltoid insertion.
2. "The painful arc" with 60–120° of abduction.
3. Pain is prominent at night.
4. Tenderness of rotator cuff lateral to the acromion, particularly in the area of the supraspinatus tendon.
5. Injection of lidocaine into the subacromial bursa relieves the pain and confirms the diagnosis.

complaints can be attributed to the periarticular structures, particularly the rotator cuff. The rotator cuff comprises of the tendons of the supraspinatus, infraspinatus, and the teres minor tendons inserting on the greater tuberosity of the humerus and the subscapularis tendon inserting on the lesser tuberosity.

The rotator cuff tendons travel underneath the anterior portion of the acromion and coricoacromial ligament to insert on the greater tuberosity. Mechanical impingement by these structures is the usual cause of rotator cuff tendonitis (RCT). RCT is particularly common in the presence of degenerative disease with osteophyte formation on the undersurface of the acromion or the acromioclavicular joint or with extensive shoulder activities that involve elevation. The supraspinatus tendon is most frequently involved; the infraspinatus tendon as well as the long-head biceps may be involved *(7)*.

Symptoms of RCT are predominantly of pain in the lateral aspect of the shoulder, particularly referred to the lateral deltoid region; RCT is characterized by a "painful arc," that is, the pain is precipitated or exacerbated by active abduction of the shoulder with pain occurring between the 60 and 120° of abduction. Abduction against resistance exacerbates pain, and passive range of motion is generally much less painful. The impingement sign (performed by the passive forward flexion of the shoulder, while stabilizing the scapula) reproduces the pain as the greater tuberosity impinges at the acromion. The diagnosis can be confirmed by injection of lidocaine into the subacromial bursa.

Therapy of RCT includes modification of shoulder activities, including lifting and other activities that place the shoulder in an elevated position, and anti-inflammatory therapy with a nonsteroidal anti-inflammatory drugs or corticosteroid injection into the subacromial bursa. A rehabilitation regimen is begun initially with passive or active assisted range of motion exercises to avoid loss of shoulder range of motion with the use of ice for pain relief and the use of heat or ultrasound therapy to aid in mobilization.

Bicipital Tendonitis

Bicipital tendonitis results from overuse and impingement of the long head of the biceps and is usually characterized by anterior shoulder pain. There is tenderness present on examination in the bicipital grove, and pain is precipitated by supination of the forearm against resistance (Yergason's test) and by flexion of the shoulder against resistance. Treatment consists of rest, application of local heat, and an NSAID, followed by a progressive exercise program after pain is controlled.

Calcific Tendonitis

Although RCT is usually caused by the mechanical and degenerative factors seen in the impingement syndrome, rotator cuff inflammation may also be related to calcium deposits in and around the rotator cuff tendons, particularly within the supraspinatus tendon. These calcium deposits (predominantly hydroxyapatite) cause local inflammation, as seen in gout and pseudogout. Although the mechanism responsible for calcium deposition is unclear, there is generally a component of degenerative change and often significant impingement. Symptoms in the acute episodes are similar to those in other forms of RCT, although sudden onset of severe pain is often seen. Shoulder X-rays reveal calcific deposits in the rotator cuff tendons or subacromial bursa. Therapy of acute calcific tendonitis is local corticosteroid injection or a nonsteroidal anti-inflammatory drug, as in other forms of RCT. In chronic cases, disruption of the calcium deposits by needling may be useful. The presence of calcium deposits radiographically, in the absence of symptoms, is relatively common in older individuals and requires no treatment.

Rotator Cuff Tear

In younger individuals, rotator cuff tears generally follow trauma. In older patients, in whom there is degenerative change occurring in the rotator cuff, tears may occur after minor trauma or even in the absence of a specific traumatic episode. Rotator cuff tears may be complete or partial and variable in size. Large acute tears are characterized by significant pain and marked weakness and are generally easily recognized. Injection of the subacromial bursa with lidocaine is often a useful diagnostic procedure. Marked weakness of the rotator cuff muscles persists after injection, despite pain relief. Large tears are associated with a positive "drop-arm" test, in which the patient is unable to maintain active abduction at 90°. Small or incomplete tears are often difficult to distinguish from RCT and are treated similarly to RCT. However, the response to subacromial corticosteroid injections is limited. Definitive diagnosis of rotator cuff tear is by MRI or arthrogram. Decisions regarding surgical repair of rotator cuff tear depend on the age, activity level, the functional needs of the patient, and the cause and size of the tear. Massive tears of the rotator cuff in elderly individuals can result in the so-called cuff tear arthropathy, with superior migration of humeral head, diminished subacromial space, and destructive changes of the glenohumeral joint. These findings are particularly seen in elderly women and may be associated with hydroxyapatite (basic calcium phosphate) in the Milwaukee shoulder syndrome (8). These elderly patients have large, often blood-tinged, shoulder effusions with few white cells. Elevated synovial fluid proteinases have been reported in some of these patients. Treatment is generally difficult because of the extensive destructive changes in the rotator cuff and glenohumeral joint. The Milwaukee shoulder syndrome may also involve other joints, particularly the knee.

Frozen Shoulder

Frozen shoulder (or adhesive capsulitis) is a syndrome of generalized shoulder pain and progressive loss of range of motion occurring in individuals over the age of 40. It may occur following a variety of shoulder problems or regional disorders or without another underlying condition (Table 4). Generalized shoulder pain and tenderness are present,

Table 4
Conditions Associated with Frozen Shoulder

1. Rotator cuff tendonitis/tear
2. Inflammatory arthritis of the shoulder
3 . Cervical spondylosis
4. Reflex sympathetic dystrophy
5. Diabetes
6. Thyroid disease
7. Prolonged immobility or diminished level of consciousness

although quite variable in severity with the loss of both active and passive range of motion in all planes. Although this disorder has sometimes been called periarthritis, fibrinous synovitis is found, affecting the entire joint on arthroscopy, with progressive adhesions forming throughout the joint space and marked contraction of the joint capsule. Arthrography shows diminished joint volume. Routine radiographs are generally normal, although the arthrogram may reveal a rotator cuff tear *(9)*.

Therapy consists of intra-articular steroids injected into the glenohumeral joint with a second simultaneous injection into the subacromial bursa, followed by aggressive physical therapy and nonsteroidal anti-inflammatory drugs. Physical therapy should begin with gentle range of motion exercises, accompanied by analgesics and heat and cold modalities with progressive stretching exercises as tolerated by the patient. The physical therapy program should be supervised by a physical therapist. Corticosteroid injections may be repeated several times at 3- to 4-wk intervals. Manipulation under anesthesia is occasionally useful in refractory cases.

Acromioclavicular Arthritis

Apart from the inflammatory arthropathies, which may affect the acromioclavicular joint, and infectious arthritis, as seen particularly in intravenous drug users, acromioclavicular joint involvement is predominantly degenerative related to joint instability from previous trauma. Acromioclavicular pain is generally localized superiorly in the shoulder but may be generalized. Tenderness may be present directly over the AC joint. Crepitus is often present, although this is often seen in asymptomatic older individuals. Elevation of the shoulder without range of motion of the glenohumeral joint is a maneuver often useful in precipitating acromioclavicular pain. Abduction of the shoulder as well as forward flexion and adduction also exacerbate acromioclavicular pain, which may falsely suggest rotator cuff involvement.

Shoulder and Arm Pain Due to Adjacent Structures

- When shoulder pain occurs with normal shoulder range of motion, which does not elicit pain, involvement of adjacent structures or referred pain should be considered.

Cervical Radiculopathy

Shoulder and arm pain commonly occurs in cervical spondylosis and radiculopathy. The upper extremity is innervated by the C4 through the T1 nerve roots *(10)*. Distribution

Table 5
Upper Extremity Symptoms and Findings of Cervical Radiculopathy

Cervical Route	Pain and Paresthesias	Motor Finding	Reflex
C5	Outer shoulder and lateral arm	Deltoid weakness	Biceps (with C6)
C6	Lateral arm, forearm, thumb, and index finger	Biceps weakness and wrist extensors (with C7)	Biceps (with C5) brachial radialis and triceps (with C7)
C7	The outer arm and middle finger	Triceps and finger	Triceps
C8	The inner arm to the 4th and 5th fingers	Finger flexor weakness extensor	None

of pain in the upper extremity is, in general, along dermatome distribution with some overlap. Distribution of symptoms and findings is shown in Table 5. Several provocative maneuvers, such as the Sperling test, may be helpful if they reproduce the pain, but are rather insensitive. The Sperling test, or cervical compression test, is performed with the patient seated by exerting downward pressure on top of the patient's head usually with the head rotated slightly toward the involved side.

Reproduction of pain suggests nerve root compression. Pain exacerbated by a Valsalva maneuver is also suggestive of radicular pain. Diagnostics include plain radiographs of the cervical spine, cervical MRI, and electrodiagnostic studies of the upper extremity. Patients in middle and older aged groups frequently have findings of cervical spondylosis as well as evidence of other degenerative or overuse conditions in the upper extremity, which may make it difficult to determine which lesion is causing the particular symptoms. In general, conditions of the shoulder may refer pain to the trapezius and rotator cuff muscles but do not refer pain to the neck proper. Local injections of lidocaine (for example, into the subacromial bursa) may be useful in differentiating the source of pain. The presence of cervical radiculopathy may potentiate the symptoms and severity of a more distal entrapment neuropathy, a condition known as the double crush syndrome.

Thoracic Outlet Syndrome

Compression of the neurovascular bundle entering the arm from the thorax is known as the thoracic outlet syndrome (11). The neurovascular bundle, consisting of the brachial plexus and the subclavian vessels, passes over the first rib between the scalene muscles, passing under the clavicle and the pectoralis minor muscle into the upper extremity. It may be compressed at multiple sites and by a variety of structures, such as a cervical rib or fibrous band at the site of a cervical rib or a long 7th cervical transverse process in addition to the above structures. Most commonly, symptomatic compression occurs by the sagging of normal musculoskeletal structures known as the "droopy shoulder" syndrome. Neurologic symptoms are far more common than vascular symptoms. Pain, paresthesias, and numbness of the ulnar aspect of the arm and hand are the most common symptoms and are typically bilateral. Symptoms are generally intermittent, varying with the posture and position and often occurring during sleep. Overhead activities frequently exacerbate the symptoms. Motor weakness is uncommon but, when present, generally affects the intrinsic muscles of the hands. Vascular symptoms include distal pallor or cyanosis in the cold or cold intolerance. Raynaud's phenomenon may occur. Claudication is very uncommon. Physical findings are generally minimal. There may be tenderness in the region of the brachial plexus. Physical diagnosis includes a number of provocative maneuvers that are neither sensitive nor specific for the presence of thoracic outlet syndrome. These rely on obliteration of the radial pulse or the reproduction of symptoms of pain and paresthesias with changes in positions of the head and shoulder. Among these is the Adson maneuver, which, if positive, produces radial pulse obliteration after deep inspiration and Valsalva maneuver with the neck extended and the head turned toward the involved side. A positive test occurs in many normal as well as symptomatic individuals. Other maneuvers include hyperabduction of the shoulder or depression of the shoulder backward and downward. A more useful maneuver is holding the arms over the head with the shoulders abducted and externally rotated for 3 min, combined with the repetitive opening and closing of the fists. Downward traction on the arm with the elbow flexed and the shoulder externally rotated may also reproduce these symptoms. Special diagnostic tests include noninvasive vascular studies and electrodiagnostic studies. Doppler ultrasonography can provide more quantitative information regarding vascular flow during the provocative maneuvers; however, their utility is limited since many normals will have some changes with these provocative maneuvers. Abnormal vascular studies are of limited value in patients who have predominantly neurologic symptoms. Nerve conduction studies and electromyography of the upper extremities are often normal in patients with symptomatic thoracic outlet syndrome but are useful in excluding cervical radiculopathy and more distal compression neuropathies.

Conservative therapy is successful in most patients with primarily neurologic symptoms. This consists primarily of physical therapy with correction of postural abnormality and sleeping position, as well as appropriate positioning for work activities. Avoidance of overhead activities is important. Gradual exercises to strengthen the neck and shoulder girdle are prescribed. NSAIDs are useful.

Reflex Sympathetic Dystrophy/Shoulder Hand Syndrome

Reflex sympathetic dystrophy (RSD) is a syndrome of severe pain and swelling of a distal extremity, associated with vasomotor changes and progressive atrophy *(12)*. It may involve either the upper or lower extremity and, in the upper extremity, is commonly called the shoulder hand syndrome. RSD generally follows trauma, which may vary from severe to trivial, and is also seen after immobilization of an extremity. The onset is usually gradual, and the predominant symptom is pain, which is usually burning or paraesthetic in character. Throbbing or aching pain also occurs. Generalized swelling of the distal extremity is usually present and there is significant hyperesthesia of the involved area. Vasomotor changes are characteristic with a cool, dusky, distal extremity. RSD may be precipitated in a susceptible individual by a wide variety of problems (Table 6). After several months, progressive brawny edema occurs with dystrophic skin changes. Burning pain and hyperesthesia persists. Finally, after 6 mo or more, progressive atrophy of the soft tissues occurs with the development of contractures.

Table 6
Precipitating Events for Shoulder Hand Syndrome

Major and minor trauma
Painful conditions of the shoulder (rotator cuff tendonitis, adhesive capsulitis)
Cervical spondylosis or radiculopathy
Myocardial infarction
Cerebrovascular accident
Peripheral nerve injury
Surgical procedures
Drugs
  Isoniazid
  Phenobarbital
  Ergotamine
  Cyclosporin

Routine laboratory studies are unrevealing. Radiographs reveal patchy osteopenia. Bone scan is the most helpful diagnostic test and reveals generalized increased uptake in the periarticular tissues.

Therapy must be vigorous and is more successful when instituted early. Pain control is critical, beginning with nonsteroidal anti-inflammatory drugs and proceeding to narcotic analgesics if necessary. A vigorous progressive physical therapy program is important. Systemic corticosteroids are indicated in all but the mildest cases, beginning with a dose of approx 60 mg of prednisone daily, tapering over 4–6 wk. Sympathetic blockade by stellate ganglion block often produces a dramatic but temporary relief of pain and may be diagnostic as well as therapeutic. Repeated sympathetic block performed every several days may be useful. A progressive physical therapy program should be continued throughout treatment. Low doses of tricyclic antidepressants may be helpful in managing the persistent pain.

PAINFUL CONDITIONS OF THE ELBOW

- Passive range of motion of the elbow is generally intact and pain-free except in articular involvement.

Except in the case of patients with a systemic iinflammatory arthritis, elbow pain is generally periarticular. Any of the inflammatory arthropathies may involve the elbow. When rheumatoid arthritis is present, and coexistent olecranon bursitis and/or rheumatoid nodules are often present. Osteoarthritis rarely involves the elbow, except in patients with a previous history of trauma or extensive occupational use such as is miners, pneumatic drill operators, or pitchers. Osteoarthritic-like changes of the elbow may be seen in calcium pyrophosphate deposition arthropathy.

Lateral Epicondylitis

Lateral epicondylitis of the elbow is one of the most common causes of elbow pain, occurring most commonly in middle-aged individuals. The lateral epicondyle is the site of insertion of the wrist extensor muscles. Lateral epicondylitis is generally precipitated by repetitive and/or vigorous gripping and grasping activity or wrist extension. It is commonly seen in racket sports and tool use and may also be precipitated by repetitively shaking hands. Pain is referred to the lateral aspect of the elbow and is exacerbated by gripping or grasping. Provocative maneuvers on examination include increased pain with resisted extension of the wrist or the middle finger. Passive stretching of the forearm extensor muscles may also produce pain. Elbow range of motion is normal. There is local tenderness at or distal to the lateral epicondyle. Pathologically, there is inflammation or tear of the common extensor tendons. Posterior interosseous nerve entrapment should be considered in different diagnosis. However, this is an uncommon syndrome and not associated with pain by the above provocative maneuvers.

Treatment of lateral epicondylitis depends particularly on limitation and modification of the precipitating activities. Initially the patient must refrain from all vigorous gripping and grasping activities. Rest of the wrist extensors is best achieved by splinting the wrist in a preformed splint, which should be removed several times daily for gentle range of motion exercises. The tennis elbow band, a nonelastic band placed distal to the epicondyle, provides general compression and is helpful in limiting forces at the site of injury or at least reminding the patient that vigorous contraction of these muscles should be avoided. Inflammation is treated with a nonsteroidal anti-inflammatory. Local icing is also helpful for pain control. An exercise regimen during the painful period should be limited to gentle range of motion and stretching followed by more vigorous stretching exercises and strengthening exercises for the wrist after the pain is adequately controlled. Returning to the usual activities should be gradual, and each session should be preceded by warm-up exercises and stretching of the wrist extensors. Local corticosteroid injections into the sites of tenderness may be helpful, although postinjection pain can be a problem and occasional soft tissue atrophy may occur. Rarely, surgery may be required in resistant cases *(13)*.

Medial Epicondylitis

Medial epicondylitis, sometimes called "golfer's elbow," is much less common than the lateral epicondylitis. The syndrome is analogous to lateral epicondylitis and involves the wrist flexors, with the local tenderness over the medial epicondyle and pain exacerbated by resisted wrist flexion or passive wrist extension. Management is similar to lateral epicondylitis.

Biceps, Insertional Tendonitis

Pain in the antecubital area may be caused by tendonitis of the insertion of the biceps tendon and is brought on by vigorous elbow flexion activity. Management is with rest and nonsteroidal anti-inflammatories, heat, or ice.

Olecranon Bursitis

The olecranon bursa, located at the extensor aspect of the olecranon process of the ulna, is commonly caused by recurrent minor trauma or pressure and is characterized by the development of a bursa effusion with some localized tenderness but relatively little pain. Elbow range of motion is normal. Aspiration of bursal fluid generally shows noninflammatory fluid, which may be hemorrhagic or blood tinged in the setting of acute trauma. Inflammatory causes of olecranon bursitis include rheumatoid arthritis, gout, and pseudogout. Both rheumatoid arthritis and gout with tophaceous deposits may be associated with olecranon bursal effusions accompanied by nodules or masses within the bursa. Aspiration of a gouty olecranon bursa will reveal large quantities of urate crystals. Significant inflammation in the olecranon bursa is most concerning for the presence of infectious bursitis, which is nearly always caused by staphylococci. Infectious bursitis is characterized by local erythema and swelling with considerable tenderness. The bursal fluid white count may be deceptively low in infectious bursitis, and white counts greater than 2000 cells/m3 should be considered characteristic of an infection rather than traumatic bursitis. Treatment of infection is by percutaneous drainage and appropriate antibiotic therapy. The differential diagnosis between septic bursitis and an underlying infectious arthritis of the elbow is assisted by the relatively normal range of motion of the elbow in infectious bursitis, in which range of motion is generally only limited by pain in significant degrees of flexion, which puts tension on the inflamed bursa. In infectious arthritis, marked loss of range of motion is evident (14).

Ulnar Nerve Entrapment at the Elbow

Ulnar nerve entrapment at the elbow is often called cubital tunnel syndrome. The ulnar nerve originates from the 8th cervical and the 1st thoracic nerve roots, which form the medial cord of the brachial plexus. The nerve extends posterior to the medial humeral epicondyle and travels through the cubital tunnel between humeral and ulnar heads of the flexor carpi ulnaris at the medial aspect of the elbow. Nerve compression at the elbow may be caused by acute or chronic recurrent trauma, repetitive elbow flexion and extension, chronic pressure on the area (such as frequently resting the elbow on hard surfaces), and by activities that keep the elbow in marked flexion for long periods (such as talking on the telephone or sleeping with the elbow in a flexed position). The most common symptoms are paresthesias in the 4th and the 5th fingers, which may be associated with sensory loss in more severe cases. Aching pain is present over the medial aspect of the elbow and may radiate distally or proximally. Intrinsic muscle weakness progressing to atrophy in severe cases may also be present. The patient may complain of weakness of the grip. In most cases, sensory findings are the predominant complaints. Physical findings indicate that they may be minimal. A positive Tinel's sign, inducing painful paresthesias by tapping at the cubital tunnel, is helpful; however, mildly positive Tinel's sign is seen in many normal patients and only a strongly positive test is helpful. Reproduction of symptoms by holding the elbow in full flexion for one minute is also useful. Nerve conduction studies are useful if the clinical diagnosis is not clear. Differential diagnosis is mainly nerve compression at other more proximal or distal sites, including C8 radiculopathy, thoracic outlet syndrome, or ulnar nerve entrapment at the wrist at Guyon's canal. Similar symptoms may also be seen in the Pancoast syndrome, in which an apical carcinoma of the lung involves the brachial plexus. The cubital tunnel syndrome may also be seen concurrently with entrapment neuropathy at another site in the double crush syndrome. This should be thought of in particular when there is a poor response to conservative therapy. Nerve conduction studies are useful in confirming the diagnosis if it is not clear clinically and particularly if conservative treatment is unsuccessful. Nerve conduction velocities may be normal in the cubital tunnel in symptomatic patients, and are particularly useful in detecting or excluding nerve compression at other sites.

Conservative therapy consists of avoiding or modifying provocative activity, in particular avoiding elbow flexion in the waking and sleeping positions. A soft night splint, such as a rolled rubber padding within a sleeve of stockinette, is useful. Padding of the elbow to avoid compression trauma against hard surfaces is important. Nonsteroidal anti-inflammatory drugs are helpful and, occasionally, local steroid injections can be used. Since there is a risk of inadvertent trauma to the nerve, injections should be performed only by experienced individuals. Surgical decompression should be performed if conservative therapy fails and the double crush syndrome, particularly due to an unrecognized cervical radiculopathy, has been excluded.

Posterior Interosseous Nerve Compression

The posterior interosseous branch of the radial nerve may be compressed in the forearm by the supinator muscles. The predominant symptom is weakness in extensor muscles, particularly of the metacarpophalangeal extensors. This is often accompanied by pain in the lateral area of the elbow or deep within the forearm. When lateral elbow pain is present, this condition is to be distinguished from lateral epicondylitis. There is frequently a history of repetitive pronation supination activities and, initially, symptoms may be transient and associated with activities. Conservative treatment consists of avoiding precipitating activities or immobilization *(15)*.

PAIN IN THE HAND AND WRIST

Entrapment Neuropathies at the Wrist

Carpal Tunnel Syndrome

Carpal tunnel syndrome is the most common entrapment neuropathy in the upper extremity and the most common cause of paresthesias in the hand. Entrapment occurs as the median nerve passes through the carpal tunnel on the volar aspect of the wrist, along with the flexor tendons. The carpal tunnel is bounded by the carpal bones and volarly by the transverse carpal ligament. A wide variety of conditions can result in an increase in carpal tunnel content, causing median nerve compression (Table 7). Most common are the chronic fibrosis and tenosynovial thickening, seen in idiopathic carpal tunnel syndrome. Rheumatoid arthritis, or other inflammatory synovitis at the wrist, is also a common cause. Pregnancy, diabetes, and hypothyroidism are also frequent causes. Occupational activity involving repetitive finger and wrist flexion clearly may precipitate or aggravate the carpal tunnel syndrome, although these activities as a sole cause are somewhat controversial (Table 7) *(16)*.

Symptoms of carpal tunnel syndrome begin with intermittent paresthesias of the hand, involving the thumb, index and long fingers, and the radial aspect of the ring finger. Often the patient will complain of symptoms throughout the hand, although most can

Table 7
Conditions Associated with Carpal Tunnel Syndrome

1. Idiopathic tenosynovitis
2. Trauma
3. Rheumatoid arthritis and other inflammatory arthropathy
4. Pregnancy
5. Osteoarthritis
6. Diabetes
7. Hypothyroidism
8. Acromegaly
9. Amyloidosis
10. Gout and pseudogout
11. Structural anomaly
12. Occupational factors

distinguish a more accurate distribution with careful observation. Paresthesias often awaken the patient at night, and subjective hand swelling is often present. Symptoms are often bilateral, the dominant hand generally being more affected. Repetitive activities of the hands and wrists exacerbate the symptoms. Physical findings are minimal, except in the later stages, when atrophy of the thenar muscle or sensory changes may be present. Tinel's sign or Phalen's sign may be present. Tinel's sign is reproduction of pain and paresthesias by tapping on the median nerve at the carpal tunnel. The Phalen test is performed with 60 s of complete wrist flexion, which produces pain and paresthesias if positive. Both false-positive and false-negative tests may occur. Abnormal tests are present in approximately two-thirds of patients with carpal tunnel syndrome. Confirmation of the diagnosis is by nerve conduction studies, which are diagnostic in more than 90% of patients. Treatment in the absence of motor findings begins with conservative therapy. The wrist is splinted in a neutral position, and provocative activities are modified or eliminated. Nonsteroidal anti-inflammatory drugs are useful. The treatment of underlying problems, such as hypothyroidism, is important. For work-related cases, assessment of ergonomic risk factors is important, and occupational therapy with modification of positions, tools, and work habits is very useful. Corticosteroid injections into the carpal tunnel are successful in most patients, at least on a temporary basis. For patients with thenar muscle weakness and atrophy, prolonged symptoms, or lack of response to conservative therapy, surgical decompression either by open carpal tunnel release or an endoscopic procedure is indicated.

Ulnar Nerve Compression at the Wrist

Ulnar nerve entrapment at the wrist can occur at Guyon's canal, beneath the volar carpal ligament at the ulnar aspect of the wrist. Symptoms are pain and paresthesias of the ulnar aspect of the wrist, the hypothenar area, and the fourth and fifth fingers. Like carpal tunnel syndrome, symptoms are often increased at night and exacerbated by complete wrist flexion or extension. Weakness of the intrinsic muscles of the hand may

Table 8
Causes of Ulnar Nerve Compression
at the Wrist

1. Trauma
2. Vibratory trauma
3. Prolonged dorsal flexion (bicyclists)
4. Ganglion and tumors
5. Arthritis (inflammatory or degenerative)
6. Structural anomalies
7. Diabetes

Table 9
Treatment of Tendonitis

1. Rest and avoidance of precipitating activities.
2. Splinting of the involved area. The splints should be removed several times daily for gentle range of motion exercises.
3. Icing is helpful for pain relief, particularly after activities.
4. Local heat may help with pain relief and immobilization.
5. Nonsteroidal anti-inflammatory drugs.
6. Local corticosteroid injections are particularly useful in several of the specific tendonitis.
7. Prolonged rest is to be avoided. Early gentle immobilization should begin as soon as inflammation subsides.
8. Gradual stretching and strengthening exercises should proceed at a pace avoiding exacerbation of pain.

occur and, in advanced cases, clawing of the fourth and fifth fingers can be seen. A number of factors may cause ulnar nerve compression (Table 8). Treatment is similar to that of carpal tunnel syndrome, with elimination of provocative activities, splinting, and anti-inflammatory medication followed by surgical decompression in those who do not respond.

Tendonitis of the Hand and Wrist

Tendonitis of the flexor and extensor tendons in the hands and wrists is a common occurrence. Although inflammatory arthritis and infection must be considered, by far the most common cause of tendonitis is the repetitive and forceful use of the involved structures, often in a nonphysiologic position. As in the entrapment neuropathies, degenerative changes, metabolic, and other systemic conditions may contribute. Localized pain and tenderness are characteristics exacerbated by the activities. There is often subjective swelling, but objective swelling on examination is much less frequent. Principals of treatment are outlined in Table 9.

Several of these specific tendonitis syndromes are as follows:

De Quervain's Tenosynovitis

De Quervain's tenosynovitis is tendonitis of the first dorsal compartment involving the abductor pollicis longus and extensor pollicis brevis. This syndrome is often precipitated by repetitive activities of the thumb and wrist. It is also common in pregnancy and frequently coexists with carpal tunnel syndrome and trigger finger. Pain is present at the area of the radial styloid, with localized tenderness and exacerbation of pain by grasping activities. A positive Finkelstein test is present (pain over the radial styloid is exacerbated by passive ulnar deviation of the wrist with the thumb held in the palm) *(13)*.

- De Quervain's tenosynovitis must be distinguished from osteoarthritis of the first carpometacarpal (basilar joint) of the thumb.

Treatment is by splinting of the thumb in a thumb spica splint along with a nonsteroidal anti-inflammatory drug. Local corticosteroid injection into the tendon sheath is helpful. In some cases, surgical decompression is necessary.

Trigger Finger/Trigger Thumb

Painful snapping at the palmar aspect of the fingers or thumb is due to development of nodular enlargement of the flexor tendon and/or constriction of the tendon sheath. The patient often notices locking of the finger in flexion, particularly at night. A nodule of the flexor tendon can be palpated to move with the tendon during flexion and extension of the digit, approximately at the level of the metacarpophalangeal joint. Etiology is generally due to repetitive movement activities and degenerative changes, although similar triggering can be seen in inflammatory arthritis, such as rheumatoid arthritis. Treatment consists of local corticosteroid injections or nonsteroidal anti-inflammatory drugs and splinting. In recurrent cases, surgical release of the proximal pulley is a simple procedure that is very effective. This should not be used in rheumatoid arthritis, in which a more extensive tenosynovectomy is required.

Hypertrophic Osteoarthropathy

Hypertrophic osteoarthropathy is a syndrome characterized by clubbing of the digits and periostitis of the distal long bones. Synovitis may be present, and polyarthralgias may be the initial manifestation in some cases. Apart from an uncommon primary form, usually beginning in childhood, hypertrophic osteoarthropathy is usually due to a systemic process, particularly pulmonary diseases (Table 10). Patients may present with clubbing of the digits, with sponginess of the nail bed. Bone pain, particularly in the distal extremities, is common and may be quite severe, but is not always present. Pain is often exacerbated by dependency of the extremity. Joint pain may be present and may be the presenting feature, particularly in some cases of bronchogenic carcinoma. Radiographs are often normal early in the disease, but the subsequent development of periostitis of the distal long bones (particularly the tibia and the fibula and the radius and ulna) is characteristic. Radionuclide bone scanning will reveal increased uptake in the periosteal areas and often at the periarticular areas as well. Laboratory findings are primarily those of the underlying process. Thorough evaluation for an underlying cause is necessary in all new cases of hypertrophic osteoarthropathy. Nonsteroidal anti-inflammatory

Table 10
Causes of Secondary Hypertrophic Osteoarthropathy

1. Pulmonary diseases
   a. Carcinoma of the lung
   b. Chronic infection (bronchiectasis or chronic bronchitis)
   c. Other chronic pulmonary condition (cystic fibrosis, pulmonary fibrosis)
2. Cardiac disease
   a. Cyanotic and congenital heart disease
   b. Infective endocarditis
3. Other inflammatory conditions
   a. Inflammatory bowel disease
   b. Hepatic cirrhosis
4. Other carcinomas
5. Thyroid disease (thyroid acropachy)

drugs are generally effective in the treatment of pain of hypertrophic osteoarthropathy. Corticosteroids and colchicine may also be useful. Treatment of the underlying condition is associated with resolution of symptoms *(12)*.

VASCULAR DISEASES

Raynaud's Phenomenon

Raynaud's phenomenon is characterized by reversible vasospasm of the hands and/ or feet in response to cold. Symptoms are classically a three-phase color change: (1) pallor of the digits associated with pain and paresthesias, followed by (2) cyanosis, which persists until (3) rewarming. Erythema of the hands occurs with rewarming due to postischemic hyperemia, associated with the resolution of pain and numbness. Not all patients will report the classical three-color change; reversible pallor or cyanosis accompanied by pain or paresthesias is likely to represent Raynaud's phenomenon. Raynaud's phenomenon may be caused by a variety of underlying conditions (Table 11). Raynaud's phenomenon in the absence of any intrinsic disease is seen in 5–10% of normal young women. Usual onset of primary Raynaud's is during adolescence. Scleroderma is the most frequently associated connective tissue disease. Raynaud's phenomenon may precede other findings of scleroderma by years and is present in nearly all patients. Features that are predictive of the future development of a connective tissue disease in patients with isolated Raynaud's include older age at onset, greater severity of Raynaud's phenomenon with digital pitting or infarcts, abnormal patterns of nail-fold capillaries, and the presence of antinuclear antibodies *(18)*.

Therapy of Raynaud's phenomenon begins with warming measures, maintaining warm temperatures of both the extremities and the core body temperature. Among the vasodilator drugs, calcium channel blockers are the preferred agents. Nifedipine is the most effective and the most widely used in a dose of 30–120 mg/d, usually in an extended release formulation. Diltiazem is also frequently used, but Verapamil, Nisoldipine, and

Table 11
Conditions Associated with Raynaud's Phenomenon

Structural Vascular Disease	Drug Associated	Blood Abnormality	Miscellaneous	Idiopathic
Connective tissue diseases	Beta blockers	Cryoglobulinemia	Hypothyroidism	
Scleroderma	Ergot	Paraproteinemia	Reflex sympathetic dystrophy	
Systemic lupus erythematosus	Methysergide	Hyperviscosity syndrome	Pheochromocytoma	
Mixed connective tissue disease		Polycythemia	Carcinoid syndrome	
Sjogren's syndrome			Primary pulmonary hypertension	
Inflammatory myopathies				
Vasculitis				
Buerger's disease				
Takayasu's arteritis				
Atherosclerosis				
Vibratory trauma				
Toxic arteriopathy				
Polyvinyl chloride				
Chemotherapy				
Extrinsic compression				
Thoracic outlet syndrome				

Nicardipane are less effective. Other sympatholytic drugs are less effective and have been associated with a steal phenomenon in the abnormal vessels and the progression of ischemic tissue damage. Smoking should be avoided. Biofeedback may sometimes be helpful.

Buerger's Disease

Buerger's disease is an indolent obliterative vasculitic disease of young smokers. It is more commonly seen in men. The distal small- and medium-sized arteries and veins are particularly commonly involved so that initial clinical involvement is distal *(19)*. Claudication of the instep of the feet is a characteristic early finding, and calf claudication is uncommon early in the disease. In the upper extremities, Raynaud's phenomenon is seen in approximately one-half of patients. Claudication may occur and digital ulcers are seen. Absence of distal pulses in the upper extremities is seen in less than half of the patients. Primary treatment is strict abstinence from tobacco in any form. Vasodilators such as calcium channel blockers or iloprost may be helpful. Because disease is predominantly distal, surgical revascularization is generally not possible.

REFERENCES

1. Mikhail IS, Alarcon GS. Nongonococcal bacterial arthritis. Rheum Dis Clin N Amer 1993; 19: 311–331.
2. Emmerson BT. The management of gout. New Engl J Med 1996; 334: 445–456.
3. Doherty M, Dieppe P. Clinical aspects of calcium pyrophosphate deposition. Rheum Dis Clin N Amer 1988; 14: 395–414.
4. Gladman DD, Shuckett R, Russell ML, et al. Psoriatic arthritis: an analysis of 220 patients. Quart J Med 1987; 62: 127–141.
5. Belhorn LR, Hess EV. Erosive osteoarthritis. Semin Arth Rheum 1993; 22: 298–306.
6. Chuang TY, Hunder GG, Ilstrup DM, Kurland LT. Polymyalgia rheumatica: a ten year epidemiologic and clinical study. Ann Int Med 1982; 97: 672–680.
7. Bland JH, Merrit JA, Bousley DR. The painful shoulder. Semin Arth Rheum 1977; 7: 21–47.
8. Halverson PB, Carrera GF, McGarty DJ. Milwaukee shoulder syndrome. 15 additional cases and a description of contributing factors. Arch Int Med 1990; 150: 677–682.
9. Biundo JJ. Frozen shoulder. Bull Rheum Dis 1994; 43: 1,2.
10. Ellenberg MR, Honet JC, Treanor WJ. Cervical radiculopathy. Arch Phys Med Rehab 1994; 75: 342–352.
11. Leffert RD. Thoracic outlet syndrome. Hand Clin 1992; 8: 285–297.
12. Kozin F. The reflex sympathetic dystrophy syndrome. Bull Rheum Dis 1986; 36: 1–8.
13. Thorson ED, Szabo RM. Tendonitis of the wrist and elbow. Occup Medicine: State-of-the-Art Reviews 1989; 4: 419–431.
14. Watrous BG, Ho G Jr. Elbow pain. Primary Care: Clinics in Office Practice 1988; 15: 725–735.
15. Peimer CA, Wheeler DR. Radial tunnel syndrome/posterior interosseous nerve compression. In: Szabo RM. Nerve Compression Syndromes-Diagnosis and Treatment, SLACK, 1989.
16. Omer GE. Median nerve compression at the wrist. Hand Clin 1992; 8: 317–324.
17. Pineda C, Fonseca C, Martinez-Lavin M. The spectrum of soft tissue and skeletal abnormalities of hypertrophic osteoarthropathy. J Rheum 1990; 17: 773–778.
18. Bolster MB, Maricq HR, Leff RI. Office evaluation and treatment of Raynaud's phenomenon. Cleveland Clin J Med 1995; 62: 51–61.
19. Olin JW. Thromboangiitis obliterans. Curr Opin Rheum 1994; 6: 44–49.

5 CHEST PAIN

WILLIAM R. LEWIS, MD
EZRA A. AMSTERDAM, MD

Key Points

- The most frequent causes of chest pain are nonlethal syndromes (musculoskeletal, gastrointestinal, panic disorder).
- The most cost-effective procedure for diagnosing the etiology of chest pain is a thorough history and physical examination.
- Patients may respond negatively when questioned about the occurrence of chest pain, despite having symptoms such as pressure, squeezing, or heaviness. Use the term "discomfort" when eliciting this aspect of the history.
- Age, gender, and risk factors are crucial determinants in establishing a differential diagnosis of chest pain that includes cardiovascular, pulmonary, and gastrointestinal etiologies.
- The discovery of coronary artery disease does not preclude another etiology as the cause of a patient's chest pain.
- The exercise treadmill test is a cost-effective method to risk-stratify patients for ischemic cardiac events. A negative test does not preclude coronary disease, but it suggests that the future risk for a coronary event is very low. A trial of medical therapy in low-risk patients is usually warranted.
- Combining clinical data (risk factors) with exercise variables in addition to the ECG affords almost comparable accuracy to imaging studies for identification of patients with high-risk CAD.
- Low-risk patients with acute chest pain can usually be identified by clinical evaluation and do not require a formal assessment by serum enzymes before undergoing immediate treadmill exercise testing.
- In a patient presenting to the emergency department with acute chest pain, an ECG should be obtained and read within 10 min.
- An abdominal process (e.g., biliary tract disease) can cause pain referred to the chest.

- The frequency of pulmonary embolism is as high as 20% in patients with low-probability V/Q scans.
- Arterial blood gases are not useful screening tests for pulmonary embolism.
- Full-dose heparin therapy should be initiated in a patient with a high clinical probability of pulmonary embolism while awaiting results of the V/Q scan.
- Unequal pressures in the arms in a patient with severe chest pain may be caused by aortic dissection.
- Aortic dissection can be accurately diagnosed by computerized tomography scan, magnetic resonance imaging, or transesophageal echocardiography, as well as aortography.
- Gastrointestinal etiologies of chest pain are typified by pain at rest and in the supine position and by dysphagia or waterbrash.
- Empirical treatment with H_2 blockers or promotility agents may be the most cost-effective therapy for gastrointestinal reflux disease.
- Mediastinal and pulmonary etiologies of chest pain typically cause pleuritic chest pain, dyspnea, and cough.

INTRODUCTION

Chest pain is one of the most frequent and challenging problems that the clinician encounters. This symptom, which can be produced by myriad disorders, may be acute or chronic and can reflect a relatively benign cause or a life-threatening process *(1–3)* (Table 1). The approach to the patient with chest pain requires a systematic evaluation that begins with the history, physical examination, and screening laboratory tests. The history is the cornerstone of the evaluation and, together with associated initial data, determines whether further investigation is indicated and what direction it should take.

The patient with acute chest pain frequently confronts the clinician with the dilemma in which misdiagnosis can result in a fatal outcome, as in myocardial infarction (MI), pulmonary embolism, or aortic dissection, while failure to initially recognize a relatively benign cause can lead to unnecessary cost and risk in evaluation and therapy. Therefore, a critical question that is often posed by the initial presentation, in addition to the etiology of the symptom, is whether the patient requires hospitalization. Proper management at this stage requires judicious decision-making based on a comprehensive assessment of the clinical data in the individual patient. In addition to the evidence for a relatively benign or more serious disorder, the answer to this difficult problem may be unduly influenced by secondary factors such as the specter of medicolegal liability.

The most common serious disorders associated with chest pain are those involving the cardiopulmonary system, whereas chest pain is most commonly produced by diseases without fatal potential, such as musculoskeletal or functional syndromes. Our limited ability to confidently diagnose the etiology of chest pain in many patients, combined with the concern for overlooking a potentially lethal process, has led to more than 2 million hospitalizations annually in this country for suspected MI. Ultimately, less than 30% of these admissions are attributable to a coronary etiology *(4)*. For these reasons,

Table 1
Diagnostic Aspects of Important Causes of Chest Pain

Cause of Acute Chest Pain	Quality	Location	Onset	Duration	Provoked By	Relieved By	Comment	Initial Dx Test
Stable angina	Pressure, constriction, burning	Retrosternal, radiates	Gradual	5–10 min	Stress	Rest, NTG	ECG:ischemia (with pain)	ETT
Unstable angina	As above	As above	Variable	>15 min	Spontaneous or stress	NTG	ECG:ischemia (with pain)	ECG
Myocardial infarction	As above	As above	Sudden	≥30 min	Spontaneous	NTG ineffective	ECG:ischemia injury, necrosis	ECG, cardiac enzymes
Mitral valve prolapse	Sharp	Anterior chest	Sudden	Fleeting	Spontaneous	Spontaneous	Midsystolic click	Echocardiogram
Aortic stenosis	As in angina	Anterior chest	Gradual	5–10 min	Stress	Rest	Also syncope or heart failure symptoms	Echocardiogram
Normal coronary-atypical chest pain syndrome (e.g., panic attack musculoskeletal disease, sensitive heart)	Sharp, lancinating, fullness	Precordial, anterior chest, variable	Variable	Seconds to days	Unpredictable	NTG ±, rest ±	ECG:no changes with pain; fluctuating clinical picture, no cardiac morbidity	Clinical (definitive-coronary angiography)
Pericarditis	Sharp or visceral, pleuritic	Anterior chest, can radiate	Variable	Hours	Respiration, supine position	Sitting, anti-inflammatory agents	ECG:ST ↑(T ↓ in later phases); ± associated with systemic illness	ECG
Aortic dissection	Same as MI ± ("tearing"), very severe	Anterior chest, back, migratory	Sudden	Hours	—	Analgesia	Unequal pulses, widened mediastinum	CT, TEE, MRI

(continued)

Table 1 *(continued)*

Cause of Acute Chest Pain	Quality	Location	Onset	Duration	Provoked By	Relieved By	Comment	Initial Dk Test
Pulmonary embolism	Same as MI, pleuritic	Variable	Sudden	Min	—	Analgesia	Tachypnea, tachycardia, pain (may be absent)	V/Q scan
Tracheobronchitis	Aching	Retrosternal	Variable	Hours to days	Respiration	Analgesia	Cough	Clinical
Pneumonitis	Aching, burning	Anterior chest	Variable	Hours to days	Respiration	Analgesia	Fever, cough, tachypnea	CXR
Mediastinitis	Sharp, pressure	Retrosternal	Gradual	Hours to days	Respiration, supine position	Analgesia	Fever, history, of esophageal or tracheal procedure	CXR
Pleuritis	Sharp, aching burning	Variable	Gradual	Hours to days	Respiration	Analgesia, splinting	Fever, dyspnea	Clinical, biopsy
Pneumothorax	Sharp	Variable	Sudden	Minutes to hours	Spontaneous coughing	Spontaneous, chest tube	Dyspnea if large	CXR
Esophageal spasm, achalasia, nutcracker esophagus, gastroesophageal reflux	Pressure, squeezing, burning	Retrosternal	Variable	5–10 min	Eating, supine position, stress, spontaneous	Nitrates, antacids Ca^{2+} antagonists	Dysphagia common	Esophagoscopy, barium swallow, motility study
Esophageal ulcer	Sharp, burning	Retrosternal	Gradual	Days	Swallowing	Antacids	Caused by some oral antibiotics	Esophagoscopy
Mallory Weiss tear, Boerhaave's syndrome	Sharp, burning	Retrosternal	Sudden	Hours	Vomiting in 75%, physical exertion	Analgesia	Hematemesis common	Esophagoscopy (water soluble contrast)
Musculoskeletal	Aching	Anterior chest, precordial	Variable	Variable	Movement of involved area	Rest, analgesia	Localized tenderness	Clinical

Neuropathic	Aching	Anterior chest, precordial	Variable	Variable	Movement of neck or trunk	Rest, analgesia	Paresthesias	Clinical
Psychologic	Variable	Variable	Variable	Variable	Variable	Variable	Usually atypical for specific organ	Clinical
Cancer	Variable	Variable	Variable	Variable	Variable	Analgesia, spontaneous		CXR
Herpes-Zoster	Burning, stabbing	Dermatomal	Gradual	Days to months	Spontaneous	Analgesia		Clinical
Pancreatitis	Dull, stabbing	Epigastric, retrosternal	Variable	Days to months	Spontaneous, eating	Analgesia	Vomiting in 80% of cases	Serum amylase, lipase
Biliary disease	Variable, colicky	Right upper quadrant, epigastric, right subscapular	Variable	Minutes to hours	Spontaneous, eating	Analgesia	Vomiting common	Serum bilirubin and alkaline phosphatase, abdominal ultrasound
Cervical spine disease	Sharp	High anterior chest, radiates to arms or shoulders	Variable	Variable	Movement of neck	Rest, analgesia	May have point tenderness on C-spine exam	Cervical spine films

All indicated tests are predicated on precise history and physical examination. CT, computer tomography; CXR, chest X-ray film; Dx, diagnostic; ECG, electrocardiogram; Echo, echocardiogram; ETT, exercise test; MRI, magnetic resonance imaging; TEE, transesophageal echocardiography; VQ, ventilation-perfusion scan; ±, variable.

the approach to chest pain continues to stimulate intensive study, which has furthered our understanding of this symptom and enhanced its management.

PATHOPHYSIOLOGY

Pain arising in the structures of the chest is produced by multiple factors that cause tissue injury, such as ischemia and inflammation. The specific pain mechanisms and mediators have been difficult to identify, but they may include factors associated with cell injury such as increased local concentration of prostaglandins, potassium ions, proteases, hydrogen ions, and kinins. The nociceptive impulses from the structures of the chest are carried by afferent fibers that enter the dorsal roots of the spinal cord at the third cervical to the ninth thoracic segments, through which they ascend to the cerebral cortex, where these impulses are perceived as pain. Cardiac afferents enter the cord at the lower cervical and first five thoracic segments. The overlapping location of symptoms produced by the structures of the thorax (and abdomen) and the basis for referred pain may be related to the neuroanatomy of these pathways. Pain fibers from many structures of the chest share common sites of entry into the spinal cord and, according to the "convergence–projection theory," impulses from these structures may converge on the same spinal neurons, confounding recognition of the origin of these impulses in the higher cortical centers *(5)*. In addition, a single spinal afferent fiber may have sensory endings on different organs. Thus, pain arising in the heart may be perceived in the left arm or jaw, and pain originating in the abdominal viscera may be localized to the chest. This phenomenon may also explain phantom limb anginal pain in an amputee with coronary artery disease (CAD) whom we treated with elimination of the phantom pain by myocardial revascularization *(6)*.

HISTORY

The history is paramount in evaluating chest pain. Chest pain is a general term and therefore may not accurately reflect the patient's experience. Chest discomfort is a more preferable descriptor and, in this chapter, chest pain will be used synonymously with discomfort. The sensation may be more specifically described by the patient as pressure, heaviness, squeezing, tightness, or burning; or it may have a sharp, sticking, lancinating, or throbbing quality. It is therefore important that the patient describe the discomfort in his/her own words. The description of the symptom should include its location, quality, duration, frequency, precipitating causes, factors that provide relief, and whether its tempo has been stable, progressive, or decreasing. It is also important to clarify whether the symptom is consistent or inconsistent in terms of its descriptors and provoking factors. Chest pain must also be assessed in the context of the patient's risk profile for a given disease. For example, in a patient under 30 yr old without coronary risk factors, chest discomfort typical of myocardial ischemia is not likely to reflect CAD. However, in this setting, it is important to be cognizant of noncoronary causes of myocardial ischemia, such as hypertrophic obstructive cardiomyopathy, aortic stenosis, and cocaine abuse. Although a well-performed initial evaluation will help to limit the number of diagnostic possibilities, diagnostic certainty is commonly not attainable without ancillary testing. The initial evaluation should afford prudent selection of the most appropriate studies indicated, thereby increasing efficiency and reducing cost.

Few causes of chest pain present in a manner that is clearly diagnostic. Indeed, the specific etiologies of chest pain may themselves have variable and inconsistent presentations. Only costochondritis, intercostal neuritis, and pleurisy cause pain that is diagnostic from their patterns of onset, location, and nature. All other etiologies may be much more elusive. Multiple disorders can produce the same type of chest pain, further complicating assessment of this symptom. For example, it is often difficult for both patient and physician to distinguish between the sensation of chest tightness that can be produced by both dyspnea and angina. The evaluation may also be confounded in many patients by the coexistence of more than one disease associated with chest pain. CAD and gastroesophageal reflux may both be present, and their symptoms can simulate each other. Further, the provoking factors for chest pain of differing etiologies may overlap. Thus, while exertional chest pain suggests angina pectoris, it can also provoke gastroesophageal reflux. In addition, treatment of one problem may ameliorate the other. Thus, nitrates or calcium channel blockers prescribed for angina may relieve occult esophageal spasm. These vasodilators may also paradoxically exacerbate the esophageal symptoms by relaxing the lower esophageal sphincter and increasing reflux. Finally, it is important to recognize that the presence of a disease that can cause chest pain is not conclusive evidence that it is responsible for the symptom. In this regard, evaluation of chest pain that results in the discovery of CAD can lead to myocardial revascularization that may not alleviate the symptom, because the etiology was an overlooked, less emergent disorder such as gastroesophageal reflux.

In a large proportion of patients presenting with acute or chronic chest pain, the etiology is psychogenic. An important disease in this category that has received increased attention is panic disorder, discussed later in this chapter. Certain aspects of the history are helpful in identifying patients with an increased probability of psychogenic symptoms, thereby obviating complex and costly evaluation for cardiac and other organic disease. Diseases of the heart, lungs, and other structures of the chest usually present with a relatively consistent pattern, whereas emotionally based symptoms are more likely to be described in terms that do not fit any organ system because of their erratic and inconsistent nature. Thus, a symptom history marked by inconsistency in quality, severity, location, duration, and provoking factors should raise the possibility of an emotional etiology. Chest pain that is chronic, severe, and frequent in the absence of objective findings on the physical examination or screening tests greatly reduces the probability of CAD or other organic cause, since such severe symptoms are usually associated with objective clinical manifestations. If the patient is assessed during an episode of chest discomfort, a complaint of severe pain associated with an appearance of relative comfort suggests a psychogenic etiology. This discordance has been referred to as *la belle indifference* and was originally applied to patients with conversion reaction (unconscious substitution of a somatic symptom for an emotional problem). Although patient assessment can suggest a psychogenic etiology of symptoms, caution must be exercised before reaching such a conclusion because of the risk of overlooking serious organic disease. Further, inconsistencies in the history may be more related to a patient's anxiety and inability as a historian than to the etiology of the symptom, which may be (after all) organically based. In addition, both organic and psychogenic pain can coexist, which can considerably confound diagnostic conclusions. Finally, some patients with disease of the heart, lungs, or other structures of the chest present with symptoms that are very atypical, whereas those without organic disease manifest symptoms that strongly suggest an organic etiology, such as angina or pericarditis. Appreciation of the value, limits, and challenges posed by the history will afford optimal yield from this basic method of evaluation.

PHYSICAL EXAMINATION

The evaluation of chest pain involves not only the physical examination of the thorax, but also of the abdomen to exclude the possibility of referred pain to the chest, and of distal vasculature disease because abnormalities distally may indicate a thoracic origin. A complete examination also requires the diagnostician to inspect, palpate, and auscultate. Skilled clinicians are as accurate as magnetic resonance imaging in estimating cardiac size *(7)* and as accurate as invasive monitoring in assessing right heart filling pressures *(8)*. Failure to perform a complete physical examination initially will lead to more expensive diagnostic testing subsequently.

The examination begins with a general assessment of the patient. Does he/she appear distressed? Are the complaints consistent with the patient's appearance, or does there appear to be less discomfort than complaint of pain? Inconsistencies in the verbalized level of pain and appearance may suggest a functional etiology. The skin of the face should also be carefully examined for pallor or flushing. The lips should be inspected for central cyanosis suggestive of pulmonary insufficiency or right-to-left intracardiac shunting. The hands and feet should be examined for pallor, poor capillary refill, or peripheral cyanosis, suggestive of circulatory insufficiency.

Vital signs consisting of temperature, respiratory rate, heart rate, and blood pressure, in both arms, are essential. Failure to perform blood pressure measurement in both arms could lead to failure to detect an aortic dissection that has compromised subclavian artery blood flow. In cases of suspected cardiac rhythm disturbance, such as atrial fibrillation or ventricular bigeminy, it is also important to measure the heart rate by cardiac auscultation to obtain the apical pulse. Cardiac arrhythmias may lead to incomplete ventricular filling during some cardiac cycles such that, during systole, an insignificant volume of blood is ejected and a peripheral pulse cannot be felt. Measurement of heart rate by palpating the peripheral pulse would therefore lead to a falsely low rate.

Inspection of the neck veins for distention and abnormal wave forms may indicate a cardiac etiology of the chest pain, such as when myocardial infarction causes ventricular dysfunction. Inspection of the thorax for abnormal pulsations or cardiac impulse may also suggest a cardiac etiology. Herpes zoster may be identified by the dermatomal rash; therefore, inspection of the skin of the chest and abdomen is also essential.

The chest wall should also be palpated, since rib fractures may be identified as point tenderness or crepitus over the fracture. Palpation of the costochondral joints along the sternum may reveal tenderness diagnostic of costochondritis. Percussion of the lung fields is also important; spontaneous pneumothorax may present with acute onset of chest pain with shortness of breath and an area of hyperresonance on percussion. In contrast, dullness to percussion would be consistent with consolidation from a pneumonia or atelectasis from bronchial obstruction by a lung mass.

The final part of the thoracic examination is auscultation. The heart should be auscultated over the aortic, pulmonic, tricuspid, and mitral areas. A late-peaking, harsh murmur over the aortic position suggests aortic stenosis as a cause of the chest pain. Mitral regurgitation murmurs or gallop rhythms may occur in acute MI. Auscultation of a sound that is scratchy or simulates the squeaking of new leather concurrent with each heartbeat is consistent with the friction rub of pericarditis. The lung fields deserve similar attention because the same squeaking sound synchronous with the respiratory cycle is diagnostic of the friction rub of pleurisy. Lack of breath sounds over an area of the chest may suggest a spontaneous pneumothorax, which is more commonly seen in younger than older adults.

It is important to examine the abdomen for causes of pain referred to the chest. A pulsatile mass may suggest an aortic aneurysm. Epigastric tenderness is consistent with pancreatitis, and right upper-quadrant tenderness associated with a Murphy's sign suggests biliary tract disease. Prior prohibition against rectal examination in MI patients has been discarded, and this evaluation is particularly important in the thrombolytic era. Guaiac positive stools suggest esophagitis, gastritis, or peptic ulcer disease as the etiology of the chest pain.

CARDIAC ETIOLOGIES OF CHEST PAIN

Ischemic Cardiac Pain—Coronary Artery Disease

CAD is the leading cause of death and a primary cause of disability in this country. Its major clinical syndromes are angina pectoris, acute MI, and sudden death. The initial presentation of CAD is acute MI in over 50% of victims, angina in approx 30%, and sudden death in 10–20%. Therefore, a majority of patients with CAD presents with a syndrome in which chest pain heralds the disease. Because of the epidemiology of CAD and its lethality, the possibility that CAD is responsible for chest pain is a foremost concern of every physician evaluating a patient with this symptom. In both acute and stable presentations of CAD, diagnostic accuracy affords therapy that not only reduces symptoms but also can increase survival. Recognition of stable angina leads to risk stratification that identifies high-risk patients who are candidates for myocardial revascularization and also indicates which patients are more appropriately treated conservatively. In acute MI, optimal management that decreases mortality is dependent on rapid diagnosis and institution of coronary reperfusion therapy. Although chest pain is the clinical hallmark of myocardial ischemia, it is important to also appreciate that a majority of ischemic episodes in angina patients are unassociated with symptoms (silent myocardial ischemia) and, in many other instances, dyspnea occurs as an anginal equivalent without chest discomfort. In addition, at least 25% of acute MIs are silent or associated with atypical symptoms. This is particularly true of elderly patients and women.

Stable Angina Pectoris

History is the primary means of diagnosing angina. In patients with typical symptoms and a positive coronary risk factor profile, the etiology is CAD with a probability approaching 90% *(9)*. Heberden's original description of anginal pain more than 200 yr ago remains unsurpassed: "...a painful and disagreeable sensation in the breast, which seems as if it would extinguish life...situated in the upper part, sometimes in the middle, sometimes at the bottom of the sternum...very frequently extends from the breast to the middle of the left arm." The most frequent site of anginal pain is the retrosternal area. The discomfort radiates bilaterally across the chest, to the ulnar and volar aspects of the left arm more frequently than to the right, and into the neck and lower jaw. Angina may sometimes be felt only in the arm or it can radiate to the chest from the arm. The discomfort is described as pressing, squeezing, crushing, or heavy and it is steady. Stable angina must be provoked by physical exertion or emotional stress, which increases the determinants of myocardial oxygen demand (heart rate, blood pressure, ventricular volume, contractility) beyond the flow reserve of a diseased coronary artery system, resulting in myocardial ischemia and its symptomatic expression, chest pain. The latter usually subsides within 5–10 min after removal of the provoking factor.

It is important to inquire as to the consistency of symptoms with a given activity or stress. Inconsistency militates against angina but, in some cases, it may reflect mixed angina or variable ambient conditions. Mixed angina describes the syndrome caused by a combination of fixed atherosclerotic coronary lesions, upon which is intermittently superimposed a variable component of additional coronary tone. This dynamic component of lesion severity accounts for the patient's differing anginal thresholds. The influence of altered ambient conditions is reflected in the more rapid rise of the determinants of myocardial oxygen demand in low temperatures than in a temperate setting. Thus, in patients with angina, exertional capacity may be reduced on a cold morning compared to a temperate afternoon. These considerations emphasize the importance of obtaining a detailed and accurate history.

Symptoms that do not represent stable angina are shooting, sharp, or throbbing pains that can last seconds or many hours, have inconsistent location, are more frequent at rest than with exertion, and have been present for years in this pattern without progression to a coronary event. Although unstable angina and vasospastic (Prinzmetal) angina are characterized by chest pain at rest, the quality of the symptom and its other characteristics are consistent with myocardial ischemic pain as previously described. Among the most common noncardiac causes of chest pain are panic disorder *(10,11)*, gastroesophageal disease *(12)*, and musculoskeletal syndromes *(13)*, which require consideration if the clinical setting of chest pain is inconsistent with CAD.

The physical examination in patients with stable angina is commonly devoid of positive cardiac findings in patients who have not had a prior MI, since left ventricular function at rest is usually normal or near normal in the absence of loss of myocardium from MI, even in the presence of severe CAD. However, during myocardial ischemia signaled by an anginal episode, the blood pressure and heart rate may be elevated, and there may be S_3 or S_4 gallops, pulmonary crackles, and a murmur of mitral regurgitation. These findings, which reflect transient mechanical dysfunction of the left ventricle, remit following the episode of ischemia. The resting electrocardiogram (ECG), which is usually normal or near normal in the absence of a prior MI, may show dynamic ST-T abnormalities of ischemia, which revert to normal following the attack. The examination may also reveal evidence of CAD risk factors such as fundascopic changes, S_4 gallop in hypertension, xanthelasma in hyperlipidemia, or bruits and diminished pulses in peripheral vascular disease. The basic laboratory findings may reveal evidence of contributing factors, such as hyperlipidemia or diabetes.

Diagnostic Tests. Noninvasive diagnostic tests provide objective data of myocardial ischemia and thereby presumptive evidence of CAD. These tests are based on the detection of several manifestations of ischemia that are absent in the control state and are induced during stress. The tests are only performed in stable patients under carefully controlled conditions. The risk of these methods is extremely small in properly selected patients who undergo testing by skilled, experienced personnel. The comparative value and limitations, including relative cost, of the following tests have been compared by Cheitlin *(14)*.

The most common method is treadmill exercise testing, which utilizes a progressive stress (speed and grade of the treadmill) to induce myocardial ischemia, detected on the ECG. Objective evidence of ischemia is 1.0 mm horizontal or downsloping ST-segment depression appearing during or immediately after exercise (Fig. 1). Interestingly, the occurrence of chest pain during the exercise test has not been a reliable predictor of CAD *(15)*. Early appearance of ST depression during the test (heart rate <120/min) and marked positivity (>2.0 mm ST depression) are associated with increased probability of a true positive result, severe CAD, and increased prognostic risk. The sensitivity (proportion of individuals with CAD who have a positive test) and specificity (proportion of normal individuals with a negative test) of the treadmill exercise test in symptomatic persons is approx 70 and 80%, respectively. However, the predictive accuracy of a positive test (proportion of positive tests that are true positives) depends on the prevalence of CAD in the population being studied, as well as the sensitivity and specificity of the test *(9)*. In patients unable to adequately perform exercise testing, Holter monitoring may be helpful in stratifying patients into high- and low-risk groups. Although the imaging tests described below are more sensitive for detecting CAD than exercise electrocardiography, consideration of both clinical and exercise variables, in addition to ST segment changes, can yield comparable results in identifying patients with severe CAD at substantially less expense *(16)*.

Cardiac ischemia can also be detected by transient myocardial perfusion abnormalities identified by nuclear scintigraphy *(17)*. Utilizing exercise or pharmacologic stress (dipyridamole or adenosine) and a radioactive tracer (thallium or sestamibi) that is taken up by the myocardium, areas of transient hypoperfusion, reflecting coronary stenoses, can be imaged noninvasively. These studies have greater sensitivity (~90%) than the exercise ECG, and their specificity has ranged from 70 to over 90%. Nuclear scintigraphy is particularly useful in patients who cannot exercise or in whom there are abnormalities in the resting ECG that preclude interpretation during exercise. It is considerably more costly than treadmill exercise testing.

Stress echocardiography *(18)* with exercise or dobutamine is also used to detect transient ischemia and thereby strengthen or reduce the likelihood of CAD. This technique is based on the development, during stress, of new segmental abnormalities of left ventricular motion in areas that are normal at rest. Its sensitivity and specificity are comparable to those of nuclear scintigraphy, and its cost is intermediate between exercise testing and scintigraphy.

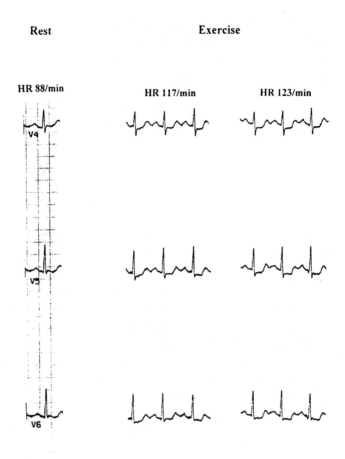

Rest   Exercise

Fig. 1. A positive exercise electrocardiogram in a 58-yr-old woman. The ST segments (leads V_4, V_5, V_6) are normal at rest and become depressed more than 1.0 mm at a heart rate (HR) of 123/min.

Coronary angiography is the definitive method for diagnosing CAD. It provides detailed analysis of the site and severity of coronary lesions and their suitability for percutaneous transluminal coronary angioplasty (PTCA) or coronary artery bypass graft surgery (CABG). This morphologic method, however, does not afford information on myocardial ischemia, a problem that particularly applies to lesions of intermediate severity (50–70% stenosis). Therefore, in patients who are candidates for revascularization procedures, angiography is often assessed in conjunction with one of the functional tests described above to confirm the presence of ischemia. Angiography is the most costly method for diagnosing CAD and it entails a minimal but finite risk of mortality (~1/1000 in stable patients), but it is indispensable when precise assessment of coronary artery anatomy is indicated.

Treatment. The management of stable angina encompasses a broad approach that includes coronary risk-factor reduction in all patients and the selection of medical therapy or myocardial revascularization, depending on the clinical findings in the individual

Table 2
Medical Therapy for Angina and Effects
on Determinants of Myocardial Oxygen Consumption

	Nitrates	β-Adrenergic Blockade	Calcium Antagonists[a]	Exercise Training
Heart rate	(↑)[b]	↓↓↓	↓ (↑)	↓
Blood pressure	↓↓	↓ (→)	↓	↓
Myocardial contractility	(↑)[b]	↓	↓	?
Ventricular volume	↓↓↓	→ (↓)	↓ (↑)	→

[a]The effects of these agents vary with the specific drug.
[b]Indirect (reflex) effect.

patient. The major reversible coronary risk factors (hypertension, smoking, hyperlipidemia) require active intervention. Recent studies confirm that risk-factor reduction retards progression and produces modest regression of CAD, but most importantly, it reduces coronary morbidity and mortality *(19)*. These patients should also receive one aspirin daily as prophylaxis against coronary thrombosis.

In most patients with stable angina, symptoms can be treated satisfactorily with medical therapy, which is based on alleviating myocardial ischemia by improving the balance between myocardial oxygen demand and supply. Oxygen demand is reduced by agents that decrease heart rate, blood pressure, contractility, and ventricular volume. These include nitrates, β-adrenergic blockers, calcium channel blockers, and exercise training (Table 2). Sublingual nitroglycerine is essential to abort acute episodes of angina and for short-interval (20 min) prophylaxis against anticipated episodes. Many patients will respond to combined therapy with two agents while some will require all three classes of drugs. The indications for CABG are (1) symptoms that are refractory to optimal medical therapy, (2) left main CAD (≥50% stenosis), and (3) 3-vessel CAD associated with decreased left ventricular function (ejection fraction <50%). In the latter two instances, CABG is indicated even in the absence of refractory symptoms because it improves survival in these high-risk patients. PTCA is superior to medical therapy in alleviating angina, and its effect on clinical outcome (myocardial infarction and mortality) is comparable to that of CABG in patients with 3-vessel CAD and preserved left ventricular function *(20)*. However, recurrent stenosis is frequent (~40%) within 6 mo of PTCA. Intracoronary stenting has reduced this problem. The comparative effects of PTCA vs CABG and vs medical therapy on survival in other subgroups of CAD patients have not been studied.

Unstable Angina

Whereas stable angina is associated with significant but quiescent coronary atherosclerotic plaques, unstable angina is usually caused by a ruptured plaque that initiates a subtotal thrombotic coronary artery occlusion. It is uncommonly the initial presentation of CAD. The quality and location of the pain parallel those of stable angina, but it is more intense, lasts longer, is more readily provoked, and frequently occurs at rest. Unstable

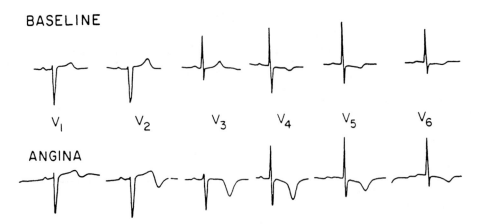

Fig. 2. Electrocardiogram of a patient hospitalized for unstable angina. During an episode of angina, there is ischemic T-wave inversion.

angina encompasses three presentations: (1) pain at rest lasting more than 10 min, (2) an increase in the tempo of previously stable angina, and (3) new-onset angina (the latter is somewhat controversial). The physical examination may be normal but is more likely to show evidence of left ventricular dysfunction than in stable angina. Unstable angina is unassociated with evidence of necrosis by ECG or cardiac serum enzymes, but the ECG may reveal ischemic ST segment and/or T-wave changes (Fig. 2). The latter findings identify a group at increased risk to progress to MI.

Diagnostic Tests. Unstable angina is diagnosed by the history *(see above)* and absence of evidence of myocardial necrosis reflected by cardiac serum enzymes and ECG. Newer cardiac markers, such as the troponins, may be positive in high-risk patients with unstable angina *(21,22)*. ECG evidence of ischemia strongly supports the diagnosis, especially when it comprises ischemic ECG changes at rest during anginal pain (Fig. 2). The noninvasive tests previously described, which can be performed after the patient has stabilized, usually show more extensive evidence of ischemia than in patients with stable angina. Coronary angiography often shows a culprit coronary lesion with a subocclusive stenosis, ulceration, and associated thrombus.

Treatment. Therapy depends on the clinical presentation *(23)*. Patients with prolonged rest angina and ECG evidence of ischemia (Fig. 2) are at high risk for complications and should be managed in a coronary care unit and treated with aspirin, heparin, nitrates, and a β-blocker. A calcium blocker can be added if necessary. In this regard, addition of nifedipine to β-blockade has reduced clinical events in unstable angina *(24)*. Over 85% of patients respond to this intensive therapy. Patients with residual ischemia on ECG and those with increased clinical risk (cardiac failure, prior MI, or previous revascularization) should undergo predischarge coronary angiography. Patients without these factors should undergo risk-stratification by noninvasive testing before discharge. Evidence of substantial ischemia on noninvasive testing is an indication for coronary angiography and myocardial revascularization if anatomy is suitable. If initial, intensive medical therapy is ineffective, prompt coronary angiography should be performed and revascularization carried out if indicated by angiography. Patients who present with progressive symptoms without rest pain should be managed on a case-by-case basis *(23)*. Some will require hospital admission for stabilization and evaluation and others may be satisfactorily managed by increasing their medical therapy (Table 2) and implementing risk-factor reduction *(19)*.

A substantial proportion of patients with severe symptoms, a low coronary risk profile, and a normal ECG (who are initially managed as unstable angina) either do not have CAD or have symptoms unrelated to coincident CAD. Because of the severity of their symptoms, it is difficult for the clinician to withhold intensive therapy. However, considerable clinical experience over the past several decades has shown that a very low-risk group with <3% probability of a coronary event can be identified among patients presenting to the emergency department with chest pain. This group is defined by atypical symptoms, a normal or near normal ECG, and no history of CAD *(4)*. In many of these patients, the etiology of their chest pain is a nonlethal process such as panic attack *(10,11)*, gastroesophageal reflux *(12)*, or musculoskeletal disease *(13)*. It is our practice to exclude myocardial ischemia in these low-risk patients by performing immediate exercise testing in the emergency department, thereby stratifying the group into those who require admission, based on a positive exercise test, and those who can be managed as outpatients, as indicated by a negative test *(4,25,25a)*. Alternatively, a short-stay unit can be utilized for these patients, with performance of exercise testing after unstable angina and myocardial infarction have been ruled out by a brief evaluation. These approaches obviate unnecessary admissions, optimize bed utilization, and reduce cost.

Myocardial Infarction

MI is the leading cause of mortality in this country, with an annual incidence of 1.5 million, of which almost 500,000 are fatal. These statistics underlie the clinician's concern in approaching the patient with chest pain in the coronary age group, and they also explain the high proportion of patients admitted to CCUs in whom evaluation for MI is negative. In almost 90% of patients with Q-wave MI, the pathophysiology is rupture of an atherosclerotic plaque that precipitates total coronary artery occlusion by thrombus. In non–Q-wave MI, the occlusion is subtotal, as in unstable angina. Other mechanisms include total coronary occlusion in a vessel supplied by collaterals or occlusion of a small coronary branch. The pain of acute MI is similar in quality and location to that of stable and unstable angina; but it is more severe and prolonged (usually >30 min to several hours) and is commonly associated with diaphoresis, nausea, and dyspnea. The physical findings depend on the extent of infarction. There may be no abnormal signs in a small, non-Q MI, whereas a large anterior MI may be associated with decreased blood pressure, tachycardia, elevated jugular venous pulse, pulmonary crackles, ectopic beats, an abnormal apical impulse, gallop rhythms, paradoxical splitting of S_2, and a mitral regurgitation murmur. Inferior MI is an indication to search for a right ventricular infarction, which is suggested by evidence of right ventricular failure (elevated jugular veins) and hypotension in the absence of left ventricular failure (clear lungs).

Diagnostic Tests. The diagnosis of acute MI is based on (1) compatible symptoms and (2) evidence of myocardial necrosis, as indicated by elevation of the MB (cardiac) fraction of serum creatine kinase and/or ECG evolution of pathologic Q waves (Fig. 3).

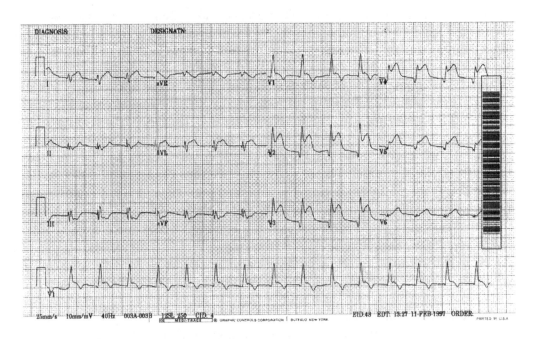

Fig. 3. Acute anterior myocardial infarction. Note ST segment elevation in anterior leads and reciprocal inferior ST segment depression.

Serum troponin levels have greater sensitivity and specificity for myocardial infarction than current cardiac markers and should therefore provide improved diagnostic accuracy *(21,22)*. In inferior MI, ST elevation in right-sided precordial leads is evidence of right ventricular infarction. The extent of myocardial dysfunction can be determined noninvasively by bedside echocardiography, which can also assess valve function, identify intracardiac shunts, and detect mural thrombi.

   Treatment. The management of uncomplicated acute MI has undergone major advances in the past decade that have reduced mortality and morbidity *(27)*. Coronary reperfusion therapy by either thrombolytic drugs or primary PTCA can increase survival and preserve myocardium. The importance of early diagnosis is underscored by the need for prompt application of these methods, since myocardial necrosis evolves rapidly. Optimal results have been attained when thrombolytic drugs have been instituted within 2 h of onset of MI. Efficacy is limited after 8 h, except in patients with ongoing evidence of ischemia. The interval for benefit from acute application of PTCA is somewhat longer. The indications for coronary reperfusion therapy in patients with acute MI are very specific and constitute ST elevation that does not normalize with nitroglycerine. Patients with non–Q-wave MI and those with unstable angina have not benefitted from thrombolytic therapy.

   Nonthrombolytic therapy also has an important role in the treatment of MI. Three agents produce benefit on early and late survival in MI patients: aspirin, β-adrenergic blockers, and angiotensin-converting enzyme inhibitors (ACEIs). Aspirin should be administered immediately and daily, and a β-blocker should be started early in the absence of contraindications. ACEIs are indicated in patients with evidence of left ventricular dysfunction. The patient's blood pressure may be a limiting factor in allowing neither or only one of the latter agents. Chest pain is an indication for nitroglycerine by topical or intravenous administration. Supplemental oxygen is routinely administered but is clearly indicated if there is evidence of hypoxemia.

In order to facilitate rapid, effective therapy of acute MI, it is important to develop a systematic method of implementation. In many facilities, this involves obtaining and interpreting an ECG and administering aspirin in the patient with chest pain within 10 min of arrival in the emergency department. If there is ST elevation unresponsive to nitroglycerine, coronary reperfusion therapy should be applied within 30 min of arrival. Chest pain is treated with nitrates and, if necessary, narcotic analgesia. A β-blocker is given if there is no cardiac failure. In the presence of failure, an ACEI is administered.

The patient with non-Q MI is treated with aspirin and a β-blocker. Diltiazem or verapamil are alternatives to the β-blocker if there is no evidence of left ventricular dysfunction, since these calcium channel blockers prevent recurrent MI in the absence of ventricular dysfunction but are associated with increased mortality in non-Q MI with ventricular dysfunction. For persistent chest pain, nitrates are added and, if necessary, narcotic analgesia.

The predischarge management of the MI patient involves prognostic stratification, by which high-risk patients are selected for coronary angiography to determine suitability for revascularization *(28)*. Cardioprotective drug therapy that increases survival includes aspirin, a β-blocker, an ACEI (patients with left ventricular dysfunction), and reduction of coronary risk factors *(19)*.

Microvascular Angina

Anginal pain in the presence of angiographically normal coronary arteries has been attributed to an impaired vasodilator capacity of the coronary microcirculation that results in an inability to increase coronary blood flow concomitant with augmented myocardial oxygen demand *(29)*. This disorder has also been referred to as cardiac syndrome X. The anginal pain is typical of that associated with CAD. In addition, objective evidence of myocardial ischemia, such as a positive exercise ECG, is part of the syndrome. A unique feature of this form of myocardial ischemia is its benign course, in terms of absence of myocardial infarction or sudden death. Diagnosis is based on a history of typical angina, objective evidence of myocardial ischemia, and documentation of impaired coronary flow reserve in the absence of angiographic CAD. The latter is measured at cardiac catheterization. Treatment consists of antianginal medication. The diagnosis of microvascular angina has sometimes been inappropriately applied to patients with chest pain atypical for angina, angiographically normal coronary arteries, and no objective evidence of myocardial ischemia. This error can be avoided by rigorous attention to the diagnostic criteria for this entity.

Ischemic Cardiac Pain—Noncoronary Etiologies

A number of conditions can cause myocardial ischemia and anginal pain in the presence of normal coronary arteries. This symptom is indistinguishable from the angina of

CAD. The major diseases in this category are aortic valve stenosis, hypertrophic obstructive cardiomyopathy, systemic hypertension, aortic valve insufficiency, and pulmonary hypertension. The mechanism of ischemia is increased myocardial oxygen demand, which outstrips the delivery capacity of normal coronary arteries. The first three entities increase oxygen demand by elevation of intraventricular pressure. Aortic insufficiency also causes inadequate diastolic coronary perfusion pressure. In addition to right ventricular ischemia, the chest discomfort of pulmonary hypertension has been attributed to pulmonary artery dilatation, but clinical studies do not support this hypothesis *(1)*.

When these conditions are severe enough to cause angina in the absence of CAD, they should be apparent from the physical examination. Critical aortic stenosis is indicated by a sustained apical impulse, a harsh, late-peaking (kite-shaped), basal, systolic ejection murmur associated with a diminished or paradoxically split A_2, S_4 gallop, and carotid pulses that are delayed and diminished. In elderly patients with critical aortic stenosis, the carotid upstroke may be normal owing to loss of vascular compliance. Hypertrophic cardiomyopathy is suggested by physical findings of left ventricular hypertrophy and an obstructive systolic ejection murmur at the apex or left sternal border that is accentuated by the Valsalva maneuver. The carotid pulses have a bifid impulse and rapid upstroke. Systemic hypertension is apparent on the physical examination, which may also reveal left ventricular hypertrophy and S_4 gallop. In addition to the characteristic early diastolic decrescendo blowing murmur at the sternal border, aortic insufficiency causes a wide arterial pulse pressure with a reduced diastolic component, bounding peripheral pulses, and a left ventricular heave. Severe pulmonary hypertension may produce peripheral cyanosis, physical findings of right ventricular hypertrophy (left parasternal lift), elevated jugular venous *a* waves, an accentuated pulmonic closing sound (audible at the apex), and murmurs of tricuspid and pulmonary insufficiency.

Diagnostic Tests

The aortic valve lesions and hypertension produce ECG evidence of left ventricular hypertrophy and repolarization changes in a majority of patients. Hypertrophic cardiomyopathy is associated with a number of ECG abnormalities, including left ventricular hypertrophy and abnormal Q waves (pseudoinfarct pattern). The foregoing conditions, especially aortic insufficiency, may show left ventricular enlargement on the chest film. In pulmonary hypertension, the ECG reveals evidence of right ventricular pressure overload: right axis deviation, right ventricular hypertrophy, and right atrial abnormality. The chest film may show enlargement of the right ventricle and main pulmonary arteries.

These lesions can be evaluated noninvasively by echocardiography, which provides detailed anatomic imaging of the abnormality, determines its severity, and assesses cardiac chamber dimensions and ventricular function. Further hemodynamic evaluation and imaging data are obtained from cardiac catheterization and angiography.

Treatment

When assessment of aortic stenosis reveals critical reduction of valve area ($<0.7 \text{ cm}^2$) associated with symptoms of angina, cardiac failure, or syncope, surgical correction is indicated. Surgery is usually performed in aortic insufficiency for symptoms of cardiac failure or, in the absence of symptoms, evidence of declining left ventricular function as indicated by a complex of parameters (e.g., falling ejection fraction or increase in left ventricular size to a critical value >5.6 cm at end systole). Medical therapy for aortic insufficiency (before this point is reached) comprises afterload reduction with an ACEI, hydralazine, or a dihydroperidine calcium channel blocker *(30)*. Hypertrophic obstructive cardiomyopathy is primarily managed with a β-blocker or calcium blocker. These agents reduce both the excessive contractility that contributes to the dynamic left ventricular outflow tract obstruction and the diastolic dysfunction that may cause pulmonary congestion. In patients with systemic hypertension, antihypertensive therapy can alleviate symptoms (e.g., angina) attributable to the excessive systemic pressure and also decreases the occurrence of MI and stroke. β-blockers and diuretics are currently recommended as first-line antihypertensive therapy, but ACEIs, calcium channel blockers, or other agents are appropriate as indicated by comorbidity. The management of secondary pulmonary hypertension consists of treating the underlying etiology (e.g., mitral stenosis, pulmonary emboli, left heart failure). Treatment of primary pulmonary hypertension has limited efficacy and includes supplemental oxygen and vasodilators such as prostacyclin, calcium blockers, or ACEIs. Lung transplant is now an option in these patients.

Nonischemic Cardiac Pain

Pericarditis

This diagnosis indicates inflammation of the pericardium, which can be caused by numerous mechanisms, including the entire spectrum of infective agents, connective tissue disease, uremia, malignancy, myocardial infarction, trauma, radiation, myxedema, and poststernotomy Dressler's syndrome. The pain of pericarditis is typically sharp; varies from mild to severe; is occasionally crushing; and is exacerbated by inspiration, coughing, movement of the trunk, swallowing, and the supine position (it may be relieved by sitting up). It is felt in the precordial or retrosternal areas with radiation to the left shoulder, arm, neck, and upper back. In contrast to the frequent absence of pain when pericarditis occurs in the course of another disease, chest pain is a prominent presenting manifestation of primary pericarditis. In the latter condition, the pain is frequently accompanied by fever, malaise, and myalgia. Only a relatively small area of the pericardium, consisting of the diaphragmatic parietal layer, has sensory fibers, which are supplied by the phrenic nerve. Inflammation of this area, therefore, produces pain referred to the neck and shoulders *(1)*. Inflammation of the remainder of the pericardium does not produce pain unless there is associated involvement of the pleura. In some patients, pericardial pain may be difficult to discern from that of myocardial ischemia. Pericardial pain usually decreases or abates when effusion develops. The cardinal sign of pericarditis is a friction rub. This finding is often transient and variable. It has a scratchy quality and up to three components, which are related to ventricular contraction, atrial contraction, and the rapid filling phase of early diastole.

Diagnostic Tests. The ECG in the early stage of pericarditis reveals characteristic ST elevation that is usually diffuse, involving all leads except aVR and V_1 (Fig. 4). In

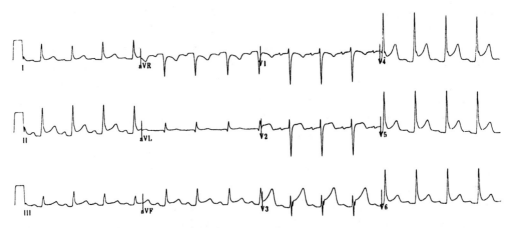

Fig. 4. Electrocardiogram in a patient with pericarditis showing characteristic diffuse ST segment elevation (except in aVR and V₁) and PR segment depression.

contrast to the findings in acute MI (Fig. 4), the upward concavity of the ST segment is preserved, there is no reciprocal ST depression, and there may be PR depression. It is important to appreciate the evolutionary changes in the ECG of pericarditis, which include return of the ST segment to baseline and symmetric T-wave inversion. For these reasons, in a patient seen several days after the onset of pericarditis, it may be difficult to distinguish the ECG changes from those of myocardial ischemia. Cardiac serum enzymes are normal unless there is associated myocardial infarction or myocarditis. The chest film and echocardiogram in the patient with painful pericarditis do not usually show an enlarged cardiac silhouette or effusion, respectively.

Treatment. Definitive treatment is that of the underlying disease. The pain of pericarditis is treated with aspirin or other nonsteroidal antiinflammatory agents. In severe pain, steroid therapy may be necessary, but it should be tapered after a week.

Mitral Valve Prolapse

This condition is the most common valve abnormality in the industrialized societies; it can be associated with chest pain that is usually atypical for angina. Further, the quality, location, and provoking factors vary from patient to patient and in the same patient at different times. The pain is often described as sharp, occurs more at rest than with exertion, and varies in duration from seconds to hours. Its mechanism is obscure. The incidence of mitral valve prolapse is higher in females than males, and it may be congenital or involve myxomatous changes such as in Marfan's syndrome. The valve leaflets are large and redundant; during late systole, one or both leaflets prolapse posteriorly into the left atrium, causing regurgitation. In addition to chest pain, atrial and ventricular arrhythmias, endocarditis, emboli, and progressive regurgitation can occur. However, these complications are very unusual in the absence of myxomatous changes. The cardiac examination typically reveals normal cardiac size and one or more nonejection, midsystolic clicks that introduce a late systolic ejection murmur at the apex. The most consistent feature of cardiac auscultation is the timing of the murmur. Maneuvers that increase heart size (supine position, squatting) cause the click to occur later in systole and diminish the murmur, while a decrease in cardiac size (induced by standing) results in earlier occurrence of the click and may increase the duration of the murmur. The ECG is usually normal but may show atrial or ventricular ectopic beats and nonspecific ST-T changes. Echocardiography reveals the characteristic posterior prolapse of the mitral valve into the left atrium during systole. If the chest pain requires treatment, β-blockers are usually used. These drugs are also useful for symptomatic arrhythmias. Antibiotic prophylaxis is indicated for patients with the systolic murmur but is not indicated for mitral prolapse detected only by echocardiography. Patients with a history of emboli, presumably from the abnormal valve, should receive antiplatelet or anticoagulant therapy.

Sensitive Heart

This recently described disorder is related to a heightened perception of stimuli within the cardiac chambers that may be sensed as chest pain *(31)*. It has been shown that, in some patients with angiographically normal coronary arteries and chest pain atypical for angina, movement of a catheter or injection of small volumes of saline or angiographic dye within the cardiac chambers reproduces their chest pain. This phenomenon is significantly less frequent in control patients with CAD or valvular heart disease. Limited experience has revealed success in treating this entity with a low dose of a tricyclic antidepressant that was felt to provide analgesia without psychotropic effects *(31)*.

MUSCULOSKELETAL ETIOLOGIES OF CHEST PAIN

Musculoskeletal abnormalities of the thoracic wall and the neck account for a substantial proportion of patients with chest pain, estimated to be as high as 20% in patients with normal coronary arteries. Musculoskeletal diseases are considered in Chapter 10; their relationship to the differential diagnosis of chest pain will be briefly reviewed here. In a recent study of the prevalence of musculoskeletal disorders in patients with chest pain and angiographically normal coronary arteries, it was found that 30% of the group had fibromyalgia and 10% had costochondritis *(13)*. In the control group of patients with CAD, only one patient had fibromyalgia and there were none with costochondritis. Fibromyalgia was diagnosed by the presence of at least eight paired tender points; additional features that supported the diagnosis included sleep disturbances, morning stiffness, fatigue, alternating diarrhea and constipation, headache, and paresthesia. The diagnosis of costochondritis was based on tenderness of the costal cartilages to palpation. Screening evaluation was also performed for related etiologies such as rheumatoid arthritis and osteoarthritis, spinal disease, rib fracture, muscle strain, and soft-tissue injury, all of which were uncommon with no statistically significant difference in the two patient populations (CAD and no CAD). Proper identification and treatment of the substantial population of patients with a musculoskeletal etiology of chest pain mistakenly considered of cardiac origin has the potential to significantly reduce the morbidity related to these syndromes. The specific therapy of these disorders is considered in Chapter 10.

VASCULAR ETIOLOGIES OF CHEST PAIN

Pulmonary Embolism

The major etiology of chest pain in this category is pulmonary embolism (PE). PE is an extremely common condition, accounting for about 50,000 deaths per year in this country. Despite its frequency and devastating consequences, it continues to be a major diagnostic challenge. The symptoms and signs of PE are multiple, but they are nonspecific, including chest pain, dyspnea, tachypnea, and tachycardia. Chest pain may be more frequent in small peripheral PE, since neural innervation is greatest at the pulmonary periphery, which is also the most likely site of infarction and associated pleural involvement. Conversely, large, proximal PE may more commonly be associated with dyspnea, syncope, cyanosis, and hypotension without pain. The chest pain of PE may simulate other conditions such as acute MI, aortic dissection, pneumothorax, rib fracture, pneumonia, and mass lesions. The key to diagnosis is a high index of suspicion based on the clinical presentation and the setting in which it occurs. The latter refers to the well-recognized risk factors for PE, which include immobilization from chronic illness, surgery or hospitalization, obesity, advanced age, cancer, pregnancy, and oral contraceptive therapy. Although PE is closely related to deep vein thrombosis in these settings, the venous process is also difficult to diagnose on the clinical examination. Therefore, when the presentation suggests PE, prompt evaluation should be initiated. If suspicion is high, therapy with intravenous heparin should be started while the evaluation progresses. The physical examination may reveal only tachycardia and tachypnea, but, in large PE, there may be evidence of right ventricular pressure overload and/or failure: elevated jugular veins, right ventricular lift, accentuated P_2, and a murmur of tricuspid insufficiency. Because most PE are relatively small, in terms of their hemodynamic effects, these physical findings are uncommon and their absence should not divert attention from this diagnosis if the overall clinical picture is compatible.

Diagnostic Tests

The chest film, ECG, and arterial blood gas are commonly normal in small PE. However, the chest film can exclude several of the conditions noted above that can simulate the symptoms of PE. In a large PE that produces acute pulmonary hypertension, the ECG may reveal right axis deviation, P pulmonale, right bundle branch block, repolarization abnormalities in leads V_{1-3}, and atrial arrhythmias. The limited value of arterial blood gases has recently caused some to advocate abandoning them, as well as the alveolar-arterial oxygen gradient, as screening tests for PE *(32)*. However, abnormal values support the presence of PE and provide an estimate of its severity. A promising screening test is the plasma D-dimer, which has shown a sensitivity of >90% in patients with angiographically documented PE *(33)*. Because of its role in the etiology of PE, detection of deep-vein thrombosis is an important element in the evaluation of the patient with suspected PE, and evaluation of the lower extremities by ultrasonography or impedance plethysmography should be performed in these patients. In large, hemodynamically compromising PE, echocardiography may reveal enlargement and depressed function of the right ventricle with tricuspid insufficiency. Massive embolism may produce

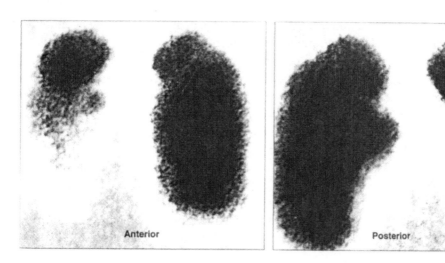

Fig. 5. Perfusion lung scans showing a large defect in the right lung, consistent with pulmonary embolism. The chest film and ventilation scan were normal. (Reprinted by permission from Cishek MB, Moser KM, Amsterdam EA. Chest pain: Fast-track assessment of urgency. J Respir Dis 1996; 17: 510–524.)

echodense structures in the main pulmonary arteries. The principal diagnostic test is the ventilation-perfusion (V-Q) scan (Fig. 5). This test is most useful if the result is normal or high probability for PE. Approximately 30% of patients with intermediate probability scans have PE, a result that ranges from <20 to >60%, depending on the patient's clinical probability of PE. Patients in this group may require pulmonary angiography, the definitive method for diagnosis of PE.

Treatment

Initial therapy for PE is heparin in full dose to achieve a partial thromboplastin time (PTT) 1.5–2. 5 times control. Oral anticoagulation with warfarin is started when the PTT is therapeutic. Heparin is continued for at least 5 d while the INR is attaining the desired level. Warfarin is usually continued for 6–12 mo. Patients with contraindications to anticoagulation or with recurrent PE despite anticoagulation are candidates for placement of an inferior vena caval filter. Thrombolytic therapy should be considered for patients in whom a large PE produces hemodynamic instability or evidence of right ventricular failure. In these high-risk patients, thrombolysis with t-PA plus heparin is superior to heparin alone in reversing right ventricular dysfunction and improving pulmonary perfusion *(34)*. Finally, prevention is critical in reducing the morbidity and mortality of PE. In patients at risk (e.g., postoperative state, prolonged bed rest), prophylactic methods include compression stockings, low-dose heparin, or a combination of the two.

Aortic Dissection

This catastrophic process had a mortality of 50% within 48 h and 90% within 3 mo before the development of effective therapy in the modern era. The advances in diagnosis and in medical and surgical therapy during the last 25 yr have achieved a current survival of over 70%. Aortic dissection is rare, with most large hospitals receiving no more than two to five cases annually; therefore, the key to recognition is a high index of suspicion. The pain is usually severe and may penetrate to the back. It may be sharp or similar to the pain of MI in quality and location. Although the pain of aortic dissection has been traditionally described as "tearing," this finding has been notable by its absence in our experience. Other important features are hypertension, absent pulses, aortic insufficiency, and evidence of end-organ vascular insufficiency (e.g., peripheral, cerebral, myocardial, renal, gastrointestinal ischemia). Hypotension suggests proximal dissection, aortic rupture, or secondary MI from retrograde dissection of a coronary artery. The ECG may be normal or show nonspecific abnormalities. Left ventricular hypertrophy is common because of the frequent history of hypertension in patients with aortic dissection. The chest film may show a widened mediastinum or increased aortic diameter in the region of the aortic knob. However, the chest film is commonly negative.

Diagnostic Tests

The goals of a diagnostic procedure in these patients are to determine the presence, origin, and extent of aortic dissection. Although aortography has been the standard approach, several noninvasive techniques now provide excellent sensitivity and specificity for detecting this disorder. These include computerized tomography (CT) scanning, magnetic resonance imaging (MRI), and transesophageal echocardiography. The specific modality utilized for diagnosis will depend on the experience, expertise, and speed with which it can be applied in a particular institution.

Treatment

Treatment is based on the patient's clinical status and the location of the dissection. Medical therapy should be instituted immediately to halt progression of the dissection during the diagnostic procedure. This entails reducing blood pressure to the lowest level compatible with organ perfusion and decreasing the rate of rise of arterial pressure. Intravenous agents should be used for precise control of therapy. Esmolol, an ultra short-acting β-adrenergic blocker, fulfills these requirements. Nitroprusside can be added if necessary for further control of blood pressure, but it should not be used without a β-blocker because of the reflex sympathetic stimulation it produces. Surgical therapy is indicated in type A (ascending aorta) dissection, whereas the results with medical therapy have equaled or exceeded of those surgery for uncomplicated type B dissection (descending aorta distal to the left subclavian artery). In the event of progression of type B dissection, surgery is indicated.

GASTROINTESTINAL ETIOLOGIES OF CHEST PAIN

It has been shown that in two-thirds of patients considered to have angina the etiology is not CAD *(12)*. In half of these patients, the cause is gastrointestinal. Furthermore, 10–30% of patients undergoing coronary arteriography have noncardiac chest pain; and, in 50% of these patients, esophageal disease is the etiology of their symptoms.

The difficulty lies in trying to distinguish a gastrointestinal etiology from a cardiac disorder. The subsequent evaluation of a patient with chest pain is usually a matter of pretest probability. In younger patients, in whom CAD is unlikely, pursuing a gastro-intestinal etiology will be most appropriate. In men over 40 and women over 50 yr of age, high-risk CAD must be excluded with a screening examination, such as a treadmill test, prior to evaluation of an esophageal etiology.

Gastroesophageal reflux disease and esophageal motility disorders (such as nutcracker esophagus, diffuse esophageal spasm, and achalasia) are the two general types of esophageal diseases commonly associated with chest pain that may be confused with cardiac etiologies. Esophageal pain typically occurs at rest, especially when a patient is in the supine position, and frequently occurs during the night. However, reflux can be provoked by exertion, confounding the distinction between a cardiac and gastrointestinal etiology to chest pain. Patients with reflux may also complain of waterbrash, a sensation of hot water, or acid, regurgitating up from their stomachs into their throats. They may also complain of a sour taste in the morning upon arising. Dysphagia may occur during meals.

Zenker's diverticulum and esophageal cysts are rare causes of chest pain. In the case of a Zenker's diverticulum, patients may complain of dysphagia as a part of the symptom complex. The pain from an esophageal cyst may be due to mass effect and is described as constant pain in the rare cases noted in the literature.

Mallory-Weiss tear and Boerhaave's syndrome are uncommon causes of chest pain and can usually be diagnosed clinically. Mallory-Weiss tear is a rent in the gastric mucosa just below the gastroesophageal junction. It usually (but not universally) presents as hematemesis following a prolonged episode of vomiting. The mucosal tear can be detected by barium swallow or endoscopy. Most tears heal with conservative therapy by endoscopic cautery; surgery is required in less than 5% of patients. Boerhaave's syndrome is a rupture of the esophagus commonly just above the gastroesophageal junction on the left side. This may also follow an episode of retching, but it can occur after any acute rise in intra-abdominal pressure, such as during a Valsalva maneuver. This diagnosis is more difficult to make and may be confused with MI or pancreatitis. Leakage of esophageal contents into the mediastinum will lead to mediastinitis, and the patient may present with chest pain and fever. Chest radiographs may demonstrate air in the mediastinum or a left hydrothorax. Barium swallow should not be performed in patients with suspected perforation of the esophagus as the leakage of barium into the mediastinum will cause mediastinitis. Water-soluble contrast swallow or endoscopy can be performed safely for diagnostic purposes. Therapy consists of immediate surgical repair of the esophagus, drainage of the mediastinum, and broad antibiotic coverage.

In other cases of febrile patients without obvious thoracic radiographic abnormalities, it is important to remember that subdiaphragmatic or liver abscesses may present with chest pain. In these cases, the etiology may only be discovered by maintaining a high degree of suspicion and evaluating the patient with abdominal ultrasound or CT scan.

Pain of other esophageal etiologies is more difficult to assess as the pain is indistinguishable from angina pectoris in its character, radiation, and even its response to treatment with nitroglycerin and calcium channel blockers. Studies have demonstrated the presence of acid-sensitive nerve endings (in cats) and mechanoreceptors (in humans) with nerve projections traveling with both vagal and sympathetic afferent fibers. Thermoreceptors have also been discovered whose afferent fibers are transmitted via the vagus nerve.

The esophageal microvasculature has also been implicated in producing pain of esophageal origin. Prolonged high-pressure contractions of the esophagus are capable of causing ischemia of the esophagus with resultant chest pain. Many patients with microvascular coronary disease have esophageal motor abnormalities, such as nutcracker esophagus, suggesting these patients have a generalized abnormality of smooth muscle.

Pain from pancreatitis and biliary disease can often be detected by measuring serum amylase, lipase, alkaline phosphatase, and total bilirubin. The incidence of myocardial ischemia is less than 5% in patients presenting acutely with normal or near normal ECGs, and it is our practice to exclude pancreatic and biliary disease in patients presenting with acute chest pain without ECG abnormalities diagnostic of myocardial injury or ischemia. In patients presenting nonacutely, it is important to consider biliary colic as an etiology, especially if the patient is a 30- to 40-yr-old woman in whom coronary disease is unlikely. Ultrasound of the gallbladder may demonstrate stones; but, as gallstones are common even in asymptomatic patients, this diagnosis is often one of exclusion.

Diagnostic Tests

In patients with probable esophageal disease, an empiric trial of antacids or H_2 blockers may be useful in establishing the diagnosis. Ambulatory monitoring of esophageal pH can be performed to assess for gastroesophageal reflux. A barium swallow may also demonstrate esophageal reflux or dysmotility. Dysmotility may best be detected with a radionuclide labeled meal. Patients with achalasia can be identified by adynamic and delayed esophageal emptying. Patients with nutcracker esophagus will demonstrate fragmentation of the bolus into several smaller components due to disordered movement of the lower esophagus. The presence of a Zenker's diverticulum can also be evaluated with barium swallow.

Endoscopy is currently the most common examination performed. Inflammation and erosion of the lower esophagus will identify patients with esophageal reflux, and biopsies may identify patients with Barrett's esophagus. Achalasia can be identified by the tightness of the esophagogastric junction and the presence of retained food. The presence of carcinoma or a Zenker's diverticulum can also be investigated. Therapeutic balloon dilation for achalasia or esophageal stricture can be guided by endoscopy.

Several provocative tests are available to evaluate for gastroesophageal reflux disease. The Bernstein test, in which 0.1 N HCl is infused into the esophagus at 6 cc/min, can evoke chest pain and is 32% sensitive and 87% specific for the diagnosis of reflux. This test has largely been replaced by 24-h pH monitoring in which a pH probe is placed into the lower esophagus that can confirm periodic acute drops in pH during reflux of stomach acid into the esophagus.

Esophageal spasm can be provoked by infusion of the short-acting inhibitor of cholinesterase activity, edrophonium chloride (80 μg/kg), or the parasympathomimetic bethanechol (50 μg/kg sc). These tests are considered positive if the patient complains of chest pain concurrently with manometrically documented esophageal spasm. The tests are plagued by relatively poor predictive accuracy.

Mechanical distention of the esophagus with a balloon 10 cm above the lower esophageal sphincter can provoke esophageal spasm. Provocation of spasm with balloon volumes of less than 8 cc is thought to be consistent with the diagnosis of pathologic esophageal spasm. Spasm occurring with balloon volumes greater than 8 cc is thought to be a normal response to mechanical stretch of the esophageal smooth muscle.

Treatment

Gastroesophageal reflux disease can be treated with lifestyle changes in less severe cases. Alcohol, smoking, caffeine, and fatty foods all lead to relaxation of the lower esophageal sphincter and resultant reflux disease. Avoidance of these substances can result in significant improvement in symptoms. Obesity increases intra-abdominal pressure, which forces gastric contents up into the esophagus; therefore weight loss is also helpful. Gravity can help keep gastric contents in the stomach, and it is important to advise patients not to have anything to eat for 3–4 h prior to going to bed and not to lie down following meals. A 4-in. block under the head of the bed can provide sufficent incline to help reduce reflux. Sleeping on numerous pillows or placing a wedge under the mattress forces the patient to sleep partially bent at the waist, which in overweight patients can increase intra-abdominal pressure and worsen reflux. If nonpharmacologic measures fail, then antacids, H_2 blockers, or motility agents such as metaclopramide or cisapride can alleviate symptoms. In severe cases, surgical procedures that attempt to restore sphincter competence by wrapping the lower end of the esophagus with a cuff of gastric fundal muscle, such as the Nissen fundoplication, can be performed. The efficacy of these procedures is unknown as there are few objective studies.

Esophageal dysmotility can be treated medically with nitroglycerin or calcium channel blockers. These agents are smooth muscle relaxants and have been demonstrated to decrease the force and duration of esophageal contractions as well as lower esophageal sphincter tone. This latter action may also worsen reflux and it is not uncommon for a patient's "angina" to worsen with calcium channel blocker or nitrate therapy owing to increased reflux. In resistant cases of esophageal dysmotility, dilation of the gastroesophageal junction with either mercury-filled bougie or balloon can disrupt the circular muscle fibers and improve symptoms. Overzealous dilation can completely disrupt the muscle fibers and lead to pathologic reflux disease. In extreme cases, esophagomyotomy, consisting of an extramucosal myotomy across the lower esophageal sphincter and proximally into the lower esophagus, can improve achalasia. Long transthoracic esophageal myotomy has been performed in medically resistant cases of nutcracker esophagus with 50% success.

Carcinoma, esophageal cyst, and Zenker's diverticulum typically require surgical intervention for relief of symptoms. Some cancers, such as lymphomas, may be radiosensitive or chemosensitive.

PULMONARY ETIOLOGIES OF CHEST PAIN

Pulmonary diseases can be separated into those of the pleura, the parenchyma, and the airways. All of these processes may present with dyspnea and chest pain, symptoms common to nearly any disorder of the chest *(35)*. Pleuritic pain, however, is very suggestive of pulmonary etiology.

Table 3 *(36)*
Transudative Pleural Fluid

Color	Straw
Protein	<3.0 gm/dL
Pleural/serum ratio	<0.5
Glucose	>60 mg/dL
Pleural/serum ratio	1.0
Lactic dehydrogenase	<200 IU/L
Pleural/serum ratio	<0.6
WBC count	<1000/mL
% neutrophils	<50%
RBC count	<5000/mL

WBC, white blood cells; RBC, red blood cells.

Pleural Disorders

The pleura is a thin membrane of mesothelial cells separated into the parietal pleura covering the chest wall, diaphragm and mediastinum, and the visceral pleura covering the entire surface of the lungs. The visceral and parietal pleural surfaces are separated by a potential space filled with about 20 cc of serous fluid. The pleura is supported by a network of lymphatics and vessels, disorders of which can lead to pleural effusions.

Pleural pain is usually unilateral and commonly arises from irritation of the parietal pleura. Because the parietal pleura is innervated by intercostal nerves, pleural pain commonly radiates to the chest wall, abdomen, neck, or shoulder. The pain is usually sharp and increases with deep respiration or coughing. Splinting may be observed while watching the patient breathe. Pain usually diminishes with the onset of pleural effusion.

On physical examination, respirations are shallow in an attempt to minimize the pleuritic pain. Patients may prefer to lie on the affected side to reduce chest-wall movement. An intercostal tenderness may be elicited and breath sounds may be decreased on the affected side. Pleural friction rub is diagnostic of pleural disease but may not be present if there is significant pleural effusion. Pleural effusion may be detected by decreases in percussion, tactile fremitus, and breath sounds. Egobronchophony (E to A change) is frequently heard at the top of the effusion.

Pleuritis is most commonly caused by painful but benign viral infections. Significant pleural effusion is uncommon in this disease, thereby allowing the pleurae to rub against each other. Significant pleural effusions are suggestive of more serious etiologies such as granulomatous diseases (tuberculosis), malignancy, collagen-vascular diseases (systemic lupus erythematosis or rheumatoid arthritis), pneumonias, pancreatitis, or heart failure *(36)*.

Pneumothorax is essentially a disease of pleural integrity. Simple spontaneous pneumothorax occurs when pleural-based blebs rupture, often after coughing or exercise. These blebs are more common in men and more common on the right side. The pneumothorax may be very small and only visible on expiratory chest radiographs, or it may be very large, but rarely does it cause a tension pneumothorax. A pneumothorax may be asymptomatic or cause

Table 4 *(36)*
Exudative Pleural Fluid

Test	Diseases
pH <7.2	Infection, malignancy
Glucose <60 mg/dL	Infection, malignancy, rheumatoid arthritis
Amylase >200 U/dL	Pancreatitis, malignancy, Boerhaave's syndrome
Rheumatoid factor, ANA	Lupus erythematosus, rheumatoid arthritis
Cytology	Malignancy, rheumatoid arthritis
RBC >5000/mL	Malignancy, trauma, pulmonary embolism
WBC >1000	Infection (PMNs: bacterial; lymphocytes; tuberculosis)

RBC, red blood cells; PMNs, polymorphonuclear neutrophils; WBC, white blood cells.

sharp lateral chest pain and acute shortness of breath. Trauma or other pulmonary disease processes such as emphysema, bronchial asthma, or pneumonia may cause pneumothorax.

Diagnostic Tests

The simplest test for evaluation of pleural-based diseases is the chest film. The presence of significant pleural effusion can be detected and the chest wall and pulmonary parenchyma can be evaluated for infection or malignancy. The presence of a pneumothorax can be adequately evaluated by on the chest film. Expiratory films may be necessary to detect a small pneumothorax.

In cases of pleural effusion in which the history and physical examination are highly suggestive of the etiology of the effusion, such as with heart failure and pancreatitis, thoracentesis is rarely useful for diagnosis. In cases in which the diagnosis is elusive, thoracentesis is indispensable. When performing thoracentesis, it is important to remove as much fluid as possible for cytologic evaluation, taking care not to remove more than 1500 cc to avoid the rare complication of re-expansion pulmonary edema. Transudates (Table 3) are suggestive of volume overload from renal or heart failure, or hypoalbuminemia. Exudates (Table 4) are suggestive of malignancy or infection, and fluid should be sent for cytology, Gram and acid-fast stains, and cultures for aerobic and anaerobic organisms. Cultures should be held long-term for fungal organisms and for acid-fast bacilli. In cases of tuberculosis and malignancy, pleural biopsy with either a hook-type needle or via open biopsy may be required to make the diagnosis.

Treatment

Treatment is disease-specific. Symptomatic large pneumothoraces can be treated with a small chest tube attached to suction or a Heimlich valve. Persistent pleural leaks may require surgery to close the defect. For large transudative pleural effusions, drainage of the pleural fluid with a needle or small catheter can improve the dyspnea. Otherwise, treatment of transudative pleural effusions is directed toward the cause of the effusion, such as heart failure, renal failure, or hypoalbuminemia.

Pleural effusions of infectious etiology need drainage with a chest tube but may require surgical drainage if loculated to prevent scarring of the pleura, formation of a pleural rind, and resultant constriction. Antibiotics specific for the infectious agent are also required. Effusions of malignant etiology may require drainage with a chest tube if they re-occur after the initial drainage. Pleurodesis for recurrent effusions can be performed chemically with tetracycline instilled into the pleural space after chest-tube drainage and removed after 1–2 h contact time. If chemical pleurodesis is unsuccessful, surgical pleurodesis can be performed as a last resort. Chemotherapy and radiation reduce the recurrence in some tumors, especially if mediastinal lymph node enlargement is contributing to the effusion.

Finally, it is important to remember that the pleura lines the diaphragm, and diseases that inflame the diaphragm may lead to pleuritic chest pain. Subdiaphragmatic abscess are such conditions. The former may cause blunting of the costophrenic angle on chest radiography from small pleural effusions, but large effusions are uncommon.

Pneumonia

Infectious etiologies include bacterial, viral, fungal, rickettsial, and protozoal (35). The chest pain is typically pleuritic, arising from inflammation of the pleura. Fever, cough, and dyspnea are also nearly universal. Sputum production is typical of bacterial processes, and a dry cough is typical of viral and protozoal etiologies. Coughing may lead to chest pain of musculoskeletal origin.

Diagnostic Tests

The clinical history and appearance of the chest radiograph may be sufficient to narrow the etiology to allow for fairly accurate diagnosis and empiric therapy without identification of the offending organism (i.e., community acquired lobar pneumonia suggesting streptococcus, or diffuse radiographic changes that appear worse than the patient's clinical status suggesting mycoplasma). Sputum Gram stain may aid in identifying the organisms present but will not detect acid-fast bacilli and protozoa. Acid-fast staining may detect tubercle bacilli, but often does not. In cases in which mycobacteria are likely, such as in AIDS patients, polymerase chain reaction amplification can be used to detect tubercle bacilli in the sputum with greater than 90% sensitivity and specificity (37). Sputum cultures are required for accurate identification of the organism and for tailoring antibiotic therapy to sensitivities. If tuberculosis or fungal etiology is expected, then cultures must be held for 6–8 wk. Cases that do not respond to initial therapy may require bronchoscopy or even open-lung biopsy for diagnosis. Pleural biopsy for detecting organisms such as mycobacteria can be performed percutaneously with a side-cutting Cope or Abrams needle.

Treatment

Therapy is specific to the suspected or confirmed etiology. Analgesia can provide temporary relief of the pleuritic pain.

Pneumonitis

Noninfectious pneumonitis or bronchitis often results from inhalation of toxic gases (Table 5) (38). In general, the more noxious the gas, the less able the patient is to deeply

Table 5
Common Causes of Industrial Pneumonitis

Agent	Setting
Ammonia	Household cleaner, refrigeration
Cadmium	Electrical conductor manufacturing, electroplating, zinc smelting
Chlorine	Swimming pools, chemical plants
Hydrocarbons	Gasoline, paint thinners
Hydrochloric acid	Swimming pools, laboratories
Isocyanates	polyurethane production, aluminum soldering flux
Mercury	Smelting, pesticide and insecticide manufacturing, instruments and lamps, neon lights, batteries
Nickel carbonyl	Nickel alloy production
Nitrogen dioxide	Corn silage decomposition, welding
Oils	Laxatives; mineral, castor, cod liver, olive; automotive oils
Ozone	Arc welding, deodorizing, flour bleaching
Phosgene	Aniline dye production, metallurgy
Radiation	Cancer therapy, industrial exposure
Smoke	Fires
Sulfur dioxide	Paper manufacturing, smelting plants
Vanadium	Steel alloy production

inhale and the more likely the injury will be localized to the upper airway. Less noxious gases may be inhaled for hours, leading predominantly to pneumonitis. Aspiration pneumonitis results from aspiration of stomach contents and direct irritation of the lung by gastric acid and food particles. Most aspirations are asymptomatic, possibly owing to the debilitated nature of most of the patients in whom aspiration is common.

Symptoms commonly include burning chest pain, cough, tachypnea, dyspnea, and fever. Chest auscultation frequently is unremarkable in acute exposures but may reveal crackles in more chronic cases. In the case of radiation exposure, symptoms may be delayed for 1–3 mo. The development of stridor in the case of any industrial exposure is an ominous sign and identifies patients likely to need mechanical ventilatory support.

Diagnostic Tests

Chest radiography is frequently misleading concerning the seriousness of the disease, as radiographic changes may lag by days, or, in the case of radiation exposure, by months. Diagnosis is made predominantly by history. In rare cases, bronchoscopy with biopsy may be helpful.

Treatment

Few of these etiologies have specific therapies, and management generally comprises supportive measures such as supplemental oxygen and intubation. Steroids have been reported to reduce the inflammation and edema in patients with marked symptoms and impending respiratory collapse. Steroids should always be used with caution, as superinfection is a common problem. In the case of nickel carbonyl inhalation, the administration of diethyl dithiocarbamate is an effective therapy. Metal fume fever is a benign and self-limiting disorder produced by the inhalation of zinc, copper, and magnesium fumes that are released from welding galvanized metals.

Atelectasis

Atelectasis is common in many types of lung diseases. Tumors or mucous plugs may obstruct bronchi leading to obstructive atelectasis. Pulmonary fibrosis may result in contraction atelectasis. Emphysematous changes may cause adjacent lung to be compressed and atelectatic. Poor respiratory effort can cause plate-like atelectasis. It is unclear if atelectasis in itself causes chest pain. This symptom is commonly associated with primary disorders known to cause chest pain, such as cancer. It has been suggested that collapse and reinflation of atelectatic portions of lung may result in fleeting sharp chest pain.

Diagnostic Tests and Treatment

Chest radiography will identify the atelectasis. If underlying malignancy is suspected, then chest CT or bronchoscopy may be needed for further investigation. Treatment is control of the underlying disease process. Atelectasis from poor respiratory effort can be treated with incentive spirometry.

Bronchitis

The etiologic agents are similar to those that involve the lung parenchyma; the same toxic gases and infectious agents may produce either pneumonitis or bronchitis. Inflammation of the bronchi can cause a burning, substernal chest pain that increases with inspiration, especially of cold, dry air. Coughing can cause musculoskeletal pain that is typically dull and increases with deep inspiration. The pain may be diffuse or localized and increases markedly when the patient is asked to cough.

Chronic Obstructive Airways Disease

Exacerbations of obstructive airway diseases, such as asthma or emphysema, can lead to dyspnea and squeezing anterior chest discomfort. This symptom complex commonly stimulates a work-up for cardiac ischemia. Because substernal chest tightness is common during exacerbations of obstructive airways disease, we do not advocate serial cardiac enzymes in the absence of ischemic ECG changes or a high coronary risk profile. In patients complaining of chest tightness in the absence of exacerbation of obstructive pulmonary disease, work-up for a cardiac etiology is indicated.

MEDIASTINAL ETIOLOGIES OF CHEST PAIN

The mediastinum is the potential space in the mid-thorax defined by the diaphragm below, the thoracic outlet above, and the two pleural cavities on either side. The mediastinum is further divided into the anterior, middle, and posterior compartments. The anterior mediastinum contains the anatomic structures from the sternum anteriorly to the pericardium posteriorly and contains the thymus, thyroid and parathyroid glands, and

Table 6 *(39)*
Location of Mediastinal Masses and Possible Etiologies

Mediastinal Compartment	Diseases
Anterior	Lipoma, thymoma, thyroidoma, parathyroidoma, lymphoma, teratoma, aneurysms, bacterial and fungal infections
Middle	Lymphoma, fungoma, bronchogenic cysts, bronchogenic cancers, esophageal diverticuli or cysts, esophageal cancer, primary cardiac tumors, aneurysms, bacterial and fungal infections
Posterior	Lymphoma, esophageal diverticuli or cysts, esophageal cancer, metastatic cancer to the spine, aortic aneurysm, neurogenic tumors, bacterial and fungal infections

lymph nodes. The middle mediastinum extends posteriorly to the anterior border of the vertebral bodies and contains the heart, great vessels, trachea, main bronchi, esophagus, phrenic and vagus nerves, and lymph nodes. The posterior mediastinum extends from the anterior vertebral bodies to the chest wall and contains the vertebral bodies, descending thoracic aorta, esophagus, thoracic duct, azygous and hemiazygous veins, inferior portion of the vagus nerve, and sympathetic chains and lymph nodes.

Mediastinal Masses

Mediastinal masses typically present with cough, hoarseness, and dyspnea, but may also present with chest pain, stridor, dysphagia, or Horner's syndrome. The chest pain may radiate anteriorly, posteriorly or straight through the chest.

Diagnostic Tests

Routine chest radiography detects the majority of mass lesions and can localize the disease process to one of the three mediastinal compartments. Knowledge of the structures contained within the compartments allows a differential diagnosis to be constructed (Table 6) *(39)*. The radiographic appearance can further narrow the differential diagnosis. CT scan or MRI may be indicated to better determine the etiology and extent of disease. When the middle mediastinum is the compartment of interest, the scans may need to be gated to the cardiac cycle to minimize motion artifact. Transthoracic and transesophageal echocardiography can be performed to examine cardiac structures but are extremely limited for examination of extracardiac structures. Bronchoscopy or esophagoscopy may be indicated to further define the anatomy of these structures and to perform biopsies.

Treatment

Therapy of mass lesions is disease-specific and requires tissue for accurate diagnosis and therapy. Mediastinoscopy or CT-guided needle biopsies are usually indicated. Surgery is usually required to alleviate the pain, typically due to mass effect compressing vital structures.

Mediastinitis

Pneumomediastinum and acute mediastinitis are rare and usually occur secondary to endoscopy, surgery, or trauma. Mediastinitis may be diagnosed by fever and widened mediastinum on chest film. Esophageal or bronchial studies with water-soluble contrast may demonstrate the perforation.

Treatment

The responsible pathogens are usually the mixed aerobic and anaerobic bacteria common to the oropharynx. Fungi, such as Actinomyces, have also been reported. Broad spectrum antibiotics to cover the mixed bacteria present constitute a requisite part of the therapy. Cases of esophageal or bronchial perforation diagnosed early can undergo primary repair. Once mediastinitis has set in, cervical esoghagostomy, gastrostomy, and drainage of the mediastinal and pleural cavities have been reported to improve survival *(40)*. Recent reports have suggested that, in cases of spontaneous esophageal rupture (such as Boerhaave's syndrome), medical therapy, consisting of nasogastric suctioning, total parenteral nutrition, and broad spectrum antibiotics, may be appropriate therapy *(41)*.

Spontaneous Mediastinitis

Spontaneous mediastinitis is rare but deserves special mention because the seriousness of antecedent events is often underestimated. Oropharyngeal infections such as exudative tonsillitis (Vincent's angina) or submandibular cellulitis (Ludwig's angina) may spread along fascial planes into the mediastinum in a condition termed descending necrotizing mediastinitis *(42)*. Diagnosis of this disorder is based on the criteria proposed by Estrera *(43)*: clinical manifestation of severe infection, characteristic radiographic features of mediastinitis, necrotizing mediastinal infection at operation or postmortem, and relationship to oropharyngeal infection with the development of the necrotizing process. The most common routes of spread are posteriorly along the esophagus (70%), anteriorly along the trachea (20%), or along the carotid artery and vagus nerves (10%). Involvement of the pericardial and pleural spaces is common; spread below the diaphragm has also been reported.

Treatment

Mortality in early series was 50%, but more recent studies have shown a 25% mortality. This decrease in mortality has been attributed to improvements in diagnosis and therapy, including the use of CT scanning to define the extent of infection, better antibiotic coverage of both aerobes and anaerobes, and more aggressive surgical drainage of all involved spaces, including the anterior neck, mediastinum, pericardium, pleura, and (rarely) intra-abdominal or retroperitoneal spaces. Tracheostomy for airway management is controversial.

Spontaneous Pneumomediastinum

Spontaneous pneumomediastinum is an unusual event and may be diagnosed by a mediastinal crunch on auscultation (Hamman's crunch) or subcutaneous emphysema in the neck. The chest film will demonstrate air contrast in the mediastinum. While pneumomediastinum secondary to trauma or iatrogenesis requires surgical intervention, spontaneous pneumomediastinum frequently is self-limited but it may require surgery if it is large and compresses vital structures.

PSYCHIATRIC ETIOLOGIES OF CHEST PAIN

Panic Disorder

The major disease in this category is panic disorder. It has recently been shown that a substantial proportion of patients with noncardiac chest pain have panic disorder. We have detected this condition in over 50% of patients admitted to the CCU in whom MI was ruled out *(10)* and in over 60% of patients with chronic chest pain and negative myocardial stress scintigraphy *(11)*. Although cardiac symptoms such as chest pain, dyspnea, and palpitations are prominent in panic disorder, the pain is usually atypical for myocardial ischemia and the patient commonly has other features suggestive of panic disorder. These include multiple and widespread somatic complaints (dizziness, choking, paresthesias, palpitations, abdominal distress, trembling) and anxiety symptoms such as agoraphobia, depersonalization, and fear of losing control. Physician recognition of this disorder in patients presenting with noncardiac chest pain is low *(44)* and may impede appropriate management. A recently described, related anxiety disorder has been termed cardiophobia *(45)*. It is characterized by a focus on chest pain and associated somatic complaints such as palpitations. There is also fear of heart attack and dying. The phobic nature of the disorder is reflected in patients' belief that they have organic heart disease despite negative objective studies. Reduction of anxiety is pursued through reassurance, avoidance of excessive use of medical facilities, and avoidance of activities associated with symptoms. Recognition of panic and other anxiety disorders presenting as chest pain is based on exclusion of a life-threatening process and awareness of the aforementioned clinical profile. Management should include referral to a mental health professional for definitive diagnosis and treatment. This approach may be facilitated by screening tools that have recently been developed for detection of panic disorder *(44)*.

SUMMARY

Chest pain continues to present a major challenge to the clinician. Its etiologies are multiple and may be acute or chronic. Cardiovascular diseases are the most common life-threatening causes of chest pain, but the most common etiologies of this symptom (gastroesophageal disease, musculoskeletal abnormalities, and panic disorder) are comparatively benign. Coronary artery disease frequently requires exclusion by noninvasive testing and, in selected patients, coronary angiography. Vigilance is also crucial for pulmonary embolic disease and aortic dissection. Although chest pain is common in diseases of the other thoracic viscera, these processes are less frequently life-threatening. The approach to the patient with chest pain begins with a precise history, complete physical examination, and screening laboratory tests, which provide a basis for further, directed pursuit of a definitive etiology. Judicious application of the most appropriate tests affords cost-effective diagnosis. Treatment should similarly follow an evidence-based approach.

ACKNOWLEDGMENT

The authors gratefully acknowledge the skilled administrative assistance of Shirl Fischer in the preparation of this chapter. Supported in part by the Preventive Cardiology Academic Award; NIH grant HL 01942-02(EAA).

REFERENCES

1. Rutledge JC, Amsterdam EA. Differential diagnosis and clinical approach to the patient with acute chest pain. Cardiology Clinics, 1984; pp. 257–268.
2. Cishek MB, Moser KM, Amsterdam EA. Chest pain: fast-track assessment of urgency. J Respir Dis 1996; 17: 510–524.
3. Cishek MB, Moser KM, Amsterdam EA. Chest pain: working up nonemergent conditions. J Respr Dis 1996; 17: 560–572.
4. Lewis WR, Amsterdam EA. Evaluation of the patient with "rule out myocardial infarction". Arch Intern Med 1996; 156: 41–45.
5. Foreman RD, Ohata CA, Gerhars KD. Neural mechanisms underlying cardiac pain. In: Schwartz PF, Brown AM, Malliani A, Zancheiit A, eds. Neural Mechanisms in Cardiac Arrhythmias. New York: Raven, 1978, 191.
6. Martin WR, Margherita A, Amsterdam EA. Phantom angina. Chest 1994; 105: 1271,1272.
7. Heckerling PS, Wiever SL, Wolfkiel CJ, Kushner MS, Dodin EM, Jelnin V, Fusman B, Chomka EV. Accuracy and reproducibility of precordial percussion and palpation for detecting increased left ventricular end-diastolic volume and mass. JAMA 1993; 270: 1943–1948.
8. Butman SM, Ewy GA, Standen JR, Kern KB, Hahn E. Bedside cardiovascular examination in patients with severe chronic heart failure: importance of rest or inducible jugular venous distension. J Amer Coll Cardiol 1993; 22: 968–974.
9. Laslett LJ, Amsterdam EA. Management of the asymptomatic patient with an abnormal exercise ECG. J Am Med Assoc 1984; 252(13): 1744–1746.
10. Carter C, Maddock R, Amsterdam EA, McCormick S, Waters C, Billett J. Panic disorder and chest pain in the coronary care unit. Psychosomatics 1992; 33: 302–309.
11. Carter C, Maddock R, Zoglio M, Lutrin C, Jella S, Amsterdam EA. Panic disorder and chest pain: a study of cardiac stress scintigraphy patients. Am J Cardiol 1994; 74: 296–298.
12. Anselmino M, Geoffrey WBC, Hinder RA. Esophageal chest pain: state of the art. Surgery Annual 1993; 25: 193–210.
13. Mukerji B, Mukerji V, Alpert MA, Selukar R. The prevalence of rheumatologic disorders in patients with chest pain and angiographically normal coronary arteries. Angiology 1995; 46: 425–430.
14. Cheitlin MD. Finding the high-risk patient with coronary artery disease. JAMA 1988; 259: 2271–2277.
15. Richardson MT, Holly RG, Amsterdam EA, Miller MF. The value of chest pain during the exercise tolerance test in predicting coronary artery disease. Diagnostic Cardiology 1992; 81: 164–171.
16. Christian TF, Miller TD, Bailey KR, Gibbons RJ. Exercise tomographic thallium-201 imaging in patients with severe coronary artery disease and normal electrocardiograms. Ann Intern Med 1994; 121: 825–832.
17. Wacker JT, Soufer R, Zaret BL. Nuclear cardiology. In: Braunwald E, ed. Heart Disease, 4th ed. Philadelphia: Saunders, 1996, pp. 273–316.
18. Afridi I, Quinones MA, Zoghibi WA, Cheirif J. Dobutamine stress echocardiography: sensitivity, specificity, and predictive value for future cardiac events. Am Heart J 1994; 127: 1510–1515.
19. Smith SC Jr, Blair SN, Criqui MH, Fletcher GF, Fuster V, Gersh BJ, Gotto AM, Gould KL, Greenland P, Grundy SM, et al. Preventing heart attack and death in patients with coronary disease. Circulation 1995; 92: 2–4.
20. The Bypass Angioplasty Revascularization Investigation (BARI) Investigators. Comparison of coronary bypass surgery with angioplasty in patients with multivessel disease. N Engl J Med 1996; 335: 217–225.
21. Ohman EM, Armstrong PW, Christenson RH, Granger CB, Katua HA, Hamm CW, O'Hanesian MA, Wagner GS, Kleiman NS, Harrell FE Jr, et al. Cardiac troponin T levels for risk stratification in acute myocardial ischemia. New Engl J Med 1996; 335: 1333–1341.

22. Antman EM, Tanasijevic MJ, Thompson B, Schactman M. Cardiac-specific troponin I levels to predict the risk of mortality in patients with acute coronary syndromes. N Engl J Med 1996; 335: 1342–1349.

23. Braunwald E, Mark DB, Jones RH, et al. Unstable Angina: Diagnosis and Management. Clinical Practice Guidelines, Number 10, Agency for Health Care Policy and Research, National Heart, Lung, and Blood Institute, 1994.

24. Report of the Holland Interuniversity Nifedipine/Metoprolol Trial (HINT) Research Group. Early treatment of unstable angina in the coronary care unit: a randomised, double blind, placebo controlled comparison of recurrent ischaemia in patients treated with nifedipine or metoprolol or both. Brit Heart J 1986; 56: 400–413.

25. Lewis WR, Amsterdam EA. Safety and utility of immediate exercise testing of low risk patients admitted to the hospital for suspected myocardial infarction. Am J Cardiol 1994; 74: 987–990.

25a. Kirk JD, Turnipseed S, Lewis WR, Amsterdam EA. Evaluation of chest pain in pow risk patients presenting to the emergency department: The role of immediate exercise testing. Am Emerg med 1997; in press.

26. Rogers WJ. Contemporary management of acute myocardial infarction. Am J Med 1995; 99: 195–206.

27. Ryan TJ, Anderson JL, Antman EM, et al. ACC/AHA guidelines for the management of patients with acute myocardial infarction: executive summary. Circulation 1996; 94: 2341–2350.

28. Deedwania PC, Amsterdam EA, Vagelos R. Evidence-based, cost-effective risk stratification and management after myocardial infarction. Arch Intern Med 1997; 157: 273–280.

29. Cannon RO 3rd, Camici PG, Epstein SE. Pathophysiological dilemma of syndrome X. Circulation 1992; 85: 883–892.

30. Levine JB, Gaasch WH. Vasoactive drugs in chronic regurgitant lesions of the mitral and aortic valves. J Am Coll Cardiol 1996; 28: 1082–1091.

31. Cannon RO 3rd. The sensitive heart. A syndrome of abnormal cardiac pain perception. JAMA 1995; 273: 883–887.

32. Goldhaber SZ. Pulmonary embolism. In: Kloner RA, ed. The Guide to Cardiology, 3rd ed. Greenwich, CT: Le Jacq Communications, 1995, pp. 627–636.

33. Goldhaber SZ, Haire WD, Feldstein ML, Miller M, Toltzis R, Smith JL, Taveira da Silva AM, Come PC, Lee RT, Parker JA, et al. Alteplase versus heparin in acute pulmonary embolism: randomised trial assessing right-ventricular function and pulmonary perfusion. Lancet 1993; 341: 507–511.

34. Goldhaber SZ, Simons GR, Elliott CG, Haire WD, Toltzis R, Blacklow SC, Doolittle MH, Weinberg DS. Quantitative plasma D-dimer levels among patients undergoing pulmonary angiography for suspected pulmonary embolism. J Amer Med Assoc 1993; 270: 2819–2822.

35. Fraser RG, Pare JAP. Diagnosis of Diseases of the Chest. 3rd ed. W.B. Saunders Company, Philadelphia, PA, 1988-[1991].

36. Light RW. Pleural Diseases. Lea & Febiger, Philadelphia, PA, 1983.

37. Ichiyama S, Iinuma Y, Tawada Y, Yarnori S, Hasegawa Y, Shimokata K, Nakashima N. Evaluation of gen-probe amplified mycobacterium tuberculosis direct test and Roche PCR-microwell plate hybridization method (Amplicor Mycobacterium) for direct detection of mycobacteria. J Clin Microbiol 1996; 4: 130–133.

38. Weill J. Occupational pulmonary diseases and acute and accidental exposures to irritant gases. In: Fishman AP, ed. Pulmonary Diseases and Disorders, 2nd ed. New York: McGraw-Hill, 1987.

39. Silverman NA, Sabiston DC. Mediastinal masses. Surg Clin North Am 1980; 60: 757.

40. Salo JA, Isolauri JO, Heikkila LJ, Markkula HT, Heikkinen LO, Kivilaakso EO, Mattila SP. Management of delayed esophageal perforation with mediastinal sepsis. Esophagectomy or primary repair? J Thoracic Cardio Surg 1993; 106: 1088–1091.

41. Slim K, Elbaz V, Pezat D, Chipponi J. Nonsurgical treatment of perforations of the thoracic esophagus. Presse Medicale 1996; 25: 154–156.

42. Alsoub H, Chacko KC. Descending necrotising mediastinitis. Postgraduate Med J 1995; 71: 98–101.

43. Estrera AS, Lundy MJ, Glusham JM, Sinn DP, Platt MR. Descending necrotizing mediastinitis. Surgery, Gynecology and Obstetrics 1983; 157: 545–552.

44. Fleet RP, Dupuis G, Marchand A, Burelle D, Arsenault A, Beitman BD. Panic disorder in emergency department chest pain patients: prevalence, comorbidity, suicidal ideation, and physician recognition. Am J Med 1996; 101: 371–380.

45. Eifert GH. Cardiophobia: a paradigmatic behavioural model of heart-focused anxiety and non-anginal chest pain. Behaviour Res Ther 1992; 4: 329–345.

6 ABDOMINAL PAIN

R. ERICK PECHA, MD
THOMAS PRINDIVILLE, MD

Key Points

- The basic types of pain are somatic, visceral, and referred.
- Innervation is associated with embryonic development: foregut, midgut, hindgut, and cloaca.
- Acute abdomen needs to be ruled out immediately.
- Cardiac pain may present with abdominal pain and should be considered early.
- Regional abdominal pains are best elucidated by history and physical examination and represent considerable overlaps requiring numerous studies.
- Pelvic structures are a frequent origin of abdominal pain in females.
- Specific overlap pain syndromes most commonly seen in the office are irritable bowel syndrome, biliary, and dyspepsia.
- The etiology of common abdominal pain syndromes such as nonulcerative dyspepsia and irritable bowel syndrome is not completely understood.
- Cost-effective use of invasive procedures for diagnosis and therapy of abdominal pain requires an understanding of the anatomy, physiology, and innervation of the abdominal viscera.

INTRODUCTION

Abdominal pain is an extremely common experience that accounts for significant disability, loss of work, and often prompts costly diagnostic work-ups, made all the more costly if accurate diagnosis and treatment is delayed. Pain perception is an entirely subjective experience that involves pathophysiologic, neurophysiologic, and psychosocial mechanisms. The variability of the perception of pain makes all-encompassing algorithmic approaches to the diagnosis of the underlying pathology a weak tool for the clinician, who must use the nuances teased from a careful interview with the patient to arrive at the appropriate next step in the work-up.

As the most frequent reason for referral to the gastroenterologist and a frequent complaint of patients seen in the primary care setting, abdominal pain stands as a singular challenge that may lead the patient and physician down dark paths of endless tests, clinic visits, and trips to the pharmacy in attempts to identify and ameliorate the noxious sensation. The clinician's attention to the patient's initial history and physical exam, in conjunction with a basic framework of knowledge of the causes and mechanisms of abdominal pain, will usually avoid trips down these costly venues.

BASIC CONSIDERATIONS

A basic understanding of the neurophysiologic mechanisms involved in pain originating in the abdomen is an important prerequisite for the clinician, who must tailor his or her interview and physical examination. Defining the vocabulary of pain is the stepping stone to this knowledge. Three basic types of pain originate in the abdomen: somatic (sometimes referred to as somatoparietal), visceral, and referred pain.

Much more is known about somatic, and especially cutaneous, pain than about abdominal visceral pain. Somatic pain, such as occurs with stimulation of the parietal peritoneum, is often described as being sharp, bright, is localized, and is clearly perceived as being pain. Somatic pain usually implies actual or potential tissue damage and induces a desire to be immobile.

Visceral pain is usually described as dull, gnawing, burning, is poorly localized and most often midline, and may be perceived as a generally disagreeable sensation such as a "sick" pain or ache. Autonomic disturbances such as nausea and vomiting, sweating, pallor, and orthostasis may accompany visceral pain. Restlessness commonly accompanies visceral pain as the patient searches for relief from this bane, which may result from stimuli that do not necessarily suggest tissue injury (e.g., vigorous contraction of a hollow viscous).

Referred pain (also known as transferred pain, or *übertageneer Schmerz* in German) combines features of somatic and visceral pain with additional qualities. It is sometimes perceived as a deep aching pain near the surface of the skin. Referred pain is localized and sometimes far away from the inciting stimulus, but in an area subserved by the same neural segment as the organ involved. Cutaneous or muscular hyperesthesia, and increased abdominal wall muscle tone, often attend the underlying visceral pain. Referred pain, due to the complex nature of the sensation, may so focus the patient's attention as to eclipse the visceral pain that is its origin. Once properly understood, referred pain may yield important clues that the clinician can use to arrive at the correct diagnosis. Table 1 summarizes qualities of these basic types of pain.

Not all processes that are destructive to the abdominal viscera result in perceived pain. For instance, Hertz in 1911 (and later others) reported that pinching, burning, stabbing, cutting, and electrical and thermal stimulation cause no pain to virtually all of the abdominal organs. Acid and alkali applied to normal gut mucosa also do not produce pain *(1–4)*. This fact is an important concept in the understanding of gastrointestinal disease.

However, four general classes of stimuli do induce abdominal pain, which is mediated by visceral afferents: (1) distention and contraction, (2) traction and torsion, (3) stretch, and (4) certain chemicals. Receptors located within the walls of hollow organs, on the

Table 1
Characteristics of the Basic Types of Abdominal Pain

Somatic Pain	Visceral Pain	Referred Pain
Sharp	Dull	Combination of sharp and dull, often with hyperesthesia of skin or muscle, increased muscle tone
Sustained	Wavering	Usually wavering
Focal, indicates site of stimulus	Poorly localized, often midline	Localized to areas remote from injury in same neural segment
Induces immobility	Restlessness a common feature	Restlessness a common feature
Unmistakably recognized as pain	Array of confusing complaints of discomfort	Burning sensation sometimes described, can eclipse visceral complaints
Usually stands alone	Autonomic disturbances common	Autonomic disturbances reflect underlying visceral stimulus

serosal surfaces of the visceral peritoneum and solid organ capsules, within the mucosa, and within mesenteric vessels and ligaments are commonly multimodal, meaning they respond to both mechanical and chemical stimuli, although mucosal receptors primarily are stimulated by chemicals *(5–8)*.

"Tension receptors" are located within the muscular layers of hollow organs and between the muscularis mucosa and the submucosa. They are functionally, if not anatomically, in series with the smooth muscle and are responsible for the response to mechanical forces. Whenever the smooth muscle containing these receptors undergoes a sufficient increase in tension, pain ensues. Gastric distention as a result of an outlet obstruction and the vigorous peristalsis that occurs consequent to a bowel obstruction are examples of forceful contractions that result in such receptor stimulation. Isometric contraction (i.e., increased muscle-cell tension occurring without a change in the diameter of the hollow viscus) also causes stimulation of these receptors. Ampullary spasm around a stone and colonic contraction around an impaction are prime examples of this phenomenon. This should be compared with the lack of pain that occurs during isotonic stretch of a hollow viscus as occurs when the rectum accommodates to a fecal bolus.

Serosal receptors, which are present within the capsule of liver and spleen, respond most readily to stretch, as occurs with the hepatic distention of congestive heart failure. Mesenteric receptors, on the other hand, respond to torsion and are activated by such clinical conditions as sigmoid or cecal volvulus, internal herniation, and ovarian torsion.

Afferent nerve fibers, which carry visceral pain sensation, can be stimulated after a variety of chemical agents are applied to abdominal structure. Chemicals or autocrines such as substance P, serotonin, histamine, and some prostaglandins are a few of the agents that have been shown to be generated as a consequence of a number of different processes including inflammation, tissue necrosis, ischemia, and hypoxia. However, bradykinin may be the most important mediator of visceral pain in this setting. Potassium chloride, hydrochloric acid, and hypertonic saline can also stimulate these visceral afferents. An explanation for the lack of consistent pain stimulation when acid is applied to the base of an ulcer crater has been suggested by recent work indicating that the mechanism of all these agents may be the induction of local smooth muscle contraction *(9)*.

NEUROPHYSIOLOGY

The skin has two types of nociceptive fibers: the myelinated A-delta fibers (which conduct impulses rapidly) and the slowly conducting unmyelinated c fibers. Cutaneous nerves have a high percentage of afferent fibers involved in pain sensation. In addition, the area that each afferent fiber serves is small compared to particular visceral afferents and are unilaterally organized into well-known dermatomal patterns. This accounts for the precise localization of cutaneous pain.

The majority of the nerves of the extensive myenteric plexus and others in the abdominal viscera, including the visceral peritoneum, have no role in the perception of pain. Many do not even project to the central nervous system (CNS) and are thought to regulate such activities as motility and secretion. Other nonnociceptive afferents are believed to carry information regarding local osmolarity, pH, the concentration of nutrients, and the state of distention and travel to the CNS along such parasympathetic tracts as the vagus nerve *(10,11)*. The parietal peritoneum is innervated by somatic nerves, accounting for the precise localization of pain associated with processes located next to or within it.

The 10% or so of visceral afferents within abdominal nerves that carry information regarding visceral pain are exclusively of the c-fiber type. They run wholly or almost wholly within the sympathetic thoracolumbar tract and serve a relatively large area compared to somatic nerves. The embryologic development of most abdominal structures begins in the midline. Visceral afferent nerves migrate with these structures and result in a lack of lateralization of most visceral pain. Patients involved in a 1949 study were usually unable to distinguish any difference in pain location when the distal esophagus, biliary tree, and upper small intestine were distended, dramatically demonstrating the fuzziness of the human visceral pain perception system *(12)*. This poor localization of visceral abdominal pain often creates great frustration for the clinician and patient, delaying correct diagnosis and sometimes masking ominous processes.

As shown in Fig. 1, painful impulses begin in the abdominal viscous, traveling afferently through the first-order neuron along vascular structures, through the regional splanchnic ganglion (e.g., celiac, hepatic, and superior mesenteric ganglions), within the splanchnic nerve toward and through the sympathetic ganglion, which is part of the sym-

Fig. 1. *(opposite)* Neuronal pathways mediating abdominal visceral pain sensation. There are three orders of neurons mediating pain sensation. The first-order neuron travels from the abdominal viscus by way of the adjacent autonomic plexus to the regional splanchnic ganglion, then along the corresponding splanchnic nerve through a ganglion of the sympathetic chain, then by way of the white ramus communicans to the spinal nerve. From there it traverses

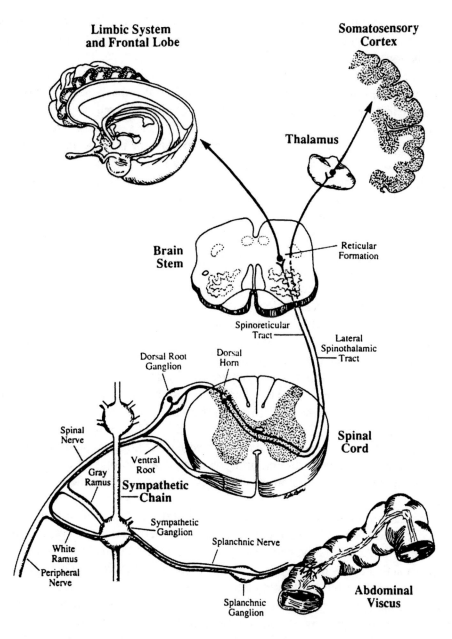

the dorsal root (its cell body lies in the dorsal root ganglion) to enter the dorsal horn of the spinal cord, where it synapses predominantly within laminae I and V. The second-order neurons leave the dorsal horn, cross the midline, and ascend primarily in two tracts. The spinothalamic tract neurons travel through the brain stem to various nuclei within the thalamus, where they synapse with third-order neurons that go predominantly to the somatosensory cortex, mediating the sensory and discriminative aspects of pain. Spinoreticular tract neurons synapse within reticular formation nuclei located primarily in the pons and medulla. From there, third-order neurons travel predominantly to the limbic system and frontal cortex, mediating aspects of pain that have to do with feelings and actions, but also make connections within the thalamus and elsewhere. (From Tadataka Tamada. Textbook of Gastroenterology. J. B. Lippincott, 1991.)

pathetic chain, and into the spinal nerve via the white ramus. The impulse enters the dorsal horn of the spinal cord after passing through the dorsal root ganglion, where the impulse is transferred to the second-order neuron via a synapse. The cell body of this nociceptive neuron lies within the dorsal root ganglion. This synapse of the first- and second-order neurons occurs within laminae I and V. This important synapse is thought to play a role in the reception of descending information, which may modify the ultimate perception of pain as suggested by the gate theory of pain explained below.

The second-order neurons, once stimulated, then send the impulse across the midline to ascend in both the lateral spinothalamic and spinoreticular tracts. The neurons traveling within the spinoreticular tract synapse within the reticular formation of the brainstem, where third-order neurons project to the limbic system and frontal cortex, areas believed to mediate feelings and action. Those neurons traveling within the spinothalamic tract synapse within the thalamus, where third-order neurons projected into the somatosensory cortex, mediating the sensory and discriminative aspects of pain. Integration of this information into perception of pain occurs as a result of less well-understood higher order synaptic processes (see Fig. 1).

In 1965, Melzack and Wall proposed that interacting factors at the site of stimulus, within the spinal cord, and in the brain determine whether peripheral stimuli will be perceived as pain (13). The "gate-control" theory they proposed involves a transmission-cell neuron in the dorsal horn of the spinal cord, which is activated (gate open) by visceral afferent nerve fibers as well as by large peripheral nerves (see Fig. 2). The inhibitory neuron in this arrangement decreases the likelihood that the transmission neuron will fire, thus tending to "close the gate" to pain transmission and thus perception. Descending signals have been identified that arise from the midbrain in areas controlled by enkephalins and opiate receptors and cause release of a variety of neurotransmitters in the dorsal horn, stimulating the inhibitory neuron, again helping to close the gate on afferent pain signals. This inhibitory neuron is also activated by the large peripheral nerves (14,15).

The efficacy of exogenous opiates in the amelioration of visceral abdominal pain is believed to result from stimulation of the descending neuronal pathways, which end in the dorsal horn. Additionally, acute pain, stress, and the administration of placebo are thought to activate this pathway (16,17). Stimulation of the skin such as occurs with transcutaneous electrical nerve stimulators (TENS units)—or even acupuncture, heat application, suction, and the "coining" practices of the orient—may decrease the perception of visceral pain by way of dorsal horn inhibitory nerve activation. Thus, the gate theory of pain is a construct that helps to unify a number of different clinical and personal experiences regarding pain.

The embryologic origin of the abdominal structures is important to the understanding of pain referred to other areas but originating in the pain fibers of the visceral peritoneum (see Table 2). Embryonic foregut is the source of the adult distal esophagus, stomach, proximal duodenum, liver, biliary tree, and pancreas. The visceral pain is usually midline and epigastric, sensed between the xiphoid process and the umbilicus. Although the gallbladder, like all organs of foregut origin, receives bilateral innervation, pain arising from this structure tends to be to the right of the midline (18).

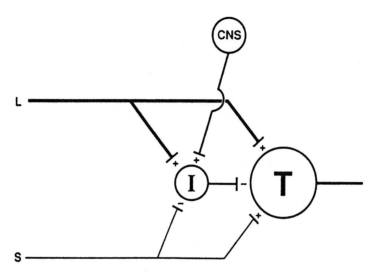

Fig. 2. The gate control theory of pain. Sensory inputs from the periphery come to the dorsal horn of the spinal cord by way of large (L) and small (S) nerve fibers. Both fiber types synapse on the second-order ("transmission cell") neurons (T); when the T-cell neurons are activated, they communicate nociceptive information to the brain. The peripheral nerve fibers also synapse on interneurons (I) within the substantia gelatinosa of the dorsal horn that, when stimulated, inhibit T-cell firing. The large neurons stimulate and the small neurons inhibit these inhibitory interneurons, thus tending to prevent and promote, respectively, central transmission of incoming nociceptive signals. "Descending inhibitory systems" arising within the central nervous system (CNS), when activated by a variety of factors, also stimulate the interneuron to inhibit T-cell firing. The balance of these excitatory and inhibitory forces determines the degree to which nociceptive information is transmitted to the brain. (+, excitatory signals; –, inhibitory signals) (From Tadataka Tamada. Textbook of Gastroenterology. J. B. Lippincott, 1991.)

The distal duodenum, remainder of the small intestine, appendix, ascending colon, and the proximal two-thirds of the transverse colon arise from the embryonic midgut. The pain of these structures is generally in a periumbilical location.

The embryonic hindgut is responsible for the development of the distal one-third of the transverse, descending, and rectosigmoid colon. Pains arising from these areas are sensed in the lower abdomen, usually between the umbilicus and the pubis, and are often perceived as midline in contrast to the bilaterally derived kidneys, ovaries, and fallopian tubes (which may be the source of severe visceral pain that is remarkably unilateral). Ascending and descending colon pain will often manifest appropriately to the right or left side of the abdomen in spite of bilateral innervation *(18)*.

The blood supply to the various structures of the abdomen follows the three basic embryonic origins: structures derived from the foregut are supplied by the celiac axis and its major branches, the midgut structures from the superior mesenteric artery, and the hindgut structures by the inferior mesenteric artery. The visceral afferents travel toward the CNS along these vessels, reflecting their origin and reinforcing the concepts of referred pain.

In the "convergence–projection" theory of referred pain, visceral afferent pain signals synapse within the dorsal horn of the spinal cord with the same second-order neurons that

Table 2
Embryologic Origins and Pain Localization of Abdominal Viscera

Embryologic Structure	Developed Structures	Location of Visceral Pain
Foregut	Distal esophagus, stomach, proximal duodenum, liver, bile ducts, gallbladder, pancreas	Between xiphoid and umbilicus
Midgut	Small intestine, appendix, ascending colon, proximal 2/3 of transverse colon	Periumbilical
Hindgut	Distal 1/3 of transverse colon, descending and sigmoid colon, rectum, superior portion of anal canal	Between umbilicus and pubis
Cloaca	Inferior 1/3 of anal canal, urinary bladder, perineum, urethra	Pelvis, perianal, or perineum

receive somatic afferent neural input. The resultant impulse is then relayed to higher CNS structures, where the perception of somatic pain occurs. Referred pain is the result of a "fooling" of the brain, which is constantly receiving somatic inputs resulting in the more familiar sensations of cutaneous pain (*see* Fig. 3).

Well-worked-out dermatomal patterns reveal the areas of the skin that correspond to the level of afferent cutaneous somatic pain fibers to the spinal cord. Using a map of cutaneous dermatomes (Fig. 4) and understanding that, because the visceral afferents from the various abdominal structures enter the spinal cord in a fashion reminiscent of their embryologic origin, it is easy to understand how gallbladder pain can cause pain over the area of the shoulder. Unfortunately, because the afferent visceral fibers from abdominal structures tend to spread (that is, enter the spinal cord at several levels), precise localization of the source of noxious abdominal pain using the referred pain as a starting point is not an exact science (*see* Table 3). Some common and well-recognized areas of referred pain during episodes of acute visceral pain are shown in Fig. 5.

APPROACH TO THE PATIENT WITH ABDOMINAL PAIN

Having the tools to understand the genesis of abdominal pain allows the clinician to direct pertinent questions regarding the characteristics of the patient's abdominal pain. Time of onset, location, intensity, quality, whether the pain is sustained or intermittent (as in colic), associations with meals, associated nausea and vomiting and the temporal relationship with the pain, presence of a fever, changes in intensity with movement or change in body position, aggravating factors, and alleviating factors such as antacids or vomiting are all time-honored pieces of information from the patient's history that should be sought at the time of the initial patient interview. Table 4 summarizes the data that should be obtained from the patient regarding his or her pain. Age and sex of the patient, underlying medical problems, ethnic background, use of medications, use of recreational drugs, and smoking history all may be important to making a correct diagnosis.

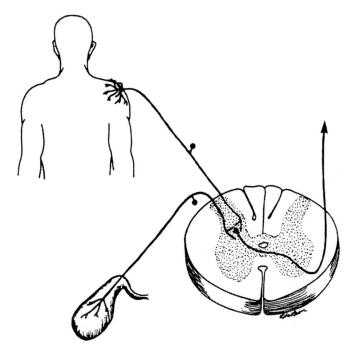

Fig. 3. Neuroanatomic basis of referred pain. According to the "convergence-projection theory," afferent nociceptive signals from abdominal visceral structures synapse within the dorsal horn of the spinal cord with the second-order neurons that receive somatic (e.g., cutaneous) input from the same spinal level. Thus, a nociceptive signal from an abdominal organ triggers firing of the same second-order neurons that would respond if noxious input were received from the corresponding somatic structure. The resulting conscious perception of pain is referred to the somatic structure, because afferent signals from this source are received more commonly than are those from the viscera. Thus, the brain is "fooled" as to the true origin of the incoming signal. (From Tadataka Tamada. Textbook of Gastroenterology. J. B. Lippincott, 1991.)

The physical examination is a critical first step in understanding a patient's abdominal pain. Oral apthous ulcers may suggest underlying Crohn's disease. Cardiac murmurs and arrhythmias may underlie an intestinal infarction from an embolus. Severe pallor may result from a bleeding ulcer or ruptured pseudoaneurysm within a pancreatic pseudocyst, whereas jaundice with pain suggests choledocholithiasis or pancreatic cancer. Bruits in the neck, chest, or abdomen can result from the atherosclerotic disease of the patient presenting with a dissecting abdominal aortic aneurysm. Bruising in the flank or around the umbilicus can result from hemorrhagic pancreatitis or other causes of retroperitoneal bleeding. The iliopsoas and obturator signs are positive in instances of retroperitoneal inflammation such as a retroperitoneal appendicitis or diverticular abscess. Presence of peritoneal irritation is best elicited by tapping the patient's heel, which causes enough movement to elicit pain without performing the sometimes agonizing and confusing maneuvers necessary to document "rebound tenderness." Table 5 lists a number of important physical signs and maneuvers involved in the work-up of abdominal pain.

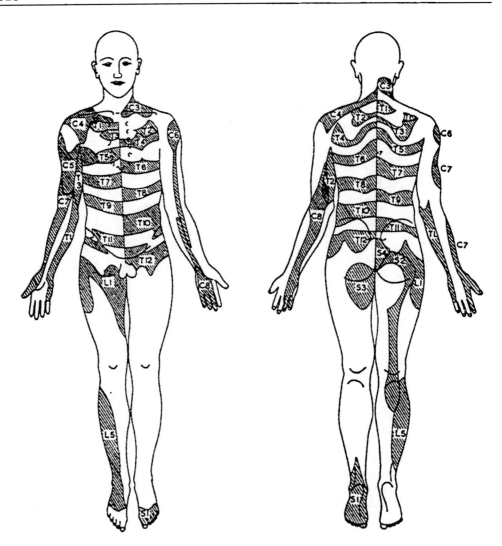

Fig. 4. Cutaneous dermatomes: Pattern of referral of pain from abdominal viscera. In general, pain is referred to the cutaneous dermatomes whose afferent nerves enter the same levels of the spinal cord as those of the affected abdominal organ. (From Lewis T. Pain. New York: Macmillan, 1942.)

Of utmost importance to the clinician evaluating a patient with abdominal pain is to determine if the underlying process is likely to be life-threatening or in need of immediate surgical attention. As Sir Zachary Cope states in his classic "Early Diagnosis of the Acute Abdomen": "the very terms 'acute abdomen' and 'abdominal emergency,' which are constantly applied to such cases, signify the need for prompt diagnosis and early treatment, by no means always surgical" *(19)*. Physical exam findings of peritoneal irritation often herald an acute abdomen, prompting further and more immediate investigation.

The abdominal cavity is lined by the parietal peritoneum, which is innervated by somatic nerves. Hence, when these nerves are stimulated, the patient develops

Table 3
Distribution of Referred Pain by Organ and Dermatome

Structure	Cutaneous Dermatomes
Foregut	
Esophagus	T4/5–T7/8
Stomach	T5–T10
Liver	T5–T10/11
Pancreas	T6–T9/10
Midgut	
Small intestine	T5–T10
Proximal colon	T8/9–L1
Hindgut	
Distal colon and rectum	T8–L1 and S2–S4
Other structures	
Diaphragm	C4
Kidney, ureter	T8/9–L3
Urinary bladder	T10/11–L1
Ovary, fallopian tube	T10–L1
Uterus	T10–L1
Cervix	T11–T12
Testicle, epididymis	T10–T12

localized, sharp pain. In the presence of an ileus, defined as lack of bowel sounds after 2 min of listening with the stethoscope, peritoneal pain suggests processes that may require rapid surgical intervention. Free air in the peritoneum must be excluded to rule out the possibility of a perforated viscous, which would require immediate surgical consultation. Table 6 lists a number of abdominal emergencies, which include such findings and demand immediate recognition and action, often surgical.

Two potentially catastrophic abdominal emergencies must be mentioned that may present in a slightly atypical manner. The first is a dissecting abdominal aortic aneurysm. Patients, usually ones at risk for atherosclerotic disease, often complain of a "ripping" type pain. Often there is no peritonitis unless the SMA is involved when bowel infarction and subsequent peritonitis can occur. Clues to this diagnosis include a palpable, pulsatile mass in the abdomen, possible acute renal failure due to involvement of the renal arteries and/or cold extremities, and generally the increased magnitude of pain. Early bowel infarction can also present with subtle findings when transmural inflammation and subsequent peritonitis have yet to develop. The patient's complaints of abdominal pain are generally far out of proportion to the physical findings, which usually include a quiet bowel and minimal peritoneal signs. Clues to the diagnosis of this devastating event include an elevated amylase with a normal lipase and air within the wall of the bowel or in the portal vein on CT scan, especially in a patient with atrial fibrillation or a hypercoagulable state.

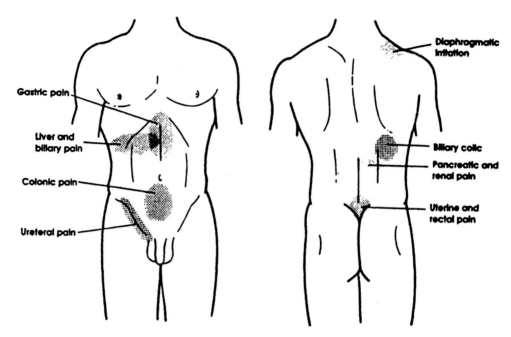

Fig. 5. Common patterns of referred pain observed in patients with acute visceral pain. (From Kelly. Textbook of Internal Medicine, 2nd Edition. T. B. Lippincott, 1992.)

Once the cloud of an impending or occurring intra-abdominal catastrophe has passed, the clinician can carefully study the patient's complaints. Attention to the physical exam should precipitate a differential diagnosis, which will then direct appropriate further studies.

DIFFERENTIAL OF ABDOMINAL PAIN BY REGION

Diffuse Abdominal Pain

The large list of potential etiologies for generalized abdominal pain makes further work-up consequent to certain historical clues. Abdominal pain occurring routinely 30 min–1 h after eating suggests the rare mesenteric ischemia (aka abdominal angina) or, if associated with nausea or vomiting, a partial small bowel obstruction. Stuttering abdominal pain in a women on birth control pills may be resultant to mesenteric venous thrombosis.

A commonly encountered entity is subacute bacterial peritonitis seen in patients with ascites. Associated peritonitis is an important clue to such diagnoses as acute cholecystitis. The presence of jaundice suggests either hepatitis or cholangitis. Metabolic diseases, including sickle-cell disease, acute intermittent porphyria, and Familial Mediterranean fever, can precipitate such complaints as well as heavy-metal poisoning such as lead or arsenic poisoning. Intestinal obstructions, early appendicitis, and acute enlargement of lymph nodes (as can occur with lymphoma) are also recognized etiologies of diffuse complaints. Severe abdominal pain, nausea, vomiting, and diarrhea occurring hours after the ingestion of food substances suggest toxin ingestion from *Staphylococcus aureus* or *Bacillus cereus* (*see* Table 7).

Table 4
Important Clues in Patient History Regarding Abdominal Pain

Descriptors Of Pain	Examples Of Patient Responses
Location	Right upper abdomen, "stomach"
Quality	Sharp, "crampy," dull, ache, burning
Intensity	Severe, 8/10
Radiation	"Wraps around to back," through to back
Onset	"In middle of night," increased over hours, severe within a minute then some better
Duration	Several minutes, hours, days, waxing and waning, cannot escape
Peritoneal signs	Pain with movement, deep breathing, passing stool, urinating
Aggravating factors	Worse after meals, worse after aspirin, increased with walking
Alleviating factors	Antacids, vomiting, passing gas/stool, belching
Changes with position	Worse with lying on back, better leaning over
Important associated factors	Fever, diarrhea, arthritis, skin rash, jaundice, change in stool color, bloody emesis or blood in stool, melena

Epigastric Pain

Distal esophagitis, nonulcer dyspepsia, gastritis, and ulcer disease followed by pancreatitis and acute cholecystitis make up the lion's share of pathologic entities causing epigastric pain. The clinician must never forget acute myocardial infarction as a cause of epigastric pain. Associated symptoms such as sweating or shortness of breath, the timing of the epigastric pain, increase with recumbent position, and relief with antacids are important clues in the history to the underlying disease process. A history of weight loss in a patient with epigastric pain demands an answer that rules out gastric or pancreatic cancer. Diabetics with gastric emptying disorders secondary to neuropathy tend to complain of epigastric pain, especially after meals as the slow-to-empty stomach stretches to accommodate the intake. Vomiting can occur with obstructive processes such as pyloric channel ulcers and high-small-bowel obstructions, infectious gastritis and gastroenteritis, acute hepatobiliary disease, acute myocardial ischemia, and pancreatitis, as well as a host of intra-abdominal processes causing a vasovagal reflex (e.g., acute appendicitis).

Lab work-up is directed toward ruling out cardiac disease (EKG, treadmill test), hepatobiliary disease (LFT's, RUQ ultrasound), pancreatic processes (amylase, lipase, and ultrasound to rule out pancreatic pseudocyst), and then intraluminal GI sources. Barium studies of the esophagus and stomach are often revealing and can give some clues as to the motility of the esophagus and stomach. Upper endoscopy, however, allows excellent visualization of inflamed mucosa, as well as the ability to perform biopsies, and is important in a negative sense since it rules out certain diseases and

Table 5
Glossary of Physical Exam Findings and Maneuvers Important
in the Evaluation of the Patient with Abdominal Pain

Abdominal sign	Ascites	Excess fluid in the peritoneal cavity
	Borborygmus	Loud bowel "rushes" suggestive of intestinal obstruction
	Courvoisier's sign	Presence of a palpable but nontender gallbladder suggestive of regional malignancy
	Cullen's sign	Bluish-green to purple discoloration around the umbilicus
	Grey Turner's sign	Nontraumatic ecchymosis on abdomen or flank
	Ileus	Paralysis of the peristaltic movement of the bowel indicated by lack of audible bowel sounds over 2 min
	Involuntary guarding	Rigidity of the abdominal wall secondary to peritoneal irritation, which the patient cannot abate
	Ladder sign	Dilated loops of bowel visible on inspection of the contour of the abdominal wall
	Rebound tenderness	Tenderness of the abdominal wall, which is greater on the sudden release of deep pressure than during the pressure itself, suggesting peritoneal irritation
	Referred tenderness	Peritoneal irritation causing pain elsewhere
	Referred rebound tenderness	Discomfort on release, remote from the site palpated
	Rub	"Leather squeak" sound on auscultation
	Tympany	Drum-like sound created by tapping over a hollow abdominal viscus
Abdominal maneuvers	Carnett's sign	Increase in pain on palpation of abdomen when abdominal musculature is tensed (as in sitting part-way up); suggestive of abdominal wall rather than visceral pathology
	Fluid wave	The tactile perception of free fluid moving within the abdominal cavity with ballottement
	Iliopsoas test (positive)	Pelvic pain produced by flexion of the thigh against resistance; suggests retroperitoneal irritation
	"Inching" the stethoscope	Moving it inch by inch over the area of the gallbladder; suggests inflammation of the gallbladder
	Murphy's sign (positive)	Arrest of inspiration with deep palpation in the area of the gallbladder; suggests inflammation of the gallbladder
	Obturator test (positive)	Pelvic pain elicited by forced rotation of the flexed hip on the ipsilateral side, suggesting retroperitoneal inflammation

Adapted from Willms J, Schneiderman H, Algranati P. Physical Diagnosis: bedside evaluation of diagnosis and function. Baltimore Williams and Wilkins, 1994.

Table 6
The Hyperacute Abdomen

Acute cholecystitis	Ectopic pregnancy
Perforated peptic ulcer	Intussusception
Acute pancreatitis	Cecal, sigmoid, or gastric volvulus
Appendicitis	Pelvic inflammatory disease
Strangulated hernia	Liver laceration
Mesenteric artery occlusion	Infection of pancreatic pseudocyst
Mesenteric venous occlusion	Splenic artery pseudoaneurysm with acute bleeding into pancreatic pseudocyst
Splenic rupture	Phlegmonous gastritis
Splenic infarction	Duodenal or colonic dissection from deceleration injury
Severe acute hepatitis	Toxic megacolon
Rupture of liver cyst or abscess	Intestinal perforation caused by ingested foreign bodies
Spontaneous hepatic rupture related to HELLP syndrome	Tiflitis (AKA cecitis) related to neutropenic states
Abdominal aortic aneurysm with or without dissection	Penetrating abdominal injuries
Intestinal perforation caused by systemic lupus erythematosis, Crohn's, Bechet's, systemic vasculitides, or helminthic infections	Gastric rupture

provides direction for future studies. CT scan can be helpful if a retrogastric pancreatic process is suspected, which may be missed using conventional transabdominal ultrasound (*see* Table 7).

Right Upper-Quadrant Pain

The painful conditions that cause pain sensed in the right upper quadrant of the abdomen generally focus the mind of the clinician on the hepatobiliary tract. This is a useful starting point, but by no means the only area of interest. In the elderly population, acute myocardial infarction may present with right upper-quadrant pain of great intensity. Associated nausea and vomiting may quickly suggest acute cholecystitis or even an obstructed biliary system yet still be a classic manifestation of myocardial ischemia. Attention to the character of the pain as well as associated symptoms is paramount.

Any history or documentation of fever associated with the onset of RUQ pain is an important clue. Peptic ulcer disease, unless associated with perforation, does not cause fever. Passage of a renal calculus, the pain of which is generally severe, is more often centered in the back or flank with radiation of pain into the groin and also does not cause fever. Congestive hepatopathy caused by, most commonly, right-sided heart failure, but also by the acute Budd-Chiari syndrome, usually is not associated with fever. The pain can be sharp and severe since Glisson's capsule, rich with nociceptive stretch fibers, is

Table 7
Causes of Abdominal Pain

Generalized Abdominal Pain	Epigastric Pain
Gastroenteritis	Gastritis
Peritonitis	Gastric ulcer
Small bowel obstruction	Gastric cancer
Small bowel infarction	Nonulcerative dyspepsia
Leukemia	Diabetic gastroparesis
Sickle-cell crisis	Pancreatitis
Early appendicitis	Pancreatic cancer
Acute abdominal lymphadenopathy	Esophagitis
Pancreatitis	Mallory-Weiss tear
Colitis	Myocardial infarction
Acute intermittent porphyria	Peritonitis
Henoch-Schonlein purpura	Boerhaave's syndrome
Black widow spider bite	Pancreatic pseudocyst
Tabes dorsalis	
Giant cell arteritis	
Intestinal ischemia due to polyarteritis nodosa, Churg-Strauss, Wegener's granulomatosis, cryoglobulinemia	
Lead poisoning	
Retroperitoneal hemorrhage	
Retroperitoneal neoplasm	
Childhood sexual abuse	
Familial Mediterranean fever	

tensed with a rapidly enlarging hepatic parenchyma. Acute cholecystitis, with or without choledocholithiasis, hepatic abscesses, infectious processes of the chest (empyema, pneumonia), pulmonary infarction, hepatic infarction (as in chemoembolization of hepatic tumors), and retrocecal appendicitis commonly have associated fever, although it may, as with many inflammatory processes, be mild or nonexistent in the elderly. Acute hepatitis can also present with fever. Hepatic tumors, unless they are infarcting or bleeding and causing associated inflammation of the serosal surface of the liver, rarely cause abdominal pain, but by virtue of humoral factors produced by some tumors, may cause fever. Likewise, processes that cause a slow obstruction of the biliary tree, as occurs with carcinoma of the head of the pancreas and ampullary carcinoma, tend not to cause the pain elicited by the resultant distention of the bile ducts.

Physical exam findings—which are of great utility in patients with right upper-quadrant pain—include observing for jaundice, eliciting peritoneal signs, and the Murphy's sign of increased pain with inspiration during deep palpation in the area of the gallbladder, which suggests inflammation. A rub over the area of the liver can occur with inflammatory processes of the liver capsule, as occurs in subcapsular bleeds and abscesses. Pulmonary infarction may also create an auscultatory rub in this area.

An upright chest X-ray, EKG, complete peripheral blood count, liver enzymes, amylase, and UA are requisite first-order tests helpful in working up right upper-quadrant pain. Whether liver enzymes were drawn during or after attacks of pain becomes an important issue in patient with suspected Sphincter of Oddi dysfunction, as triaging of these patients is necessary for deciding which patients should undergo endoscopic retrograde cholangiogram with manometry. Transcutaneous ultrasonography probably has the highest yield for any second-order lab or imaging work, as hepatobiliary and renal pathology is often evident using this very noninvasive modality. Increasing in order of cost, upper endoscopy, HIDA scan with or without CCK, and computed tomography represent the next level of diagnostic tests for the work-up of right upper-quadrant pain followed by ERCP, abdominal MRI, and liver sulfur-colloid scan. In the case of abnormal liver function studies the clinical assessment has the highest level of accuracy for predicting whether the abnormalities are intra- or extrahepatic. In the case of an intrahepatic process or, if a question arises, transcutaneous ultrasonography has a significant yield for demonstrating lesions and no dilated intrahepatic ducts. With cholestatic enzymes and a supportive history of extrahepatic biliary tract obstruction, an ERCP is the procedure of choice, since it is both diagnostic and therapeutic. Upper GI endoscopy, abdominal MRI, and liver sulfur-colloid scans are usually reserved for the patient with recurrent and enigmatic pain. Ten percent of the population of the United States has cholelithiasis, and approx 1.2% of these patients have bouts of right upper-quadrant pain attributed to their stones each year. In the case of ultrasound-demonstrated stones diseases, an HIDA scan with or without CCK will confirm cystic duct dysfunction secondary to stone inclusion or other anatomic processes (*see* Table 8).

Left Upper-Quadrant Pain

Pain in the abdomen isolated to the left upper quadrant is not a particularly common complaint. After ruling out an intrathoracic source of the pain, such as myocardial ischemia, pneumonia, and empyema, gastric ulcer and pancreatitis should be considered. Chronic abdominal pain in this region may be caused by a pancreatic pseudocyst. The spleen is found in this area; and splenic infarction, abscess, or acute congestion due to the onset of portal hypertension or acute splenic vein thrombosis may present with left upper-quadrant pain. The presence of a splenic friction rub suggests some inflammation of the splenic capsule. Infections such as mononucleosis or acute human immunodeficiency virus may cause acute splenomegaly, and the clinician should gingerly palpate the abdomen in such patients or risk precipitating splenic rupture. Lymphoma and acute leukemia can cause splenomegaly, but the degree of pain elicited (as in hepatomegaly) is more likely if the enlargement occurred over a short time. Table 8 provides a differential as to possible causes of left upper-quadrant pain.

Work-up of such pain, particularly if acute, includes the CXR, EKG, CBC, liver enzymes, amylase, and lipase. Ultrasound, especially with Doppler capability, can rapidly diagnose splenic vein thrombosis. Abdominal CT is another excellent modality to evaluate the splenic parenchyma, and to identify pancreatic processes and pseudocysts.

Table 8
Causes of Abdominal Pain

Right upper-quadrant pain	Left upper-quadrant pain
Acute cholecystitis	Gastritis
Cholangitis	Gastric volvulus
Hepatitis	Pancreatitis
Peptic ulcer	Pancreatic cancer
Retrocecal appendicitis	Pancreatic pseudocyst
Hepatic abscess	Myocardial infarction
Hepatoma with necrosis	Splenic infarction
Focal nodular hyperplasia with necrosis	Splenic rupture
Subcapsular hepatic hematoma	Splenic abscess
Hepatomegaly from congestive heart failure	Splenomegaly caused by
Acute Budd-Chiari	mononucleosis
Myocardial ischemia	HIV
Pericarditis	splenic vein thrombosis
Pneumonia	cirrhosis
Empyema	lymphoma
Nephritis	Pneumonia
Perinephric abscess	Empyema
Renal colic	Nephritis
	Perinephric abscess
	Renal colic
Right lower-quadrant pain	Left lower-quadrant pain
Appendicitis, acute or chronic	Diverticulitis
Ileitis secondary to	Constipation or obstruction
Crohn's disease	Acute infectious colitis
Yersinea infection	Ulcerative colitis
Diverticulitis	Ischemic colitis
Intra-abdominal abscess	Colon cancer
Ogilvie's syndrome	Irritable bowel disease
Psoas abscess	Pelvic inflammatory disease
Cholecystitis	Endometriosis
Perforated ulcer	Ureteral calculi
Leaking aneurysm	Testicular torsion
Meckel's diverticulitis	Epididymitis
Intussusception	Mittelschmerz
Cecal volvulus	Ovarian cyst or torsion
Irritable bowel disease	Ectopic pregnancy
Pelvic inflammatory disease	Leaking aneurysm
Ureteral calculi	Intestinal obstruction
Testicular torsion	Cystitis
Epididymitis	Bladder outlet obstruction
Mittelschmerz	
Ovarian cyst or torsion	
Ectopic pregnancy	
Endometriosis	
Leaking aneurysm	
Intestinal obstruction	
Cystitis	
Bladder outlet obstruction	
Colon cancer	

Right Lower-Quadrant Pain

Acute and chronic appendicitis are classic causes of right lower-quadrant pain, causing localization by virtue of the concomitant local peritoneal irritation. The terminal ileum is a luminal structure in this vicinity, and inflammatory conditions of it often result in pain in this area. Such common diseases of the terminal ileum include Crohn's disease (with or without associated abdominal abscesses) and ulcerative colitis with so-called backwash ileitis. Patients with iron-overload states, such as chronic hemolytic anemias (sickle cell, thalassemia, hemochromatosis), and alcoholics (with consequent hemosiderosis) are at particular risk for Yersinia infection, which can present with complaints of right lower-quadrant pain caused by colitis and acute mesenteric lymphadenopathy. Mycobacterium tuberculosis, when involving the bowel, is most likely to affect the ileocecal valve. Amoeba infections of the bowel can be limited to the region of the cecum as can cytomegalovirus infections seen in immunodeficient states such as AIDS. The ileocecal valve is usually in this anatomic location, and its presence should be remembered in patients with a history of ingesting foreign bodies as perforation of the bowel tends to occur here and at the pylorus.

Psoas abscesses can occur consequent to diverticulitis, chronic appendicitis, and fistulous diseases of the bowel, such as Crohn's disease. While some patients present with right lower-quadrant pain, the presence of a psoas or obturator sign may be the only clues to complaints of vague abdominal pain increased by walking in the setting of fever or lab suggestion of inflammation (e.g., elevated white count, ESR).

Pelvic organs in female patients can be a source of right lower-quadrant pain; and one who is attempting to distinguish between right lower-quadrant abdominal pain and pelvic pain can be frustrated by the expanded differential in women with such complaints. Female patients of childbearing age must have a pregnancy test; and a careful pelvic exam is critical in the work-up of such patients, since pelvic inflammatory disease, ectopic pregnancy, endometriosis, ovarian cysts, and the pain of Mittelsschmerz are not uncommon etiologies of right lower-quadrant pain in female patients.

Appropriate lab work is dictated by the overall history and physical exam. Complete blood count, pregnancy tests in females, and upright CXR and KUB to evaluate free air, the air fluid levels of an abscess, and in the acutely presenting patient an Ogilvie's syndrome, intussusception, or cecal volvulus are appropriate starting points. LFT's and amylase occasionally will reveal a brewing cholecystitis or pancreatitis in patients with right lower-quadrant pain; but if the amylase and not the lipase is elevated, an ovarian source may be to blame. While transabdominal ultrasound has been investigated as a modality to diagnose appendicitis, the sensitivity remains poor. Its great value in the work-up of right lower-quadrant pain is for visualization of pelvic organs. Abdominal and pelvic CT is an invaluable method for identifying the presence of an abscess, especially when retroperitoneal. A urinalysis may reveal an atypical presentation of cystitis or passage of a kidney stone, but other patient complaints will suggest these.

Left Lower Abdominal Pain

Common etiologies of left lower-quadrant abdominal pain include diverticulitis, constipation, infectious colitis, ischemic colitis in the at-risk elderly patient with underlying vascular disease, and pelvic sources in the female. Ulcerative colitis and urogenital sources of pain also deserve consideration. The history of onset and associated complaints of diarrhea (bloody or nonbloody) are critical in determining the next steps in diagnosis and management.

Complete blood count, upright KUB, and urinalysis to rule out large bowel obstruction, sigmoid volvulus, and the air fluid levels of a diverticular abscess are important starting points in the work-up. As in right lower-quadrant abdominal pain, a pelvic exam for female patients is mandatory. Flexible sigmoidoscopy is a relatively benign and reasonably high-yield procedure, which can rapidly bring to light the presence of pseudomembranous colitis, inflammatory bowel disease, colonic tumors that have invaded local pelvic structures, and ischemic colitis with its bloody edematous mucosa and sharply defined border. In patients with irritable bowel disease, the extreme discomfort initiated by the procedure may in itself be a clue to the underlying disorder. However, caution must be exercised before employing this modality as diverticulitis may be worsened with the increased intraluminal pressure the procedure creates. Therefore, in the case of anorexia, focal abdominal pain, elevated white count, and fever, a course of broad spectrum antibiotic therapy prior to contrast studies is the preferred approach. After the course of antibiotic therapy a barium enema is the first-line diagnostic test. As mentioned, the utility of ultrasound is greatest in investigating pelvic etiologies of pain. Abdominal CT may reveal diverticular or psoas abscesses; but in many cases of diverticulitis, intramural colonic air with edema and narrowing of the lumen may be the findings, suggesting microabscesses.

SPECIFIC PAIN SYNDROMES

The various pathologies of abdominal pain are protean; it is important to review the most common diagnoses encountered by the clinician. The etiologies of the hyperacute abdomen should be recognized by the clinician early. The severity of pain and the rapidity of the decline in these patients tends to make the diagnosis evident. However, the office-based clinician will not regularly encounter such patients. In this section we attempt to outline the more common etiologies of abdominal pain and arrange them by the frequency of encounter in the primary care setting.

Irritable Bowel Syndrome

The irritable bowel syndrome (IBS) is one of the most commonly encountered abdominal pain syndromes that the clinician faces. Indeed, it is the most common cause for referral to gastroenterologists, constituting 20–50% of referred patients (20); and estimates of the prevalence of IBS in the general population are in the neighborhood of 15% or more (21,22). The IBS is considered to be a motor disorder consisting of altered bowel habits, abdominal pain, and the absence of detectable organic pathology (23). Female-to-male prevalence is approx 2:1 (although the reverse may be true in India), and there is a higher incidence among whites than nonwhites. This, combined with a study showing that up to 44% of patients diagnosed with IBS report sexual abuse as children, suggests that the experience of IBS is related to life experiences (22,24,25).

The IBS comprises two variants: the pain predominant and diarrhea predominant forms. The pain is thought to be a result of vigorous contractions of the colon, often noted

Table 9
Features of Irritable Bowel Syndrome (IBS)

Consistent with a Diagnosis IBS	Not Associated with IBS

1. Lower abdominal pain
  a. Aggravated by meals
  b. Relieved by defecation
  c. More frequent bowel movement with
    onset of pain
  d. Looser stools with onset of pain
  e. Does not awaken patient
2. Visible abdominal distention
3. Small stools (with constipation or diarrhea)
4. Chronic symptoms consistent in pattern
  but variable in severity
5. Symptoms worse with periods of stress
	1. Onset in old age
	2. Steady progressive course
	3. Frequent awakening by symptoms
	4. Fever
	5. Weight loss
	6. Rectal bleeding from other than
	  fissures or hemorrhoids
	7. Steatorrhea
	8. Dehydration
	9. New symptoms after a long period

Adapted from Sleisenger and Fordtran. Gastrointestinal Disease. W. B. Saunders, 1993.

on barium enema studies and flexible sigmoidoscopy of these patients. The term spastic colon or spastic bowel syndrome is often used synonymously for this disorder. Manometric studies suggest small bowel and even gastric motility abnormalities in these patients, making irritable bowel syndrome a more inclusive term *(26)*. Manometric studies, however, suggest that patients with IBS have markedly diminished high-amplitude peristaltic contractions (HAPCs), which normally occur after meals, and increased powerful colonic segmenting contractions, both of which contribute to constipation and pain *(27–30)*.

Differentiating IBS from organic disease is a challenge for the clinician, and reports of delays in diagnosing serious disease in patients who were previously labeled as having IBS abound. Four symptoms present in IBS that may be helpful in this discernment: (1) visible abdominal distention, (2) relief of abdominal pain by bowel movement, (3) more frequent bowel movements with the onset of pain, and (4) looser stools with onset of pain. Some 91% of patients with IBS, but only 30% with organic disease, have two or more of these complaints *(23,30)*. Table 9 outlines important features of IBS in distinguishing it from organic disease.

Complaints of abdominal pain are varied, ranging from bloating, crampy, aching, and dull to burning, knife-like, sharp, or steady. The pain can be acute and intermittent or superimposed on chronic pain. While the pain is most often sensed in the left lower quadrant and the lower abdomen in general, it may be sensed anywhere in the abdomen; and experimental balloon distention reveals that the trigger points for a particular patient's abdominal pain may be anywhere from the esophagus to the distal colon *(31)*. One particularly vexing and common source of abdominal pain in patients with IBS originates from distention of the colon at the splenic flexure, which, for unclear reasons (perhaps local stretch, tension, and stimulation of somatic parietal pain receptors), may produce pain in the RUQ or the precordium. This type of chest pain, however, is relieved by passing gas. To make matters more complicated, balloon distention within the colon itself may produce complaints of pain nearly everywhere in the abdomen (*see*

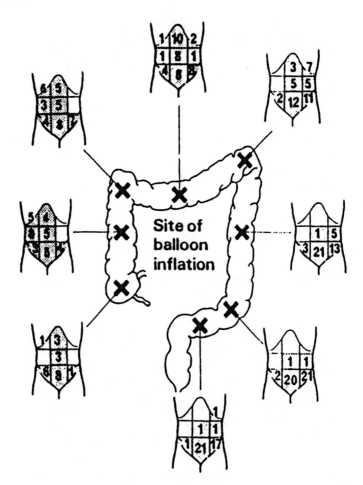

Fig. 6. Distribution of abdominal pain induced by balloon inflations when the balloon was inflated in the indicated locations in 48 patients investigated for abdominal pain. (From Swarbrick ET, Hegarty JE, Bat L, Williams CB, Dawson AM. Site of pain from the irritable bowel. Lancet 1980; 2: 443.)

Fig. 6). Radiation of the pain is considered unusual, but radiation may occur to the lower back.

Abnormal psychologic features, including depression, anxiety, and somatization, have been reported in 70–90% of patients with IBS *(32)*; and while emotional stress can trigger hypermotility in normal subjects as well as in patients with IBS, the threshold is lower in IBS patients *(33)*. IBS patients often have a preoccupation with illness and, with the variety of symptom complaints, may present a formidable challenge to the clinician in the new medical world order of managed care and cost containment.

Reasonable work-up for patients with suspected IBS is aimed at quickly eliminating more ominous pathology. Basic blood work to rule out anemia and underlying inflammation is requisite, as is a good basic physical exam with rectal examination and stool hemoccult. Flexible sigmoidoscopy is easily performed in the outpatient setting and is associated with very low risk; the exaggerated pain it may produce in patients with IBS

Table 10
Recommended Laboratory Investigations for Suspected IBS

All Patients	Individualized
Complete blood count	Stool culture, C. diff toxin, ova and parasite
Erythrocyte sedimentation rate	Colonoscopy
Flexible sigmoidoscopy	Esophagogastroduodenoscopy
Lactose withdrawal and rechallenge	Hydrogen breath test
Stool for WBC's, spot fecal fat, Giardia EIA	Small bowel follow-through
	Rectal manometry
	Colonic inertia studies

may be valuable information and should be performed. A lactose withdrawal and challenge is inexpensive, detects a common disorder (which often manifests in the third decade), and may obviate further and more expensive testing. Testing the stool for WBCs and Giardia EIA is reasonable, because the presence of the former demands further work-up for colitis and the latter may expose a common and treatable infection, which may present subclinically and occasionally chronically. Other modalities of investigation should be pursued on a case-by-case basis (see Table 10). Patients with leukocytosis, elevated ESR, blood, white cells, fat in the stool, stool weight exceeding 200 g/d, persistent diarrhea in spite of a 48-h fast, hypokalemia, or lack of a spastic response to rectal stimulation during rectal manometry are unlikely to have IBS (23).

Frequent office visits to initially establish patient trust, high-fiber diets, avoidance of narcotics, tranquilizers, and antispasmodics such as dicyclomine (Bentyl) or hyoscyamine (Levsin) are basic mainstays of therapy. Few randomized control trials of therapy exist, and all are characterized by a high placebo effect. Promotility agents, Lupron and Lactobacillus, have demonstrated beneficial effects (34). Some clinicians feel that physical exercise may improve the symptoms of IBS, possibly through release of endorphin, in addition to improving the overall sense of well-being, an important modifier in the perception of pain (35).

Dyspepsia

Dyspepsia is a term used to describe a combination of symptoms including persistent or recurrent epigastric or upper abdominal pain or discomfort. Belching, eructations, flatulence, nausea, and heartburn may be present, but the only consistent feature is the localization of symptoms to the upper abdomen. Three classes of dyspepsia have been proposed: (1) those with an identifiable cause for symptoms, which improve if the disease is eradicated (e.g., PUD, GERD, cancer, hepatobiliary disease); (2) those with identifiable abnormalities of unclear relevance (Helicobactor pylori infection, gastritis, histologic duodenitis, gastroparesis, or gastroduodenal or small bowel dysmotility); and (3) those with no cause recognizable by current technologies. The latter two categories constitute functional dyspepsia (or idiopathic, essential) (36). Nonulcer dyspepsia constitutes a subgroup in which the symptoms are most like those of peptic ulcer disease, but no ulcer is found. Organic causes of dyspepsia predominate in the elderly, while the reverse is true for the young.

Table 11
Symptoms of Gastric and Duodenal Ulcers and Nonulcer Dyspepsia

Symptom	Gastric Ulcer, %	Duodenal Ulcer, %	Nonulcer Dyspepsia, %
Pain/discomfort[a]	100	100	100
Features of the pain			
Primary pain			
Epigastric	67	61–86	52–73
Right hypochondrium	6	7–17	4
Left hypochondrium	6	3–5	5
Frequently severe	68	53	37
Within 30 min of food	20	5	32
Gnawing pain	13	16	6
Increased by food	24	10–40	45
Clusters (episodic)	16	56	35
Relieved by alkali	36–87	39–86	26–75
Food relief	2–48	20–63	4–32
Occurs at night	32–43	50–88	24–32
Not related to food or variable	22–53	21–49	22–65
Radiation to back	34	20–31	24–28
Increased appetite		19	
Anorexia	46–57	25–36	26–36
Weight loss	24–61	19–45	18–32
Nausea	54–70	49–59	43–60
Vomiting	38–73	25–57	26–34
Heartburn	19	27–59	28
Nondyspeptic symptoms	2	8	18
Fatty food intolerance		41–72	53
Bloating	55	49	52
Belching	48	59	60

[a]Patients were ascertained for these series by dyspepsia or upper abdominal pain presenting in a hospital setting. It is obvious that the symptoms' complexes are usually not specific.
Adapted from Sleisenger and Fordtran. Gastrointestinal Disease. W. B. Saunders, 1993.

   While the details of the patient complaints regarding dyspepsia may suggest GERD in the patient with associated heartburn and exacerbations at night, there exits considerable overlap with ulcer disease as well as biliary tract disease. Endoscopy is very often necessary to identify the exact cause of the pain. Tables 11 and 12 highlight these difficulties.
   There exist a host of uncommon diseases that can cause dyspepsia including Crohn's disease, gastric syphilis, eosinophilic gastritis, tuberculosis, Menetrier's disease, sarcoidosis, and celiac sprue, which cannot be accurately identified without endoscopy and biopsy. NSAIDs, antibiotics (such as tetracyline), drugs such as digitalis, KCL, theophylline, and ethanol can cause dyspepsia by way of inducing mucosal injury and will resolve after withdrawal of the offending agent. Metabolic disturbances, such as diabetic

Table 12
Endoscopic Diagnoses of Patients with Dyspepsia (*n* = 3667 Dyspeptics)[a]

Normal	Reflux	Duodenitis/Gastritis	Ulcer	Cancer
1232	878	765	729	74
(33.6%)	(23.9%)	(20.9%)	(19.9%)	(2.0%)

[a]Data from the United Kingdom.
Adapted from Sleisenger and Fordtran. Gastrointestinal Disease. W. B. Saunders, 1993.

ketoacidosis or diabetic neuropathy, hyperparathyroidism, and hyper- and hypothyroidism, can cause dyspepsia. Biliary pain is often manifest by dyspepsia and is discussed below.

The role of *Helicobacter pylori* infection in the etiology of nonulcerative dyspepsia remains unclear. Some 50% of patients with nonulcerative dyspepsia are infected with *H. pylori*, but this number approaches that found in the general population when matched for age *(37,38)*. Tally evaluated some 24 published studies and found that methodological limitations including failure of randomization, lack of an adequate definition of dyspepsia, lack of blinding in patients treated with bismuth, lack of proof of eradication of *H. pylori*, and follow-up problems (among others) prevent a definitive recommendation concerning the relationship between the chronic antritis caused by *H. pylori* and nonulcerative dyspepsia *(39)*. Sixteen of the 24 studies examined showed improvement of symptoms with treatment for *H. pylori* infection. Indeed, if a definitive link exits between the two, the term functional dyspepsia can no longer be applied to *H. pylori* positive patients with nonulcerative dyspepsia.

Work-up for patients with dyspepsia revolves around rapidly eliminating serious organic pathology. EKG and/or exercise treadmill testing, evaluation for blood in the stool, palpation for abdominal masses, the elimination of potential offending medications and alcohol, and a short trial of antacids or H2 blockers is a useful starting point. Any history of weight loss, unremitting or recurrent pain, or GI blood loss implies a need for upper endoscopy. Other tests to exclude biliary disease are discussed below.

Treatment of dyspepsia caused by organic disease is aimed at the underlying cause. In patients with nonulcerative dyspepsia, while convincing proof that *H. pylori* is the cause of the pain does not yet exist, the WHO classification of *H. pylori* as a carcinogen makes it wise for the clinician who diagnoses the infection by biopsy or serology to prescribe an effective course of antibiotics for *H. pylori* infection. There exist, as with the *H. pylori* data, diverging studies concerning the utility of such promotility agents as metaclopramide, cisapride, and the as-yet unavailable domperidone in the resolution of the pain of nonulcerative dyspepsia. Given the high cost of cisapride and the potential for neurological side effects, especially in the elderly, with metaclopramide, it would be useful to document a delay in gastric emptying with a nuclear medicine gastric emptying time prior to a trial of these agents. Other agents such as pirenzepine and sucralfate have been studied for their utility in nonulcerative dyspepsia, but the results are mixed.

Biliary Pain

Defining biliary colic is an important starting point when discussing biliary tract pain. Colic generally refers to the intermittent, crampy pain of rapid onset, high intensity, short

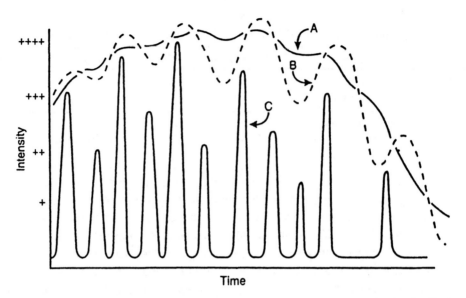

Fig. 7. Various patterns of acute pain. According to an analysis of 100 cases of colic (half biliary, half renal) by French and Robb, A, a sustained pattern was more typical of biliary pain; B, an undulating pattern was more typical of renal pain; and C, an intermittent pattern (true colic) was rarely described by patients with either biliary or renal pain. (From Bockus. Gastroenterology, 5th ed. W. B. Saunders, 1995.)

duration (on the order of minutes), and intermittent remissions as caused classically by colonic spasm, or gaseous distention of the colon or small bowel. Biliary colic, conversely, is of slower onset to peak intensity (10–60 min), and can last for hours. Peaks and valleys to the pain are not a predominant feature. Figure 7 illustrates the different characteristics of biliary, renal, and classic colic.

Biliary pain is caused by the stimulation of stretch or chemical receptors within the biliary tree and gallbladder and is most often a result of gallstone related events. The precipitation of biliary pain, by ingestion of a fatty meal is unproven, though the concept of gallbladder contraction with subsequent elevation of intrabiliary pressures caused by the elevation of CCK (which occurs especially after a high-fat meal) is alluring. Development of evening or nocturnal pain, however, is common. Nausea and vomiting may accompany biliary pain, and the "indigestion" is very often unimproved by antacids. Biliary pain often begins in the midline but shifts to the right upper quadrant, especially in the event of associated local peritonitis, as may occur with acute cholecystitis. Reference of pain to the back and right shoulder is not uncommon. Biliary pain may manifest in the chest or even the left upper quadrant, though this is less common.

Hemobilia, as may occur after a liver biopsy or rupture of a hepatic artery, produces similar intense pain. Sphincter of Oddi dysfunction (SOD), more common in women and variously associated with sphincter stenosis, can give rise to biliary pain with or without concomitant liver enzyme abnormalities and in the absence of gallstones and variously responds to such smooth muscle relaxants as nitrates and calcium channel blockers. SOD is diagnosed by manometry during endoscopic retrograde cholangiography and is remedi-

Table 13
Suggested Tests in the Work-Up of Biliary Pain

Acute unremitting biliary pain	Complete blood count
	Liver enzymes including direct and indirect bilirubin
	Amylase, lipase
	EKG
	Urinalysis
	Pulse oximetry
	Right upper-quadrant ultrasound
	Upright KUB and CXR
	Consider HIDA scan and upper endoscopy, ERCP
Intermittent biliary pain	Liver enzymes including direct and indirect bilirubin– most helpful with episodes of pain
	Amylase, lipase—most helpful with episodes of pain
	Urinalysis
	EKG and/or exercise treadmill test
	Right upper-quadrant ultrasound
	Consider upper endoscopy
	Consider ERCP with or without manometry

able by sphincterotomy, which can be performed at that time. Malignancies, such as ampullary tumors, pancreatic carcinoma, Klatskin tumors, hepatomas, and metastatic tumors, often cause no pain, possibly owing to the accommodation of the biliary stretch receptors.

Cholangitis is a potentially life-threatening infection of an obstructed biliary system. Charcot's triad of fever, right upper-quadrant abdominal pain, and jaundice are classic clinical indicators of the presence of cholangitis. Antibiotics, early definition as to the nature of the obstruction, and drainage of the obstructed biliary tree are crucial management steps in the care of these very ill patients.

The work-up of patients depends on the nature of presentation. Acute onset, unremitting biliary type pain, or fever is indication for immediate blood work and imaging studies. Ruling out a cardiac source cannot be over-emphasized. Presence of an elevated alkaline phosphatase and direct bilirubin (the innocuous Gilbert's disorder produces an elevated indirect bilirubin) is generally considered the liver enzyme pattern of an obstructed biliary system, but transaminase elevation is common and a normal aspartate transaminase (AST) is unlikely in acute biliary processes. Serum amylase may be elevated in acute cholecystitis, but the serum lipase should be significantly elevated only with pancreatitis, which may or may not be related to gallstone disease. Transabdominal ultrasound is an attractive noninvasive test that will reveal the presence of gallstones, the existence and extent of biliary duct dilation, presence of air within the gallbladder wall in the emphysematous gallbladder of the diabetic, and some information regarding the size and function of the gallbladder. Fluid around a flaccid gallbladder may suggest acalculous cholecystitis. The sonographic Murphy's sign is of questionable sensitivity and utility for suspected acute cholecystitis and is operator- and patient-dependent. HIDA scanning will highlight the presence of an obstructed cystic duct. X-rays will reveal gallstone some 15% of the time, a figure that represents the presence of calcium. ERCP is best for defining the structure and pathologies involved in biliary diseases. Perhaps more significantly, ERCP allows for stone removal from the common bile duct, immediate biliary drainage, bile sampling for culture, manometric studies, ampullary and biliary biopsy, and brushing for malignancy. The role of the purely diagnostic and emerging new technology, MRC (magnetic resonance cholangiography), is undefined; in the work-up of biliary pain its cost and lack of therapeutic limb may ultimately limit its widespread usefulness.

With intermittent biliary-type pain, knowledge of the presence of gallstones within the gallbladder is helpful but by no means proof of the cause of the pain, which may very well be a duodenal ulcer. Liver enzymes and amylase and lipase drawn during attacks of pain are very helpful in determining the next appropriate test. Table 13 outlines the laboratory approach to biliary pain. Cholecystectomy is often carried out on patients with known gallstone and attacks of pain suspicious for biliary tract origin. Similar pain may occur after surgery and may be functional in nature (postcholecystectomy syndrome) or due to retained stones within the bile duct or the occasional formation of gallstones years later in the cystic duct stump or the common bile duct itself. Intraoperative cholangiograms may miss 4–10% of the stones. Often combined imaging, endoscopic, and surgical approaches are employed to identify and rectify biliary pain.

REFERENCES

1. Hertz AF. The sensibility of the alimentary canal in health and disease. Lancet 1911; 1: 1051–1054.
2. Ray BS, Neill CL. Abdominal visceral sensation in man. Ann Surg 1947; 126: 709–724.
3. Bentley FH. Observations on visceral pain. Ann Surg 1948; 128: 881–887.
4. Wolf S. Gastric sensibility. In: Wolf S, ed. The Stomach. New York: Oxford University Press, 1965: 88–97.
5. Leek BF. Abdominal and pelvic visceral receptors. Br Med Bull 1977; 33: 163–168.
6. Higashi H. Pharmacological aspects of visceral sensory receptors. In: Cervero F, Morrison JFB, eds. Visceral sensation. Amsterdam: Elsevier, 1986: 149.
7. Lepkin M, Sleisenter MH. Studies of visceral pain: measurements of stimulus intensity and duration associated with the onset of pain in esophagus, ileum, and colon. J Clin Invest 1958; 37: 28–34.
8. Klein KB, Mellinkoff SM. Approach to the patient with abdominal pain. In: Yamada T, ed. Textbook of Gastroenterology. Philadelphia: J. B. Lippincott, 1991: 660–681.
9. Harrison A, Isenberg JI, Schapira M, Hagie L. Most patients with active symptomatic duodenal ulcers fail to develop ulcer-type pain in response to gastroduodenal acidification. J Clin Gastroenterol 1982; 4: 105–107.
10. Iggo A. Afferent C-fibers and visceral sensation. In: Cervero F, Morrison JFB, eds. Visceral Sensation. Amsterdam: Elsevier, 1986: 149.
11. Andrews PLR. Vagal afferent innervation of the gastrointestinal tract. In: Cervero F, Morrison JFB, eds. Visceral Sensation. Amsterdam: Elsevier, 1986: 65.
12. Chapman WP, Herrera R, Jones CM. A comparison of pain produced experimentally in lower esophagus, common bile duct, and upper small intestine with pain experienced by patients with diseases of biliary tract and pancreas. Surg Gynecol Obstet 1949; 89: 573–582.
13. Melzack R, Wall PD. Pain mechanisms: a new theory of pain. Science 1965; 150: 971–979.
14. Melzack R, Wall PD. Gate-control and other mechanism. In: The challenge of pain, ed 2. London: Penguin Books, 1988: 165–182.
15. Lumb BM. Brainstem control of visceral afferent pathways in the spinal cord. In: Cervero F, Morrison JFB, eds. Visceral Sensation. Amsterdam: Elsevier, 1986: 279.
16. Frenk H, Cannon JT, Lewis JW, Liebeskind JC. Neural and neurochemical mechanisms of pain inhibition. In: Sternbach RA, ed. The Psychology of Pain, ed 2. New York: Raven, 1986: 25–48.

17. Fields HL. Neurophysiology of pain and pain modulation. Am J Med 1984; 77(Suppl 3A): 2–8.
18. Janig W, Morrison JFB. Functional properties of spinal visceral afferents supplying abdominal and pelvic organs, with special emphasis on visceral nociception. In: Cervero F, Morrison JFB, eds. Visceral sensation. New York: Elsevier, 1986: 87.
19. Cope Z. Cope's Early Diagnosis of the Acute Abdomen. Revised by Silen W, 18th ed. New York: Oxford University Press, 1991.
20. Harvey, RF, Salih, SY, Read, E. Organic and functional disorders among 200 outpatients. Lancet 1983; 1: 632–634.
21. Talley NJ, Zinsmeister AR, Van Dyke C, Melton LJ. Epidemiology of colonic symptoms and irritable bowel syndrome. Gastroenterol 1991; 101: 927–934.
22. Ferguson A, Sircus W, Eastwood M. Frequency of "functional" gastrointestinal disorders. Lancet 1977; 2: 613,614.
23. Schuster MM. Irritable bowel syndrome. In: Sleisenger MH, Fordtran JS, eds. Gastrointestinal Disease: Pathophysiology, Diagnosis, Management, 5th ed. Philadelphia: WB Saunders, 1993; 917–913.
24. Pimparkear BD. Irritable bowel syndrome. J Int Med Assoc 1970; 54: 95. 1–3.
25. Drossman DA, Lesserman J, Nachman G, et al. Sexual and physical abuse in women with functional or organic gastrointestinal disorder. Ann Int Med 1990; 113: 828–833.
26. Horowitz L, Farrar JT. Intraluminal small intestinal pressure in normal patients and in patients with functional gastrointestinal disorders. Gastroenterology 1962; 42: 455–464.
27. Chaudhary NA, Truelove SC. Human colonic motility: A comparative study of normal subjects, patients with ulcerative colitis and patients with irritable bowel syndrome. Gastroenterology 1961; 40: 1–17.
28. Narducci F, Bassotti, G, Bagurri M, Morell A. Twenty-four-hour manometric recording of colonic motor activity in healthy man. Gut 1987; 28: 17–25.
29. Connell AM, Jones FA, Rowlands EN. Motility of the pelvic colon. IV. Abdominal pain associated with colonic hypermotility after meals. Gut 1965; 6: 105–112.
30. Manning AP, Thompson WG, Heaton KW, Morris AF. Towards positive diagnosis of the irritable bowel. Br Med J 1978; 280: 633–653.
31. Moriarty KJ, Dawson AM. Functional abdominal pain: further evidence that whole gut is affected. Br J med 1982; 284: 1670–1672.
32. Welch GW, Hillman LC, Pomare EW. Psychoneurotic symptomatology in the irritable bowel syndrome: A study of reporters and non-reporters. Br Med J 1985; 291: 1382–1384.
33. Wangle AG, Deller DJ. Intestinal motility in man: III. mechanisms of constipation and diarrhea with particular reference to the irritable colon syndrome. Gastroentero 1965; 48: 69–84.
34. Halpern GM, Prindiville TP, Blankenburg M, Hsia T, Gershwin ME. Treatment of irritable bowel syndrome with lacteol fort: a randomized, double-blind, cross-over trial. Am J of Gastro 1996; 91: 2. 1579–1585.
35. Abstract from DDW 1996 on IBS and exercise from U. Tennessee.
36. Talley NJ, Colin-Jones D, Koch KL, Koch M, Nyren O, Stanghellini V. Functional dyspepsia: a classification with guidelines for diagnosis and management. Gastroenterol Int 1991; 4: 145–149.
37. Dooley CP, Cohen H, Fitzgibbons P, Bauer M, Appleman MD, Perez-Perez GI, Blaser MJ. Prevalence of Helicobacter pylori and histologic gastritis in asymptomatic persons. N Eng J Med 1989; 322: 1562–1566.
38. Bernersen B, Johnsen R, Bostad L, Straume B, Sommer Al Burhol PG. Is Helicobacter pylori the cause of dyspepsia? Br Med J 1992; 304: 1276–1278.
39. Talley NJ. A critique of therapeutic trials in Helicobacter pylori-positive functional dyspepsia. Gastroenterol 1994; 106: 1174–1183.

7 PELVIC, PERINEAL, AND GENITAL PAIN

ANTHONY R. STONE, MBCHB, FRCS (ED)
JAE H. KIM, MD

Key Points

- The etiology of pelvic pain is poorly understood.
- Diagnosis is based on exclusion, and is generally based on most prominent symptom.
- This gives rise to many named conditions associated with pelvic pain.
- Treatment is often directed at this prominent symptom, so that results are poor and few good outcome studies are available.
- Many of these conditions have associated bladder/bowel dysfunction, suggesting a common etiological link.
- Evidence exists to implicate abnormal pelvic floor function as the key etiologic factor.
- This opens the door to alternative and possibly better therapy, e.g., biofeedback, neuromodulation.

INTRODUCTION

Pelvic, perineal, and genital pain is poorly understood and consequently poorly managed by the majority of physicians. In a typical urology or gynecology practice, a significant number of patients may be seen whose symptoms include pelvic pain. This will be associated with a wide variety of problems, including voiding dysfunction, bowel problems, sexual dysfunction, and constitutional symptoms. Clinicians will often focus on the organ system they understand best and manage the patient accordingly, without any true understanding of the etiology of the problem.

This process has lead to a proliferation of diagnoses that have no sound pathophysiologic basis and hence treatment is often empiric (Fig. 1). Female patients seen by a urologist will be diagnosed as having interstitial cystitis, urethral syndrome, or urethrotrigonitis. If the patient has been evaluated by a gynecologist, she may be characterized as having vulvodynia, vulvar vestibulitis, vaginismus, or endometriosis. The male patient is not excluded from this process, as many patients will be characterized as

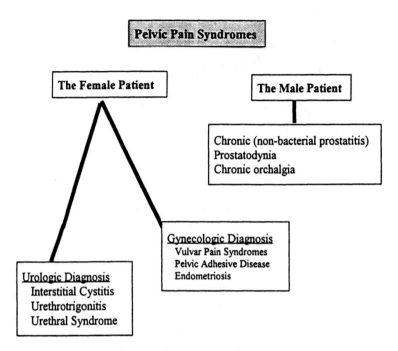

Fig. 1. Pelvic pain syndromes.

having prostatitis, abacterial prostatitis, prostatodynia, or chronic orchalgia. If these patients are questioned carefully, they often have associated bowel problems, namely chronic constipation, irritable bowel syndrome, or rectal pain. As with any chronic pain syndrome, patients will often have a significant element of depression or psychoneurosis clouding the issue. It is unclear in these situations whether these phenomena are the cause or the effect of the pelvic pain. Patients will often have seen multiple doctors and are frequently labeled as "crazy" to counteract the lack of a clear diagnosis.

As one would expect, results of therapies directed at the most prominent symptom are often no better than placebo. Also outcome analysis of treatment in the literature is virtually nonexistent. There are few studies on the economic consequences of this problem and the overall cost to the health care system. Despite this, patients every day are consuming millions of dollars worth of drugs and are allowing themselves to undergo operations that have never proven to be effective.

This chapter will thus focus on the problem of chronic pelvic pain. Common acute problems such as dysmenorrhea, mittelschmerz, bacterial cystitis pain, and childbirth are not discussed. These problems are managed by treatment of the cause, which is well-understood and adequately dealt with in conventional texts. The specific diagnoses associated with chronic pelvic pain, for which adequate etiologic and pathophysiologic explanations are unclear, will be discussed in both males and females. The traditional treatments of these problems and published results will be described. We will attempt to critique this organ-focused approach and suggest a more rational etiologic basis, providing a link between many of these syndromes. Based on this analysis, newer and developing treatments will be described.

THE FEMALE PATIENT

For the purposes of this chapter, pain syndromes will all be referred to as pelvic in origin. Distinction between pelvic, perineal, and genital pain in the female patient is often impossible and will therefore be ignored.

All the diagnoses to be described have five prominent components; namely, pain, voiding and bowel problems, sexual dysfunction, constitutional symptoms, and psychogenic abnormalities. The contribution of these in each diagnosis or syndrome and in individual patients will vary considerably. However, understanding these components will allow the reader to identify a common thread between these so-called different diagnoses.

Interstitial Cystitis

Interstitial cystitis is an idiopathic, chronic bladder disorder characterized by varying degrees of suprapubic pain, dyspareunia, urinary urgency, and frequency without demonstrable infection. The pain is classically related to bladder filling and relieved by voiding, although some patients experience pain at the end of voiding. Incontinence is generally uncommon. The typical patient has usually seen three to five physicians before being labeled with the diagnosis. The National Institute of Health Criteria for diagnosis of interstitial cystitis require: (1) the presence of Hunner's ulcers at cystoscopy, (2) the presence of glomerulations on bladder filling under anesthesia, (3) the presence of pain and irritative voiding symptoms for over 9 mo, and (4) exclusion of known bladder diseases.

Epidemiology

Epidemiologic characteristics of the disorder in the United States have been lacking, but a recent study demonstrated that there may be as many as 43,500 women in the United States with interstitial cystitis (1). The disease mainly affects Caucasians, but may be seen in blacks and other ethnic minorities. Men comprise approximately 10% of interstitial cystitis patients whose symptoms may mimic those of prostatitis or prostatodynia.

Etiology and Pathogenesis

Although numerous theories of pathogenesis have been proposed, the etiology of interstitial cystitis is still unknown. The proposed causes of interstitial cystitis include infectious, autoimmune, endocrinologic, neurogenic, and psychoneurotic pathologies.

A history of UTI is twice as common among interstitial cystitis patients as controls, and by the time the diagnosis is made, most patients have generally been treated with a variety of antibiotics for suspected bacterial UTIs. Fastidious organisms such as Gardinella vaginalis, Lactobacillus, and Salmonella have been cited in the literature as potential infective agents in interstitial cystitis (2). In addition, histological findings of epithelial ulceration, submucosal inflammation and presence of mast cells, and increased permeability of the epithelium seen in interstitial cystitis are similar to those of recurrent bacterial cystitis. Electron microscopic examinations also have shown embedded microorganisms in the bladder walls of interstitial cystitis patients (3). Despite the continued effort, however, no microorganism has been clearly identified as a known cause of interstitial cystitis. The failure to respond to multiple antimicrobial agents also makes an infectious etiology unlikely.

Interest in autoimmune disorder as a potential cause of interstitial cystitis was stimulated by Silk in 1970 *(4)*, although IC had previously been compared with other diseases associated with immune dysfunction. In 1938, Fister suggested that there were certain similarities between IC and systemic lupus erythematosus (SLE), although at that time SLE was thought to be caused by absorption of bacterial toxins *(5)*. By the late 1940s, SLE and other "collagen diseases" were known to be linked to abnormalities of the immune system. Hand proposed that the higher incidence of various allergies in his IC patients probably indicated some underlying disturbance of their immune regulation, possibly causing their IC *(6)*. Shipton reported a small series of IC patients who had concomitant features of other autoimmune diseases *(7)*. Recent studies have examined the role of circulating antibladder antibodies, nonorgan specific antibodies (e.g., rheumatoid factor, antinuclear, and antimitochondrial antibodies), fixed immunoglobulins in the bladder tissue, HLA-tissue typing, and altered immunoglobulin and complement levels in the development of IC. However, evidence to date has failed to confirm a primary autoimmune etiology for IC.

The mucous lining of the bladder epithelium, with its high content of glycosaminoglycans (GAG), is thought to act as an important defense mechanism between the urothelial cells and harmful substances in the urine. One hypothesis of pathophysiology for IC involves the quantitative and qualitative alteration of this protective layer, allowing toxic substances to initiate and perpetuate an inflammatory response in the deeper layer of the bladder. Studies have suggested that patients with IC demonstrate decreased urinary excretion of GAG in comparison to controls, and biochemical composition of the GAGs in the mucous lining may also be altered in patients with IC *(8)*. Ultrastructural studies of the bladder epithelium, however, so far have not demonstrated differences between IC patients and controls *(9)*, and the mechanism of defective glycocalyx with a permeable urothelium still remains speculative.

Pathophysiologic role of mast cells in interstitial cystitis was first suggested by Simmons in 1950s, and subsequent studies have provided further support for this hypothesis *(10)*. Mast cells play a crucial role in the development of allergic reactions by releasing preformed molecules such as histamine, proteases, cytokines, vasoactive peptides (VIP), tumor necrosis factor (TNF), and many others. These agents promote leukocyte migration, erythema, vasodilation, and fibrosis, which are all features of interstitial cystitis. Recent studies have documented the presence of mast-cell infiltrates in the bladders of interstitial cystitis; elevated mast-cell counts have been demonstrated in the lamina propria as well as the detrusor layers, and electron microscopic evaluation of these tissues has shown different stages of secretory degranulation within the mast cells. Mastocystosis, however, is not a pathognomonic finding of interstitial cystitis and may also be seen in a variety of inflammatory and neuroendocrine disorders.

Recent electron microscopic studies have demonstrated that mast cells are closely associated with sensory nerve fibers in the bladder. These unmyelinated sensory afferent fibers and their neurotransmitters can directly promote local inflammation as well as by activation and degranulation of mast cells. Proliferation of these nerve fibers in the submucosa of bladder biopsies from interstitial cystitis patients has been demonstrated, providing further support for a neurogenic pathogenesis of interstitial cystitis.

Treatment

The lack of knowledge regarding the pathophysiology of IC has led to numerous non-specific and empiric therapies. The evaluation of efficacy of various treatment modalities is further complicated by subjective manifestations (pain, urgency, frequency) of IC.

Current therapy consists of hydraulic bladder distention under a light general anesthetic. Many patients may also benefit from the use of the tricyclic antidepressant amitriptyline (25–75 mg qhs). Not only does this drug improve symptoms by its central effects, but it is thought to have a stabilizing effect on mast cells. Recently, sodium pentosan polysulfate (Elmiron) has been approved for use in IC. Experimentally this drug is thought to enhance the protective glycosaminoglycan layer of the transitional epithelium. Clinical trials have been mixed in their results with responses of no better than 37%.

Nalmefene, an opiate antagonist capable of preventing mast-cell degranulation experimentally, is presently undergoing clinical trials. Additional uncontrolled trials have been reported using the antihistamine hydroxyzine and the calcium channel blocker nifedipine. Results are as yet scarce and seem to be no better than placebo.

Conventionally, if these measures do not work, intravesical therapy is used. Dimethyl-sulfoxide is the most commonly used agent. This has anti-inflammatory, analgesic, and anesthetic properties. It may be combined with sodium bicarbonate, steroids, and heparin, all with the hope of decreasing the bladder "inflammation." This therapy is usually repeated at weekly intervals over a period of 6–8 wk. A 50–60% response rate is reported, but duration is quite variable and controlled trials have not been carried out. Clorpactin (WWCS-90) in a 0.4% concentration has also been used intravesically. This agent is painful, requiring an anesthetic to administer. Results are similar to DMSO. Silver nitrate has also been used, but is mentioned here for historic purposes only.

Other therapies used include trancutaneous electrical stimulation (TENS), and specific ulcers have been fulgurated or excised by electrocautery or laser. Results of these modalities are also quite variable.

Many patients whose symptoms are unremitting have subjected themselves to excisional surgery. Classically a supratrigonal cystectomy and reconstruction by cecocystoplasty was advocated. Success rates of up to 75% have been reported, but these are generally short-lived, with pain returning in some form or another. This has lead to the use of cystectomy and bladder replacement, either to the urethra, or in conjunction with a continent catheterizeable stoma. Ileal conduit following cystectomy and urethrectomy is advocated by some. The results of all these procedures are generally poor. The occasional patient may obtain a good result; however many will have recurrence of pain, often in a slightly different site. For this reason, surgery is generally not recommended. Occasionally a patient may present who genuinely has a small contracted bladder. In this situation, a surgical procedure may be considered.

Urethral Syndrome

Urethral syndrome is a diagnosis of exclusion. This clinical entity describes urinary frequency, urgency, and dysuria in the absence of bacteriuria in both initial and midstream urine. Pyuria may be an infrequent finding in the urinalysis. The diagnosis of urethral syndrome can only be made once UTI, stones, tumors, trauma, radiation injury, neurogenic disorder, and other pathologic processes have been ruled out.

Epidemiology

Absence of strict diagnostic criteria in the past has resulted in a lack of clear understanding of the disorder. The syndrome is mostly associated with women during the reproductive years, but similar conditions may be found in men and children of either sex.

Etiology

Various etiologies of the urethral syndrome have been proposed with scant evidence. Intracoital and lower urinary tract colonization by fecal bacteria and fastidious organisms have been investigated with inconclusive results (11). The failure of various antimicrobials to improve the symptoms also questions the infectious etiology. Urethral stenosis and obstruction have also been implicated in the pathogenesis of the disorder. Although symptomatic improvements of the patients with urethral dilations have been reported (12), anatomic urethral obstruction has not been demonstrated in the majority of patients with urethral syndrome. Urodynamic examination of the urethral syndrome patients has demonstrated prolonged flow phase and increased external sphincter tone, suggesting a neurogenic component of the disorder.

Treatment

Numerous forms of treatment for urethral syndrome have been advocated in the past, including ingestion of cranberry juice, antispasmodics, sitz baths, sedatives, antidepressants, estrogen, and resection of urethral mucosa. Although the use of sounds and antimicrobials have been the most popular form of treatment, no therapy so far has been consistently successful nor proven to be superior to others. Absence of clear etiology and persistence of symptoms without development of organic changes have led some to attribute the condition to neurosis and suggest that the treatment should only be supportive and noninvasive.

Urethrotrigonitis

This "condition" may also be diagnosed in women with similar irritative symptoms. Classically, as with the urethral syndrome, the patient will present with episodic frequency, urgency, and suprapubic discomfort without evidence of an overt urinary tract infection. Cystoscopic examination may provide evidence of trigonal inflammation. It should be remembered that the trigonal epithelium in the female is under estrogenic influence and may normally exhibit the appearance of squamous metaplasia.

Treatment classically consists of a combination of urethral dilatation and trigonal fulguration. No rational basis exists for these therapies and, as expected, good outcome studies are absent.

Vulvar Pain Syndrome

In 1983, the Seventh Congress for the International Society for the Study of Vulvar Disease (ISSVD) defined vulvodynia as chronic vulvar discomfort characterized by burning, stinging, irritation, and rawness *(13)*. Vulvar vestibulitis, a subset of vulvodynia, was also defined as a syndrome with severe pain on vestibular touch or attempted vaginal entry and physical findings confined to vulvar erythema of various degrees. Vulvodynia, vulvar vestibulitis, and other disorders known as vaginismus and burning vulvar syndrome share several common symptoms and may be better characterized by the generic term, vulvar pain syndrome.

Although the actual incidence of vulvar pain syndrome is unknown, it may be as high as 15% percent among women seen in a general gynecologic practice *(14)*. The disorder is most commonly associated with nulliparous white females in their fourth decade. Higher incidence of allergy, human papilloma virus and candidal infection, and history of sexual abuse have been associated with the patients with vulvar pain syndrome.

Etiology

The etiology of vulvar pain syndrome continues to be controversial. Proposed pathophysiologies of vulvar pain syndrome include infections, allergic or autoimmune reactions, and psychogenic processes. In the older literature, human papillomavirus (HPV) was implied as the most likely etiology of the vulvar pain syndrome. Several studies reported higher incidence of HPV virus in the vulvar tissue of women with the syndrome. Subsequent studies, however, have failed to identify specific HPV types associated with the syndrome, and subclinical HPV infection in the pathogenesis of vulvar pain syndrome to date has never been proved *(15)*. History of recurrent candidal infections in many patients with vulvar pain syndrome suggests fungal infection as a potential agent in the development of vulvar pain syndrome. Although a cause–effect relationship has not been firmly established, in practice many patients are empirically treated with topical antifungal agents without culture diagnosis. Others have proposed crossreactivity between the antigens of *Candida albicans* and vulvovaginal tissues of the patients as an underlying etiology *(16)*. According to this theory, the hosts' immune response may perpetuate local inflammation and pain in the vulvar tissues. A significant prevalence of sexual abuse history, somatization disorders, and depression among the patients with vulvar pain syndrome indicate that psychologic stresses may in part be responsible for vulvar pain syndrome *(17)*.

Treatment

The optimal therapy for vulvar pain syndrome remains elusive. Conservative therapies such as sitz baths, antibiotics, antimycotics, anti-inflammatory agents, topical steroids, and lubrications have not been effective. Topical anesthetic agents also have been used to provide temporary relief to allow coitus. Relief of pain and dyspareunia have been reported with the use of interferon for the treatment of condyloma acuminatum. Complete relief has been reported with intralesional interferon-α injection therapy with varying success rate *(18)*.

Endometriosis

Endometriosis is a benign condition in which endometrial glands are present outside the endometrial cavity. Symptoms attributable to endometriosis include generalized pelvic pain, dysmenorrhea, anal dyspareunia. In a significant proportion of the patients undergoing gynecologic evaluation for chronic pelvic pain, the disorder has been attributed to endometriosis. Recent laparoscopic evaluations have reported that the incidence of endometriosis may be as high as 51% in women seeking evaluation for pelvic pain (19).

Pelvic pain secondary to endometriosis may be related to sequential swelling of endometrial implants and the extravasation of blood and debris into surrounding tissues. Peritoneal irritation and scarring by the lesion may contribute to the production of pain. It also has been postulated that endometrial lesions may secrete inflammatory mediators such as prostaglandins and interleukin to promote local inflammation and production of pain.

Medical therapy for pain relief in endometriosis includes progesterone, Danazol, androgenic steroids, and synthetic GnRH agonist. Although the medical therapies provide symptomatic relief in a majority of patients during the treatment period, recurrence of symptoms commonly occurs following the discontinuation of therapies. Extirpative surgical therapy is the only available treatment offering the possibility of permanent cure. In advanced cases of endometriosis, total abdominal hysterectomy combined with salpingo-oophorectomy has been associated with the best success rate. Conservative surgical excision at laparotomy, presacral neurectomy, laparoscopic laser or electrocoagulation, and ablation of uterosacral ligament have been associated with varied results (20). In general, combination medical and surgical therapy has not demonstrated additional benefits for the treatment of endometriosis-associated pelvic pain.

Although endometriosis appears to be more frequent in chronic pelvic pain patients than in asymptomatic population, severity of pain does not appear to be related to the amount of lesions present. In his study, Vercellini reported that endometriosis was found in 41 of 126 women (32.5%) examined by laparoscopy for chronic pelvic pain (21). Fedele et al. (22), on the other hand, reported that no relationship is found between the severity of pain and the stage of endometrial lesions. In addition, a large number of patients with endometriosis do not complain of pelvic pain, regardless of the stage of endometrioses. This lack of correlation between the extent of endometriosis and pelvic pain disputes the causal relationship and questions the use of extirpative surgery to eliminate endometriosis in the treatment of chronic pelvic pain.

Pelvic Adhesive Disease

Pelvic adhesive disease is not a diagnostic entity, like the above-mentioned conditions, but is often quoted by gynecologists as a frequent finding in women with chronic pelvic pain. It occurs postoperatively or as a consequence of pelvic inflammatory disease. As with endometriosis, adhesions are found laparoscopically in up to 40% of women with this problem. Unfortunately, it is also found in many patients without pelvic pain and there is no quantitative relationship between the presence of adhesions and pain (23).

Although the author feels the association of this entity with pain may be due to the prevalence of laparoscopy as a diagnostic tool, results of adhesiolysis are encouraging. Up to 85% of patients have been reported to be improved following this procedure. Most studies have rather short follow-up periods; patients with a long history of pain fared less well.

THE MALE PATIENT

As interstitial cystitis and syndromes involving sexual dysfunction are more common in females, pelvic pain syndromes are not traditionally associated with the male patient. However, in community urologic practice, many patients are diagnosed as having chronic prostatitis. This is characterized by the presence of chronic perineal and suprapubic discomfort and ejaculatory pain. Stamey and Meares classified these syndromes further by a fastidious search for bacterial infection in the prostatic fluid. They divided prostatitis into subtypes; namely, chronic bacterial, chronic abacterial, and prostatodynia, depending on the characteristics of the expressed prostatic secretions. Many of these patients have no evidence of bacterial infection, thus, as in the female patient, treatment is often unsatisfactory. The nature of these conditions will be described.

Chronic (nonbacterial) Prostatitis

Chronic prostatitis is one of the most common urologic conditions, affecting men of all ages. The disorder is characterized by painful symptoms referable to prostate, including perineal and suprapubic discomfort/pain. In addition, urinary frequency and urgency and pain on ejaculation are frequent symptoms. The recent National Institute for Diabetes and Digestive and Kidney Disease consensus classifies chronic prostatitis into (1) chronic bacterial prostatitis, (2) chronic prostatitis (chronic pelvic pain syndrome), and (3) asymptomatic chronic prostatitis. Nonbacterial chronic prostatitis is about eight times more common than bacterial prostatitis.

The most commonly used diagnostic method for chronic prostatitis is the Stamey localization procedure, which examines fractionations of urine specimen with expressed prostatic secretion. Patients with nonbacterial prostatitis must have 10 or more white blood cells per high-power field and no bacterial growth in the cultures of prostatic secretion.

Attempts to identify etiologic bacterial organisms for chronic prostatitis have been unsuccessful. The clinical observation that approximately one-third of the patients with nonbacterial prostatitis have associated urethritis suggests that Chlamydia trichomatis may be an etiologic agent. Isolation of Chlamydia in the aspiration cytology of the prostate has been reported by Poletti *(24)*. Mardh et al., on the other hand, reported that Chlamydia trichomatis was isolated in only one of 53 patients with nonbacterial prostatitis *(25)*. Ureaplasma urealyticum has also been cultured at a higher rate from the urethra of the patients with prostatitis in a few studies. Other infectious organisms such as anaerobes, fungi, and viral agents have also been implicated without conclusive results.

Increased concentration of creatinine, urate, and white blood cells expressed in prostatic secretion have been reported in patients with chronic prostatitis, suggesting the role of urinary reflux into the prostatic ducts initiating a chemical inflammation. Based on urodynamic findings and symptomatic relief with $\alpha 1$-antagonist therapy, Kaplan et al. have also suggested that many men who are diagnosed as having refractory chronic nonbacterial prostatitis may have bladder outlet obstruction *(26)*. Psychological factors may have a role in the symptomatology of chronic prostatitis: de la Rosette and others have reported that 50–60% of the patients have associated history of anxiety, depression, hypochondria, and sexual dysfunction *(27)*.

As the etiology of the condition is unknown, various forms of empirical therapy have been proposed. A clinical trial with antimicrobial therapy probably has been the most commonly used mode of treatment. After 1–3 wk of therapy, subjective improvement and expressed prostatic secretion inflammatory infiltrate should be monitored. Nonsteroidal anti-inflammatory agents may be effective in alleviating symptoms, but relapse is common. α1-Adrenergic antagonists have also provided subjective improvement, particularly in those patients with voiding difficulties. Nickel et al. recently reported that the use of transrectal hyperthermia is associated with symptomatic relief in the patients with chronic prostatitis *(28)*. Hot sitz bath and therapeutic prostatic massage are occasionally beneficial.

Prostatodynia

Prostatodynia and nonbacterial chronic prostatitis are similar entities; symptoms of prostatodynia include urinary frequency, urgency, and dysuria associated with pelvic and perineal pain. The patient will often complain of pain after ejaculation. The diagnosis is differentiated from abacterial prostatitis by a lack of significant leukocytosis in the expressed prostatic secretion. In a large study, nearly a third of 597 "prostatitis" patients were diagnosed with prostatodynia *(29)*. As with prostatitis, infectious, musculoskeletal, and psychological etiologies have been associated with prostatodynia. Most patients will have been tried on several courses of antibiotics despite the lack of bacterial evidence.

As with all these conditions, the treatment of prostatodynia has been unsatisfactory. Apart from antibiotics, patients may undergo prostatic massage, or be managed with α-blockers, nonsteroidal anti-inflammatory agents, or other analgesics.

Chronic Orchalgia

Chronic orchalgia has been defined as intermittent or constant testicular pain that lasts 3 mo or longer and interferes with normal daily activities *(30)*. This condition has previously been named as orchiodynia, orchidalgia, and testalgia. Chronic testicular pain is associated with various etiologies, such as infection, trauma, hydrocele, varicocele, and testicular tumor. Pain in the testis can also be referred from other sites, such as obstructing stone in the ureter, genitofemoral and ilioinguinal nerve stimulation by an inguinal hernia, or entrapment neuropathy following hernia repair. However, in about 25% of patients with chronic testicular pain, no obvious pathology is found, making diagnosis and management a difficult clinical problem. When thorough history and physical examination demonstrate no objective physical finding, chronic orchalgia should be considered as the diagnosis.

Because of its elusive etiology, finding appropriate treatment modalities for chronic orchalgia has been difficult. Initial course of action should be nonsurgical and conservative. Nonsurgical management should include antibiotics, anti-inflammatory agents, and psychologic evaluation in appropriate patients. In most patients, spermatic cord block and transcutaneous electrical nerve stimulation provide at least temporary relief. The spermatic cord block consists of an injection of long-acting local anesthetic agents, most commonly bupivacaine hydrochloride without epinephrine, in combination with corticosteroid methylprednisolone. If the pain originates in the testis, epididymis, or spermatic cord, an injection brings prompt pain relief, which may last from several hours to weeks. In patients with good response, periodic cord block may be maintained. Transcutaneous electrical nerve stimulation has been used successfully in other chronic pelvic pain syndromes, and a 1- to 3-mo trial may produce relief from orchalgia with minimal side effects.

When above measures fail to provide sufficient pain relief, the next course of therapy is no longer unanimous, and various surgical procedures have been proposed including epididymectomy and scrotal or inguinal orchiectomy. Davis and Noble reported that inguinal orchiectomy was the most successful surgical option, with 75% of the patients reporting complete pain relief. Costable et al., on the other hand, reported that 80% of the patients continued to have significant pain after orchiectomy *(31)*. Similar variability in response has been reported regarding the efficacy of epididymectomy in relieving intractable epididymal pain. Recently, microsurgical denervation of the spermatic cord has been proposed as an effective treatment of chronic orchalgia and has been gaining more attention as an organ-sparing alternative.

PELVIC PAIN—A CRITICAL OVERVIEW

This description of these specific diagnoses, associated with pelvic and genital pain, will reinforce the conviction that, in most of these conditions, a suitable etiology remains elusive and treatment is accordingly empirical. Clearly this a clinical area that needs to be rethought.

The remainder of this chapter will therefore describe and evaluate evidence of a common pathway in the pathogenesis of pain in many of these patients, and explore additional and possible more rational methods of treatment.

The Role of the Pelvic-Floor Musculature in Pelvic Pain Syndromes

Anatomic Definitions

There are several commonly used terms for the pelvic structures that provide support and sphincteric function. The most commonly used are pelvic or urogenital diaphragm. For the purposes of this chapter, the term pelvic floor will be used to include all the structures that contribute to these functions.

The major muscular component of the pelvic floor is levator ani, which forms a broad skeletal muscle "cradle," extending from the inner surface of the pubis anteriorly to the ischial spines posteriorly. Laterally it is attached to the tendinous arch of the obturator fascia; medially, it forms a median rapine, with the contralateral muscle, between the rectum and coccyx.

The levator is subdivided into three portions: pubococcygeus, iliococcygeus, and ischiococcygeus. The most medial and inferior fibers of pubococcygeus are often referred to as puborectalis.

This muscular cradle is invested above and below with fascia; superiorly this is referred to as the endopelvic fascia, and certain portions of this endopelvic/levator fascia are condensed together to form specific ligaments with important supportive roles.

These include the pubourethral ligaments, the urethropelvic ligaments, and the pubocervical fascia, providing support to the urethra, bladder base, and anterior vagina. The uterus and vaginal vault are supported by the cardinal and sacrouterine ligaments and the posterior vagina and rectum by the rectovaginal septum. In the midline between the anus and vagina is a tendinous structure known as the perineal body. Additional muscular structures are found beneath this, namely ischiocavernosus, bulbocavernosus, the transverse perineal muscles, and the urogenital diaphragm.

Neuroanatomy and Physiology

The coordination of the pelvic floor with the vesicourethral unit, anal sphincter, and genital organs requires the complex interaction of multiple neural pathways. In considering bladder function, classically these pathways have been described as loops (Bradley and Sundin). Conceptually these may be considered as a series of reflex arcs that are inhibited or facilitated by various descending pathways. These may be traced from the frontal lobes to the nucleus ceruleus in the pons, the pontine micturition center.

Descending pathways are located in the reticulospinal pathways synapsing with detrusor motor nuclei in the intermediolateral nuclei of the sacral cord at S2-S4. Postganglionic fibers then travel via the pelvic nerves to the detrusor. Additional descending pathways are found in the corticospinal tract that synapse with the pudendal nuclei in the gray matter of the sacral spinal cord. Postsynaptic fibers exit as the pudendal nerve to innervate the pelvic floor striated muscle and external sphincter.

The detrusor motor nuclei and the pudendal nuclei are separate entities in the sacral cord. They are able to function in an interdependent fashion due to the presence of interneurons which allow the somatic and autonomic components of the pelvis and pelvic floor to act in a coordinated manner.

The origin of sensory impulses in the pelvis and pelvic viscera is poorly understood. Most investigators agree that there is an extensive plexus of nerve fibers in the lamina propria of the urethra and bladder. Specialized nerve endings have not been described in these areas, although substance P has been demonstrated by immunofluorescence in association with these nerves. The pelvic floor musculature does contain muscle spindles, but these are not seen in the rest of the urinary tract.

Sensory impulses from the pelvic organs are transmitted to the sacral spinal cord via both the pudendal nerve and the pelvic nerves. The hypogastric plexus also plays some part in this afferent pathway, although its exact role is unknown. Bladder and urethral sensation ascends in the spinothalamic tract. Sensory impulses associated with urethral function are transmitted via the dorsal columns.

This afferent activity clearly plays a significant role in micturition and anal sphincter control. However, its role in producing pelvic pain is complicated. Stimulation of the pudendal nerves, comprising contributions from sacral nerves S2-4, produces contraction in the pelvic floor musculature. More importantly, referred sensation will be elicited in those areas also supplied by these dermatomes: scrotum/vagina, penis, rectal area, thigh, groin, ankles, and feet. Stimulation of S3 specifically will produce visible contraction of the levator muscle along with the sensation of pressure deep in the pelvis, along with discomfort in the rectum and scrotum.

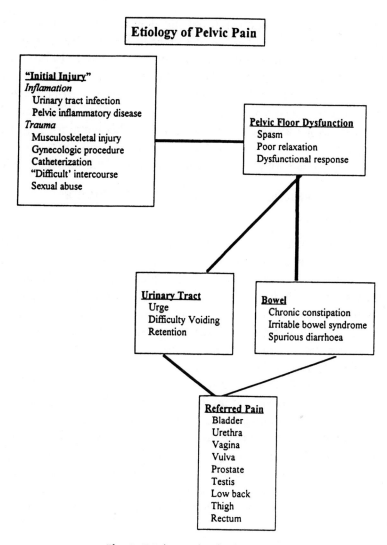

Fig. 2. Etiology of pelvic pain.

Thus it can be appreciated that abnormal or dysfunctional activity of the pelvic musculature may be associated with referred pain in those areas with similar innervation. Although this may be a gross oversimplification, it allows a concept of pelvic pain to be evolved (Fig. 2).

Functional Considerations

The pelvic floor is a unique structure in that, despite its voluntary characteristics, skeletal muscle composition, and inert fascial components, it takes part in several vital autonomic functions. These include the storage and elimination of urine and feces, sexual function (in both males and females), and childbirth. Along with these, the pelvic floor maintains the support of the pelvic and abdominal viscera.

Many of these functions, as described above, require the involvement of multiple, complex reflex arcs with various levels of neurological integration and modulation.

Conceptually, the reader will appreciate that any degree of dysfunction in this muscular complex will give rise to functional changes in the viscera it subserves. In addition, one pain may be produced, which will be perceived by the patient to be originating at a specific site or in a specific organ or related to the functional change. The clinician will also interpret this as an organ-related problem. For instance, one of the "classic" symptoms of urethral syndrome is a burning pain in the urethral area. Exhaustive studies have failed to consistently identify a urethral lesion causing this symptom. Despite this, treatment is always directed at the urethra. Many of these patients, on the other hand, may benefit from simple behavioral modification involving retraining the pelvic floor.

Evidence for a Neuromuscular Etiology

Urodynamic Evidence

In our own experience and in the experience of others, it has become clear that many pelvic and perineal pain syndromes include symptoms of voiding dysfunction. These range from frequency of micturition to complete urinary retention. In our own urodynamic laboratory this has been correlated with various abnormal patterns of detrusor and sphincter behavior. The detrusor abnormalities are seen most commonly in the voiding phase: they include poorly sustained or low-pressure detrusor contraction. In some cases, inappropriate detrusor contractions during the filling phase (detrusor instability) may be perceived by the patient as pelvic pain.

Sphincteric abnormalities seen in these cases include incomplete outlet relaxation, dyssynergic sphincter activity, and urethral instability. The symptoms related to these findings are intermittent voiding, incomplete emptying and straining to void.

The student of urodynamics will realize that these findings can be related to abnormal pelvic-floor activity. Normal voiding or volitional detrusor contraction is initiated by relaxation of the pelvic floor. Failure to appropriately relax this muscle will thus impact on voiding efficiency. Also, abnormal detrusor contractility can be inhibited by pelvic-floor activity. If this is deficient, the detrusor may contract inappropriately (detrusor instability).

Clinical Evidence

Many of the conditions described in this chapter are associated with visceral dysfunction. Bladder symptoms go hand in hand with interstitial cystitis, urethral syndrome, and prostatic syndromes. Careful history will often elicit associated bowel dysfunction.

In addition, attention to the pelvic or rectal exam in these patients will identify abnormalities of the pelvic-floor musculature. Areas of tenderness in the levators are common. This may be lateralized by the patient because of pain originating along the pelvic insertion of this muscle. Levator spasm may be evident and, most significantly, inability to contract this muscle is very common. Patients will often contract the abdominal, gluteal, or thigh muscles when asked to specifically contract the pelvic floor. If the pelvic floor is chronically contracted, they may be unable to contract this further; so it is important to note the differences between the contracted and relaxed state, if any.

Therapeutic Evidence

Treatment of pelvic floor dysfunction in the management of pelvic pain is becoming increasingly more popular. These fall into three broad categories; namely, (1) simple behavioral modification, (2) specific biofeedback techniques, and (3) neuromodulation.

Behavioral Modification

Bladder training and timed voiding protocols are established in both urologic and gynecologic practice. They have traditionally been used for urinary frequency and urge syndromes, with reasonable reported efficacy. These techniques rely on the patient's ability to suppress either the sensation of urgency or an unstable detrusor contraction. They require that the patient be able to contract the pelvic floor in order to achieve this. This is the same contraction used in Kegel's exercises, popularized in the early 1950s by Dr. Kegel, to improve pubococcygeus function in the treatment of stress incontinence.

This approach has been used successfully in the treatment of pelvic pain *(32)*. Chaiken et al. applied behavioral therapy to a group of 42 women with a diagnosis of interstitial cystitis. The protocol consisted of a voiding diary, timed voiding, controlled fluid intake, and pelvic-floor training techniques. All patients had failed traditional therapeutic measures. Using a global assessment scale, 50% of the patients were markedly improved, and over 80% had some positive change in symptoms. The authors emphasize the importance of the relaxation phase of the pelvic-floor exercises in the success of this treatment.

Biofeedback

Clearly, these simple measures will not work if the patient cannot isolate the pelvic floor and consequently is unable to contract and relax this muscle appropriately. In these situations, attempts to "re-educate" the pelvic floor must be used. The most commonly used technique, in this situation, utilizes electromyographic measurements of pelvic-floor activity. In most protocols a vaginal probe will be used, although a rectal probe can be substituted in male patients. In the clinic situation the patient's pelvic-floor activity will be monitored at rest and during a contraction. EMG activity is displayed on a screen, so that the patient may assess his or her performance. Multiple sessions may be required to improve the patients ability to isolate the pelvic-floor activity from surrounding muscle groups. These sessions may be required to also improve the patient's ability to relax the pelvic floor. A portable device may be used to maximize the effectiveness of the therapy.

Glazer et al. used EMG biofeedback in a group of 33 women with the diagnosis of vulvar vestibulitis syndrome *(33)*. In this report, subjective improvement in pain averaged 83%. In addition, 28 of 33 women resumed intercourse by the end of treatment. It should be noted that, along with this improvement, pelvic-floor contractions increased by 95.4%, and resting pelvic-floor tension decreased by 68%.

Neuromodulation Techniques

Despite these simple measures, there will always remain a group who are resistant to this conservative treatment. In these cases, a more direct approach at modifying the neuromuscular dysfunction may be required. The literature is full of techniques directed at denervation of the bladder.

Hydrodistention, cystolysis, cystocystoplasty, sacral rhizotomy, and subtrigonal phenol injection were used mostly to reduce bladder hyperactivity by peripheral denervation. In general, these techniques do not work. They have also been used to modify "bladder" pain with similar lack of success.

Attempts to stimulate the pelvic nerves to control the bladder have also been used. Methods used include stimulation of the spinal cord, cauda equina, pelvic nerves, pudendal nerve, detrusor muscle, and pelvic floor, also with varying degrees of success.

At the present time, the method that seems to have the most promise is stimulation of the sacral roots, most commonly S3 (34). The technique consists of acute stimulation, followed by a short period of evaluation leading to implantation of a permanent neurostimulator.

In the acute phase, the sacral roots are accessed percutaneously with a hollow needle passed into the sacral foramen through the overlying skin of the sacral area. Stimulation of this needle will confirm its proximity to the appropriate sacral root (S3) by a tingling sensation in the rectum, vagina, or scrotum. This will be accompanied by a deepening of the buttocks groove ("bellows" response) and planter flexion of the great toe only. When this response is achieved, a pacing wire is passed through the needle so that stimulation may continue in the subchronic evaluation period. The patient is sent home with the temporary pacing wire connected to an external nerve stimulator device. During this time the patient is instructed to maintain the maximum comfortable level of stimulation. Also during this time, 3–5 d, the patient is asked to keep a diary on voiding and incontinent events, and the level of pain.

If a 50% or greater symptomatic response is achieved during the subchronic evaluation, a permanent neurostimulation device may be implanted. This, of course, requires a general anesthetic and an open surgical procedure. A permanent electrode is placed in the sacral foramen via a midline sacral incision. The electrode is secured to the periosteum of the adjacent sacrum to prevent migration. The neurostimulator is placed in a subcutaneous pocket in the lower abdominal wall so that belts or clothing will not put pressure on this area. This also allows the stimulation parameters to be set by an external computer. This interphases with the neurostimulator through the skin and subcutaneous tissue.

Tanagho and Schmidt have pioneered these techniques over the past 10 yr. During this time they have reported their results in a significant number of patients with both voiding dysfunction and pelvic pain. As a reflection of' the complexity of this problem, this technique has never gained wide acceptance and is still being performed under the auspices of a clinical trial at this time.

Away from the rigors of the FDA, several European centers have used these methods with good success and have incorporated them into their standard management of pelvic pain.

Recently, renewed interest has been shown in the use of acupuncture to treat pelvic pain. This modality has been used for centuries to treat pain of all types. A site just above the medial malleolus has been shown to have reasonable effects in these patients (35).

The Pain Clinic Approach

The above discussion will go to emphasize the complexity of management of the pelvic pain patient. Associated problems such as depression, anxiety, and drug addiction have not been touched on. Clearly some patients will need the benefits of the multidisciplinary approach afforded by a comprehensive pain clinic, including the services of an anesthesiologist, psychologist, physiotherapist, and social worker.

CONCLUSION

The etiology of most cases of pelvic pain remains elusive. Hopefully the lack of success in targeting specific organ sites will encourage physicians to explore the neuromuscular dysfunctional theories expounded in this chapter. In this way our understanding of this problem will improve, leading to less inappropriate surgical procedures and hopefully better results overall. It is accepted that pelvic floor or neuromuscular dysfunction are not the cause of every case of pelvic pain seen and, clearly, many aspects need to be better understood. However, several questions remain: Is the associated pelvic floor dysfunction a primary event or secondary? If it is the latter, what is the nature of the initiating stimulus, and how does this produce the neuromuscular dysfunction, how is it perpetuated, and how does it produce pain? Having answered these questions, will we develop effective treatments to treat these patients? In this era of cost containment in health care, will enough resources be available to treat this rather unfashionable, but very costly problem? As clinicians managing these patients, it is important for us to educate the insurance industry of the fact that new treatments must be developed and to justify this by providing outcome data on the traditional methods, showing lack of effectiveness and considerable cost to both patient and health care provider.

The number of patients with this problem is considerable, and clinicians in many disciplines will have some contact. It is therefore imperative that doctors have an understanding of these problems and treat the patient with appropriate care.

REFERENCES

1. Held PJ, Hanno PM, Wein AJ, et al. Epidemiology of interstitial cystitis: 2. In: Hanno PM, Staskin DR, Krane RJ, et al., eds. Interstitial Cystitis. London, 1990, p. 29.
2. Knight IT, Shults S, Kaspar CW. Direct detection of salmonella spp. in estuaries by using a DNA probe. Appl Environ Microbiol 1990; 56: 1059–1063.
3. Elliot T, Reed L, Slack R. Bacteriology and ultrastructure of the bladder in patients with urinary tract infections. J Infect 1985; 11: 191–196.
4. Silk MR. Bladder antibodies in interstitial cystitis. J Urol 1970; 103: 307–309.
5. Fister GM. Similarity of interstitial cystitis to lupus erythematosus. J Urol 1938; 40: 37–51.
6. Hand JR. Interstitial cystitis: report of 223 Cases. J Urol 1949; 61: 291–310.
7. Shipton EA. Hunner's ulcer (chronic interstitial cystitis). A manifestation of collagen disease. Br J Urol 1965; 37: 443–449.
8. Sant GR, Ucci AA, Alroy J. Bladder Surgace Glycosaminoglycans (GAGs) in Interstitial Cystitis. J Urol 1986; 135: 175A.
9. Dixon JS, Hald T. Morphological studies of the bladder wall in interstitial cystitis. In: George NJR, Gosling JA, eds. Sensory Disorders of the Bladder and Urethra. Heidelberg: Springer-Verlag, 1986, p. 63.
10. Simmons JL. Interstitial cystitis: an explanation for beneficial effect of an antihistamine. J Urol 1961; 85: 149–155.
11. Stamm WE, Wagner KF, Amsel R. Causes of the acute urethral syndrome in women. N Engl J Med 1980; 303: 409–418.
12. Mabry EW, Carson CC, Older RA. Evaluation of women with chronic voiding discomfort. Urology 1981; 18: 244–246.

13. ISSVD: Burning vulvar syndrome: report of the ISSVD. J Reprod Med 1984; 29: 457–463.

14. Getsch MF. Vulvar vestibulitis: prevalence and historic features in a general gynecologic preactive population. Am J Obstet Gynecol 1991; 164: 1609–1616.

15. Peckham BM, Maki DG, Patterson JJ. Focal vulvitis: a characteristic syndrome and cause of dyspareunia. Am J Obstet Gynecol 1986; 154: 855–864.

16. Ashman RB, Ott AK. Autoimmunity as a factor in recurrent vaginal Candidiasis and the minor vestibular gland syndrome. J Reprod Med 1989; 34: 264–266.

17. Stout AL, Steege JF. Psychosocial and behavioral self-reports of chronic pelvic pain patients. Paper presented at the meeting of the American Society for Psychosomatic Obstetrics and Gynecology; Houston, TX, March 1991.

18. Marinoff SC, Turner ML, Hirsch RP. Intralesional alpha-interferon: cost-effective therapy for vulvar vestibulitis syndrome. J Reprod Med 1993; 38: 19–24.

19. Stout AL Steege JF, Dodson WC. Relationship of laparoscopic findings to self-report of pelvic pain. Am J Obstet Gynecol 1991; 164: 73–79.

20. Puolakka J, Kauppila A, Ronnberg L. Results in the operative treatment of pelvic endometriosis. Acta Obstet Gynecol Scan 1980; 59: 429–434.

21. Vercellini P, Fidele L, Molterri P, Arcaini L, Candiani GB. Laparoscopy in the diagnosis of chronic pelvic pain in adolescent women. J Reprod Med 1989; 34: 827–830.

22. Fidele L, Parazzini F, Bianchi S, Archaini L, Candiani CB. Stage and localization of pelvic endometriosis and pain. Fertil Steril 1990; 53: 155–158.

23. Stout AL, Steege JF. Psychological assessment of women seeking treatment for premenstrual syndrome. J Psychosom Res 1985; 29: 621–627.

24. Poletti F, Medici MC, Alinovi A. Isolation of Chlamydia trichomatis from the prostatic cells in patients affected by non-acute abacterial prostatitis. J Urol 1985; 134: 691–693.

25. Mardh PA, Ripa KT, Collen S, Treharne JD, Darougar S. Role of Chlamydia trachomatis in non-acute prostatitis. Br J Vener Dis 1978; 54: 330–334.

26. Kaplan SA, Alexis TE, Jacobs BZ. Urodynamic evidence of vesical neck obstruction in men with misdiagnosed chronic nonbacterial prostatitis and the therapeutic role of endoscopic incision of the bladder neck. J Urol 1994; 152: 2063–2065.

27. de la Rosette JJ, Hubregtse MR, Karthaus HF, Debruyne FM. Results of a questionnaire among Dutch urologists and general peactionaers concerning diagnostics and treatment of patients with prostatitis syndrome. Eur Urol 1992; 22: 14–18.

28. Nickel JC, Sorenson R. Transurethral microwave thermotherapy for nonbacterial prostatitis: a randomized double blind sham controlled study using new prostatitis specific assessment questionnaire. J Urol 1996; 155: 1950–1955.

29. Brunner G, Weidner W, Schiefer HG. Studies on the role of ureaplasma urealyticum and mycoplasma hominis in prostatitis. J Infect Dis 1983; 147: 807–813.

30. Davis B, Noble M, Weigel J, Foret H, Mebust W. Analysis and management of chronic testicular pain. J Urol 1990; 143: 936–939.

31. Constabile R, Hahn M, McLeod D. Chronic orchalgia in the pain prone patient: the clinical perspective. J Urol 1991; 146: 1571–1574.

32. Chaiken DC, Blaivas JG, Blaivas ST. Behavioral therapy for the treatment of refractory interstitial cystitis. J Urol 1993; 149: 1445–1448.

33. Glazer HI, Rodke G, Swencionis C, Hertz R, Young AW. Treatment of vulvar vestibulitis syndrome with electromyographic biofeedback of pelvic floor musculature. J Reprod Med 1995; 4: 283–290.

34. Siegel SW. Management of voiding dysfunction with an implantable neuroprosthesis. Urol Clin North Am 1992; 19: 163–170.

35. Stoller ML, Copeland S, Millard RJ, Murnaghan GF. The efficacy of acupuncture in reversing the unstable bladder in pig-tailed monkeys. J Urol 1987; 137: 104A.

8 Low Back Pain: Diagnosis and Management

E. Ralph Johnson, MD
Viviane Ugalde, MD

Key Points

- The management of low back pain is an essential part of most medical practices; the annual cost for diagnosis and treatment exceeds $24 billion.
- Although low back pain is a common disorder, there are several red flags that should alert the clinician that a more extensive work-up is required.
- The common red flags suggesting an immediate work-up include progressive neurological deficit, bowel or bladder control problems, back pain (which increases in the supine position), fever and chills associated with back pain, an immunocompromised patient, a recent history of cancer, or of recent intravenous drug use.
- For most acute musculotendinous injuries, the most common recommended treatment options are rest, ice packs, and analgesics.
- Myofacial pain syndrome is a complex with no specific pathophysiology that requires early intervention, including possible use of trigger point injections.
- Exercise and physical therapy are essential components in the treatment of chronic low back syndrome. Low back pain, even with neural impingement, is often amenable to nonoperative treatment.
- Even though chronic low back pain is a common disorder, it should be taken seriously and each patient should be individually evaluated.

INTRODUCTION

Management of low back pain (LBP) is an essential part of most medical practices. The annual directs costs for the diagnosis and treatment of LBP in the United States exceeds $24 billion. There are 2.4 million Americans permanently disabled with LBP. Effective management of low back disorders requires timely and appropriate evaluation, diagnostic testing, and proven treatment techniques in order to ensure cost-effective outcomes.

Competent management of acute LBP begins with a solid pathophysiologic working diagnosis. Such a diagnosis directs appropriate evaluation and treatment techniques and provides a natural history framework to monitor recovery. This chapter will present specific diagnoses for LBP, the ICD9 code for that disorder, treatment for the disorder, the natural history of the disorder, and any red flags or *caveats* that might change the treatment process.

There are general red flags which should be familiar to all clinicians dealing with LBP *(1)*. These red flags alert the clinician that consideration should be given to additional workup such as immediate diagnostic imaging to exclude conditions such as epidural abscess, epidural hematoma, neoplasm, or central disk herniation, which may require immediate surgery. Those red flags are:

1. Progressive neurologic deficit.
2. Bowel or bladder control problems.
3. Back pain that increases in the supine position.
4. Fever and chills associated with back pain.
5. An immunocompromised patient.
6. A recent history of cancer.
7. History of recent iv drug use.

Most of the information in this chapter will deal with acute LBP. However, chronic low back syndromes will also be discussed. For the purpose of this chapter, chronic pain will be described as any pain that persists for 6 mo after definitive diagnosis and treatment. If a definitive diagnosis has not been made or definitive treatment not done, the pain syndrome will be designated as an acute pain.

Recommendations for treatment were derived from literature review and personal-experience. There has been a great deal of literature published regarding evaluation and treatment of LBP, but there have been few randomized controlled studies. Most of the controlled studies are hampered by low sample size, poor randomization methodology, poor descriptions of drop outs, lack of placebo, the presence of confusing cointerventions, lack of blindedness for patients and therapists, and lack of a pathophysiologic diagnosis *(2)*. In the absence of convincing literature, conservative management is indicated *(3)*.

A review by Shekelle and colleagues indicates that spinal manipulation is of short-term benefit in some patients, particularly those with uncomplicated, acute LBP *(4)*. Spinal manipulation for LBP is usually performed by an osteopathic physician, a chiropractor, or a physical therapist with specific training and skills in manipulation. Neurologic injuries do occur with spinal manipulation. A review of the indications and techniques of spinal manipulation is beyond the scope of this chapter.

Those who wish a more comprehensive review of the evaluation and treatment of LBP are referred to the excellent text by Borenstein *(5)*.

MUSCULOTENDINOUS DISORDERS (ENSETHOPATHIES) PRODUCING LBP

Acute Musculotendinous Strains

Acute musculotendinous strains (ICD9 720.1) are partial tears of the musculotendinous junction producing disruption and tears of myofibrils, microhemorrhage, and inflammatory cell infiltrates. Sixty percent of all LBP presenting in a general medical office are in this diagnostic category. The natural history shows that the pathophysiologic disorder is healed within 30 d if no further injury is sustained; that is, the microscopic changes resolve, the injured myofibrils regenerate, the microhemorrhage clears, and the inflammatory infiltrate disappears within that period.

Diagnosis

- Physical examination reveals muscular pain and tenderness in the lumbosacral paraspinous muscles and decreased range of motion without neurological deficit. Often patients will complain of pain during direct palpation of the injured structure and experience increased pain with passive stretch or active resisted motion of the involved muscle/tendon.
- There are no specific diagnostic tests that verify the diagnosis; however, the diagnosis can be made with a competent clinical history and physical examination.
- Lumbosacral low back X-rays are not indicated unless there is history of recent major trauma or the presence of one of the red flags described in the introduction.

Treatment

- During the first 3 d of modified rest at home, ice packs and analgesics are recommended.
- Although NSAIDs are acceptable, acetaminophen is preferred during the first few days (if there is no history of liver disease) since there is one animal model report that NSAIDs given in the first few days may inhibit the natural healing process.
- Muscle relaxants such as cyclobenzaprine (Flexeril®) (10 mg TID) or methocarbamol (Robaxin®) (750 mg QID) may be helpful if marked muscle spasm is present (6).
- Bed rest should not extend beyond 3 d (7).
- After the first 3 d, graded return to functional and work activities is indicated with the provision that no additional injury be initiated by the activity.
- Specific referral to a physical therapist is rarely indicated during the first 30 d following the injury.
- Aggressive exercises run the risk of reinjury. However, walking and swimming (in pools with water temp >80°F) are useful in preventing muscular and cardiovascular deconditioning until recovery is complete.
- Lumbosacral bracing is not required.
- Referral to a specialist may be indicated if the back pain persists for longer than 30 d.

Caveat

Aggressive stretching or strengthening exercises early in therapy may aggravate the injury.

Acute Lumbosacral Sprains

Acute lumbosacral sprains (ICD9 846.0) are tears of the supporting ligaments of the lower spine. There are no specific criteria for grading a lumbosacral sprain as there are for an ankle or knee sprain. However, if the degree of trauma involved in the sprain is severe or if instability is suspected from physical examination, lumbosacral X-rays, including cautious flexion/extension films (preferably under the supervision of a radiologist), are indicated. If there is any radiographic instability, orthopedic referral should be immediately obtained.

Diagnosis

Same as acute lumbosacral strain *(see above)*.

Treatment

- Treatment of an uncomplicated ligamentous lumbosacral sprain without instability is similar to that of a musculotendinous strain.
- However, modified bed rest may be required beyond 3 d.
- If the sprain is more severe, protective lumbosacral bracing may be needed. Any lumbosacral sprain pain lasting more than 30 d should be referred to an orthopedic surgeon.

Caveat

Aggressive stretching or strengthening exercises early in therapy may aggravate the injury.

Fibromyalgia Syndrome

Fibromyalgia syndrome (ICD 9 729.1) is a symptom complex that includes muscle pain and tenderness, tender points, fatigue, depression, and insomnia *(8–10)*. The problem is frequently chronic with prolonged periods of pain, which limit occupational and family activities. There is no generally acceptable pathophysiology for the diagnosis of this entity. Although there are numerous reports of biochemical, electrodiagnostic, and microscopic changes in muscle, none have been reproducible.

Diagnosis

- The symptom complex includes the findings listed in the diagnostic criteria below:
  1. History of widespread pain for at least 3 mo.
  2. Pain in 11 of 18 tender points on digital palpation. (Approximate force of 4 kg. Subject must state that point is "painful," not just "tender".)
  3. Associated symptoms:
     a. Nonrestorative sleep.
     b. Modulation of symptoms with activity.
     c. Alleviation of symptoms with heat (or sometimes ice).
     d. Intensity of symptoms with anxiety or stress.
     e. Type A personality.
  4. Exclusion criteria (absence of):
     a. Elevated muscle enzymes or erythrocyte sedimentation rate.
     b. Presence of another disorder that can explain symptoms (i.e., bursitis, tendinitis, arthritis).

Treatment

- As might be expected with a disease entity with no specific pathophysiology, treatment regimens are varied and numerous.

- Acceptable treatment includes muscle relaxants, antidepressive medications, and analgesics (NSAID or acetaminophen).
- Tender point injections with lidocaine can relieve pain if completed with proper technique.
- Physical modalities such as massage and stretching are important.
- Spray and stretch techniques with Fluori-Methane® can be taught to family members for home therapy.
- Biofeedback and relaxation techniques.
- Ergonomic adjustments at home and workplace.
- Return to work and social activities early.

Caveat

Ongoing treatment for this difficult disorder requires commitment from patient, family, and physician. Fibromyalgia support groups are a great help in providing psychological and social support.

Myofascial Pain Syndrome

Myofascial pain syndrome *(11,12)* (ICD9 724.2) is another pain complex with no specific pathophysiology. Early intervention is important.

Diagnosis

- Five major criteria must be present for diagnosis:
    1. Localized spontaneous pain.
    2. Spontaneous pain or altered sensation in expected referred pain area for given trigger points.
    3. Taut, palpable band in accessible muscle.
    4. Exquisite, localized tenderness in a precise point along the taut band.
    5. Some measurable degree of reduced range of movement.

One of three minor criteria must also be present:

1. Reproduction of spontaneously perceived pain and altered sensations by pressure on trigger point.
2. Elicitation of a local twitch response of muscular fibers by transverse "snapping" palpation or by needle insertion into a trigger point.
3. Pain relief obtained by muscle stretching or injection of trigger point.

Treatment

- Education regarding potentiating factors such as caffeine and fatigue.
- Medications:
    NSAID or acetaminophen (NSAIDs more effective for exacerbations).
    Tricyclic antidepressants improve stage III sleep patterns and decrease uptake of serotonin in ascending afferent pain fibers.
    Cyclobenzaprine modulates muscle tension by reducing gamma afferent activity.
- Trigger point injections.
- Spray and stretch after icing or Fluori-Methane® (home program).

- Physical therapy:
    Isometric contraction–relaxation.
    Deep kneading friction massage.
- Trancutaneous electrical neurostimulation (TENS) may be beneficial in some patients with chronic LBP even though there are concerns that there are no statistically significant benefits from TENS *(43)*.
- Instruction in body mechanics and work-site ergonomics.
- Aerobic exercise improves ATP levels, enhances growth hormone secretion and protein synthesis, improves endurance, and decreases fatigue.
- Exercise must be in a graded program.

ARTICULAR DISORDERS ASSOCIATED WITH LBP: INFLAMMATORY ARTHRITIDES

Ankylosing Spondylitis

Ankylosing spondylitis *(14,15)* (ICD9 720.0) is an inflammatory spondyloarthropathy producing low back, neck, sacroiliac, and hip pain. Early diagnosis is imperative to prevent severe disabling deformities. The natural history of ankylosing spondylitis includes ankylosis of the spine with calcification of the anterior and posterior longitudinal ligaments, both producing marked restriction of range of motion, and ankylosis of the costovertebral joints with resultant restrictive lung disease. If ankylosis occurs with joint deformity in a nonfunctional position, disability is profound. If ankylosis occurs in a functional position, the disability associated with ankylosing spondylitis is significantly limited.

Diagnosis

- Ankylosing spondylitis should be suspected in any patient older than 20 yr with LBP or neck pain who presents with tenderness over the sacroiliac joints.
- Early diagnosis is verified by an elevated erythrocyte sedimentation rate or sclerosis at the sacroiliac joints on pelvic X-rays.
- If ankylosing spondylitis is suspected but sacroiliac plain X-rays are normal, a bone scan or CT scan may verify the diagnosis.
- HLA-B27 is present in 90% of Caucasians with ankylosing spondylitis but is not specifically diagnostic.

Treatment

- Anti-inflammatory medication such as indomethacin (Indocin®) beginning with 25 mg po TID and progressing to 75 mg po TID.
- Immediate referral to a physical therapist for instruction in deformity preventing exercises and positions such as thoracic extension exercises, range of motion exercises, and deep breathing exercises (to limit restrictive lung disease).
- Modifications of workplace to prevent deformity.
- Evaluation every 6 mo to ensure compliance with deformity-preventing techniques and reinforcement of the importance of those techniques.

- If the pain is not controlled by the above or if deformity begins, referral to a rheumatologist.

Caveat

If early diagnosis and aggressive treatment do not occur, significant limiting deformity may occur within 2 yr of onset of this disease.

Rheumatoid Arthritis

Rheumatoid arthritis (ICD9 714.0) is a complex rheumatologic disorder producing multiple joint inflammatory arthropathy. Although LBP is reported in rheumatoid arthritis, the pathophysiology is not well-understood. Nonrheumatoid LBP factors may be involved. Facet joint involvement from rheumatoid synovitis does not appear to be prominent in etiology *(16)*. The treatment of LBP in rheumatoid arthritis involves control of the multijoint inflammatory process. Rest is beneficial. Physical therapy may include heat to the low back in the form of hydrocollator packs. For multijoint involvement, Hubbard tank hydrotherapy for 20 min at 98–102°F (water temperature depends on the patient's age and cardiovascular status) may be helpful. Swimming pool exercise therapy with water temperature above 80°F allows low back nonload exercise.

Reiter's Spondyloarthropathy

Reiter's spondyloarthropathy (ICD9 711.8) is a syndrome associated with arthritis, urethritis, and conjunctivitis *(17)*. It is most commonly seen in young men and primarily affects the low back and lower extremities. Three percent of individuals with nonspecific urethritis develop Reiter's syndrome. The conjunctivitis is usually mild. Back pain is a frequent symptom.

Diagnosis

- Laboratory findings are nonspecific and may include:
  Elevated erythrocyte sedimentation rate (in 70–80%). A positive HLA-B27 is helpful in differentiating Reiter's from rheumatoid arthritis but not from other spondyloarthropathies.
- Decreased ROM of lumbar spine.
- X-ray findings:
  There may be joint destruction on X-ray, most severely in the feet. Periosteal new bone formation occurs at the attachment of the planter fascia and Achilles tendon into the calcaneus.

Treatment

- Indomethacin (Indocin®) 25 mg po TID.
- Muscle relaxant.
- Antibiotic for specific urethritis organisms.

Caveat

Special care should be given to recommend low-intensity exercise and gentle stretching, since these patients are more susceptible to musculotendinous injuries.

Spondyloarthropathy Associated with Inflammatory Bowel Disease

Spondyloarthropathy associated with inflammatory bowel disease such as ulcerative colitis (ICD9 713.1/556.0) or regional ileitis (ICD9 713.1/ 555.9) produces an articular involvement of the spine similar in course to ankylosing spondylitis.

Diagnosis

- Spondyloarthropathy in association with ulcerative colitis or Crohn's disease.

Treatment

- Pharmacologic control of underlying bowel disease *(18)*.

Caveat

Spinal involvement is independent of the bowel inflammatory activity and may antedate the symptoms of the bowel disease. Special care should be given to recommend low-intensity exercise and gentle stretching, since these patients are more susceptible to musculotendinous injuries.

Psoriatic Arthritis

Psoriatic arthritis (ICD9 696.0) is an arthritic disorder associated with the skin manifestations of psoriasis *(19)*. The basic pathophysiology is unknown. Axial skeletal disease is usually associated with men with late onset psoriasis.

Diagnosis

- Classic distal phalangeal erosive appearance on X-ray.
- Psoriatic skin and nail disease
- Increased erythrocyte sedimentation rate.
- 50% are HLA-B27–positive.

Treatment

- Sulfasalazine.
- Corticosteroids.
- Immunosuppressives such as methotrexate.
- Photochemotherapy for skin.

Caveat

The clinical course may be unpredictable. Special care should be given to recommend low-intensity exercise and gentle stretching, since these patients are more susceptible to musculotendinous injuries.

ARTERIAL DISORDERS ASSOCIATED WITH LBP: DEGENERATIVE ARTHRITIDES

Osteoarthritis of Spine

Osteoarthritis of spine (ICD9 721.90) is a degenerative disorder producing LBP through either joint surface incongruity or the development of spurs and/or posterior disk bars that produce nerve impingement *(20)*. Neural impingement will be discussed in a section below. The pathophysiology is still under investigation but may involve proteoglycans in the cartilage matrix that are altered by time and stress. The cartilage matrix is disrupted, producing joint incongruity. The disease process is associated with aging, although it is seen at times in younger patients.

Diagnosis

- Develops slowly.
- Early morning stiffness.
- Articular degeneration on X-ray with subchondral sclerosis and decreased joint space.
- Normal erythrocyte sedimentation rate, serum calcium, and alkaline phosphatase.

Treatment

- NSAID or acetaminophen.
- Home exercise program to include range of motion, stretching, and functional exercises such as stationary bicycle or walking.
- Pool therapy with water temperature >80°F.
- Lumbosacral support belt or corset.

Diffuse Idiopathic Skeletal Hyperostosis

Diffuse idiopathic skeletal hyperostosis (ICD9 721.6) is a source of aching LBP in the older age population. It is also given the names DISH, vertebral osteophytosis, and ankylosing hyperostosis of Forestier.

Diagnosis

- Spinal stiffness and aching in 80%.
- Pain usually mild and intermittent.
- Extensive calcification of anterolateral aspect of vertebrae.
- Bridging osteophytes of contiguous vertebrae on X-ray.
- Enthesis calcification (at attachment of muscle/tendon).
- Natural course benign and develops slowly.

Treatment

- NSAID or acetaminophen.
- Home exercise program (*see* section on Osteoarthritis, *above*).

Caveat

There may be no early radiographic findings, only low back stiffness and aching.

Lumbar Spondylosis

Lumbar spondylosis without nerve impingement (ICD9 721.3) is a form of degenerative osteoarthritis producing spurs and bars at multiple levels that have not developed to the point of neural impingement *(21)*.

Diagnosis

- Symptoms same as degenerative osteoarthritis.
- Pain is aching in quality.
- Usually occurs after the age of 40.
- Osteoarthritic spurs may be evident on X-rays.

Treatment

- Treatment is nonsurgical when no nerve impingement is present.
- Pharmacologic and physical therapy treatment are generally the same as degenerative arthritis.
- Acutely may require hydrocodone or oxycodone rather than NSAID or acetaminophen for pain relief.
- Corset or chair back type brace may be helpful for structural support.
- Back school *(22)*.

Degenerative Disk Disorder

Degenerative disk disorder (ICD9 722.52) is a common etiology for LBP *(23)*. The pathophysiology of the disorder involves loss of up to 30% of the water content of the annulus fibrosus after 18 yr of age. The annulus is weakened, allowing bulging of the disk. Although degenerative disk disease may produce aching LBP, it is frequently asymptomatic.

Diagnosis

- General aching LBP.
- Radiographic evidence of loss of disk space.
- Pain aggravated by lifting, twisting, or long periods of sitting (intradiskal pressure is greater in the sitting position than it is in the supine or standing position).

Treatment

- NSAID or acetaminophen.
- Physical therapy for abdominal and back strengthening exercises.
- Instruction in body and back mechanics.
- Lumbosacral support belt (canvas type with Velcro closure).
- Back school *(22)*.

Facet Syndrome

Facet syndrome (ICD9 721.90) is a form of degenerative arthritis that alters the function of spinal facet articulations and their smooth capsules *(24)*. Capsular stresses produce osteoarthritis and hypermobility producing articular pain.

Diagnosis

- Reproducible specific point pain on twist of the spine.
- CT scan may show articular changes.

Treatment

- NSAID or acetaminophen.
- Facet injection with 1% lidocaine and/or a corticosteroid *(25)*.
- Facet denervation under fluoroscopy with phenol or radiofrequency.

Spondylolisthesis

Spondylolisthesis (ICD9 738.4) is a subluxation of a vertebral body on its supportive base, either the sacrum or the vertebra below. The pathophysiology usually involves dissolution (spondylolysis) of the pars interarticularis of the posterior arch, which allows the vetebral body to slip, usually in the anterior direction.

Diagnosis

- Frequently occurs in young adults.
- Leg pain may be present.
- LBP aggravated by activity and relieved by rest.
- Step sign on palpating spinous processes.
- Radiographic evidence of subluxation.

Treatment

- Low back flexion exercises.
- Lumbosacral support belt or antilordotic thoracolumbosacral plastic orthosis *(26)*.
- NSAID or acetaminophen.
- Surgical stabilization if pain persists and subluxation >25% of the contiguous surface (Grade II or worse).

Scoliosis

Scoliosis (ICD9 737.30) is a lateral curvature of the spine associated with rotation of the vertebral body that may produce LBP *(27,28)*. Clinically significant scoliosis is usually associated with a curvature greater than 10°. The etiology and pathophysiology of scoliosis are varied. Most are idiopathic; however, dysplastic vertebrae, muscular dystrophy, and neurological disorders may be involved.

Diagnosis

- Pain is worse on ambulation and decreases when patient is supine.
- Pain is usually worse at or just below the apex of the curve.
- Radiographic evidence of lateral curvature greater than 10° is usually associated with vertebral rotation.

Treatment

- NSAID or acetaminophen.
- Bracing.
- Scoliosis exercises with physical therapist.
- Swimming and cycling are recommended.
- Surgical correction with spinal fusion.

Caveats

Surgical correction should be done by the time the curvature is 40°.

Coccydynia

Coccydynia (ICD9 724.79) is pain originating from the coccyx secondary to a traumatic injury to the coccyx.

Diagnosis

- Pain on sitting, especially on hard surfaces.
- Relieved on standing and walking.
- Pain at end of coccyx on rectal exam.
- May be radiographic evidence of coccygeal fracture.

Treatment

- NSAID or acetaminophen.
- Circular cushion or pillow.
- Lidocaine injection.
- Pelvic stabilization and hip flexibility program.
- Surgery.

LBP WITH NEURAL IMPINGEMENT

Herniated Disk

Herniated disk (ICD9 724.4) with an acute lumbosacral root compression (radiculopathy) is a common cause of both dull aching and sharp lancinating LBP frequently radiating down the leg. A degenerated annulus fibrosus weakens and allows herniation of the mucopolysaccharide nucleus pulposus, which usually herniates posterolaterally into the area of the intervertebral foramen and its nerve root. Many herniated disks are amenable to nonoperative treatment *(29)*.

Diagnosis

- Sharp lancinating pain with or without radiation to the leg.
- Pain aggravated by cough, sneeze, or straining at stool.
- Neurologic evidence of root compression in the form of a focal decreased deep tendon reflex or muscle weakness on manual muscle test.
- Evidence of image defect on CT, MRI, or myelogram.
- Evidence of acute nerve root impingement on electromyogram.

Treatment

- Bed rest initially (may require more than the 3 d suggested for musculotendinous strains/sprains), then a graded increase in exercise including walking.
- NSAID or acetaminophen, but acutely may require short-term hydrocodone or oxycodone for pain relief.
- Lumbosacral support belt or corset.
- Physical therapy:

Hydrocollator packs.
Sedative massage.
Exercises with emphasis on dynamic stabilization.
- Pool therapy.
- Epidural steroids *(30)*.
- Surgery:
  Best results in a patient under 40 yr of age with a single image defect and a neurological deficit at the same level on physical or electromyographic exam.

Caveats

Any loss of urinary bladder or bowel control associated with LBP may be a symptom of central disk herniation with spinal cord or cauda equina compression requiring immediate imaging and surgical decompression. Moderately large herniated disks may respond to conservative management and not require surgery. Successful surgery will resolve or significantly reduce the sharp lancinating pain, but the dull aching pain may persist. Lumbar fusion is indicated only if there is evidence of instability.

Lumbar Spondylosis with Spinal Stenosis

Lumbar spondylosis with spinal stenosis (ICD9 724.02) is an advanced degenerative arthritic disorder that may produce LBP and spinal cord or cauda equina compression with neurologic sequelae similar to a central disk herniation *(31–33)*.

Diagnosis

- Advanced degenerative arthritis on X-ray.
- Pronounced LBP.
- Bilateral leg pain with activity.

Treatment

- Analgesics such as a NSAID or acetaminophen (may need hydrocodone or oxycodone for brief periods).
- Pool therapy.
- Instruction in body and back mechanics.
- Lumbar brace or corset *(34)*.
- Surgery if symptoms are severe or progressive neurological deficit.

Caveat

Same as for central disk herniation.

Piriformis Syndrome

Piriformis syndrome (ICD9 355.0) is an unusual segmental compressive neuropathy of the sciatic nerve in which all or part of the sciatic nerve passes through the piriformis muscle, a short external rotator of the hip *(35)*. This disorder produces LBP and mimics a lumbar radiculopathy.

Diagnosis

- LBP radiating down the leg.
- Negative straight leg raising test.
- Frequently involves the peroneal portion of the sciatic nerve.
- Positive Freiburg's sign: pain aggravated by internal hip rotation.
- Electrodiagnosis *(36)*.

Treatment

- NSAID or acetaminophen.
- Gentle stretch of piriformis by internal hip rotation.
- Physical therapy for tension release techniques and instruction in a pelvic stabilization program.
- Surgical decompression.

Caveat

Surgical decompression should be delayed until conservative therapy has failed, since the surgical approach is difficult.

Epidural Abscess and Hematoma

Epidural abscess *(37)* (ICD9 324.1) and hematoma (ICD9 336.9) are disorders producing severe LBP and requiring emergency surgery for evacuation. Predisposing factors include alcoholism, cirrhosis, and iv drug use. Speed in diagnosis is critical since late diagnosis may result in permanent neurological motor and sensory deficits.

Diagnosis

- Severe LBP unrelieved by rest.
- Increased erythrocyte sedimentation rate, positive CSF or blood culture, leukocytosis for epidural abscess.
- Image defect on MRI.

Treatment

- Surgical evacuation and decompression.
- Intravenous antibiotics for abscess.

Disk Space Infection

Disk space infection (ICD9 722.93) is a source of severe sharp LBP. It is one complication of disk surgery. The natural course of treated disk infection in children is relatively benign. Fever is not commonly present. Most recover from the infection.

Diagnosis

- Severe localized back pain.
- Elevated erythrocyte sedimention rate in 75%.
- Elevated C-reactive protein.
- MR with Gadolinium sensitive for early diagnosis.

Treatment

- Bed rest.
- Immobilization with cast or brace.
- Severe pain may require morphine, including epidural morphine.
- Surgical exploration if signs of spinal cord compression develop.

BONE

Osteoporosis with Compression Fracture

Osteoporosis with compression fracture (ICD9 733.00) is a metabolic disorder of bone mass per unit volume *(38)*. The ratio of bone mineral content to bone matrix is normal. Back pain is uncommon in the absence of fracture, but compression fractures with back pain are common and can occur with minimal trauma. Pain is increased with movement, especially flexion. The etiology of osteoporosis is multifactorial. It is present in 29% of women and 18% of men between the ages of 45 and 79 yr and present in 50% of women over the age of 50 yr.

Diagnosis

- X-ray evidence of osteoporosis and fracture.
- Bone scan may help identify fracture.
- Bone-density studies positive for loss of bone mass.
- Serum calcium, phosphorus, alkaline phosphatase, and urinary hydroxyproline are normal.

Treatment

- NSAID or acetaminophen.
- Acutely may require hydocodone or oxycodone for relief.
- If pain severe on flexion, a Knight-Taylor brace to limit thoracic flexion may be helpful in controlling pain.
- Pharmacologic treatment of osteoporosis:
    Calcium supplements.
    Vit D.
    Estrogen in postmenopausal women.
    Calcitonin.
    Etidronate.
    Alendronate (Fosamax®).
- Regular exercise with emphasis on extension and weight-bearing activities *(39,40)*. Exercise alone has been shown to decrease the rate of bone mineral loss, but, when combined with hormone replacement, exercise can produce an increase in bone mineral density. Pectoral stretching and reinforcement of upright posture is helpful in preventing kyphosis.
- Avoid excess protein, alcohol, caffeine, and smoking.
- Pool therapy.
- Avoid excess protein, alcohol, caffeine, and smoking.

Caveat

An exercise program is required that does not produce compressive vertebral stress. Lumbar flexion exercises produce vertebral compression stress.

Osteomalacia

Osteomalacia (ICD9 268.2) is a metabolic disorder of bone mineralization associated with loss of bone mass/unit volume and with a decrease in the ratio of bone mineral to bone matrix *(41)*. Multiple etiologies are associated with osteomalacia, including vitamin D deficiency, genetic mineral defects, and calcium deficiency. The major complaint is bone pain. In nutritional osteomalacia, backache with spine tenderness is present in 90%. Fractures of the spine usually do not occur unless there is concomitant osteoporosis.

Diagnosis

- X-ray evidence of demineralization.
- Laboratory abnormalities dependent on etiology.
- Urinary calcium excretion < 75 mg/d.
- Pain worse with activity or increased standing.
- Bone biopsy with tetracycline fluorescence.

Treatment

- Directed to basic underlying disease, may include:
    Vit D supplement.
    Pancreatic enzyme supplement.
    Phosphate supplement.
- Back support or brace.

Paget's Disease of Bone

Paget's disease of bone (ICD9 731.0) is a disorder producing foci of bone resorption and irregular new bone formation, which occurs in 3% of individuals over 40 yr of age and 10% of those over 80 yr of age *(42)*. The pathogenesis is unknown, but there is increased osteoblastic resorption of bone producing accelerated remodeling and highly vascular bone, which is structurally weak. Most individuals with this disorder are asymptomatic. However, there is spine involvement in 35% and LBP in 12% of those with Paget's disease of bone. Neurological complications are uncommon.

Diagnosis

- Deep boring pain.
- Pain not related to activity.
- No increase in pain at night.
- Not relieved by rest or NSAID.
- Increased alkaline phosphatase.
- Increased 24-h total urinary hydroxyproline.
- Erythrocyte sedimentation rate and serum calcium are normal.
- Osteoclastic absorption of bone in pelvis, spine, and skull on X-ray.

Treatment

- Diphosphonate such as etidronate disodium (Didronel®), 5 mg/kg/d po for 6 mo of year, or pamidronate disodium (Aredia®), 30 mg/d iv for 3 consecutive days.
- Calcitonin to decrease bone resorption.

Caveat

Osteosarcoma or fibrosarcoma develops in 1%.

Osteomyelitis of Vertebra

Osteomyelitis of vertebra (ICD9 730.8) is an infection involving spinal bone *(37,43)*. Fifty-two percent of individuals with vertebral osteomyelitis are over 50 yr of age. The primary symptom is LBP.

Diagnosis

- Sharp LBP.
- Fever and general malaise.
- Leukocytosis and elevated erythrocyte sedimentation rate.
- Subchondral bone loss on X-ray.
- Blood culture positive in 50%.
- Bone aspiration or surgical biopsy may be helpful.

Treatment

- Antibiotics (Staphylococcus is the most common organism, but Pseudomonas is becoming more common).
- Immobilization.

Caveat

Diagnosis is frequently made late.

Vertebral Epiphysitis

Vertebral epiphysitis (ICD9 732.0), also called vertebral osteochondritis or Scheurmann's disease, produces irregularity of ossification and endochondral growth primarily in the thoracic spine in teenagers. If untreated, there is back pain and progressive kyphosis.

Diagnosis

- Increasing wedging of vertebrae (T8 most involved usually).
- Schmorl's nodes.
- Kyphosis.

Treatment

- Rest and decreased activity during rapid growth years.
- Physical therapy re: back extension exercises.
- Spinal bracing until growth completed.

Spinal Column Tumors

Spinal column tumors (ICD9 239.2) include multiple myeloma; osteoid osteoma; giant cell tumor; osteoblastoma; osteosarcoma; and metastatic lung, breast, or prostate carcinoma *(44,45)*. Back pain is the presenting symptom in 75% of spinal tumors. Osteochondroma is an uncommon source of LBP.

Diagnosis3

- Pain increased in supine position.
- History of primary carcinoma known to metastasize to bone.
- X-ray or bone scan evidence of neoplasm (plain X-rays demonstrate the spinal lesion in over 90%).
- Elevated serum alkaline phosphatase.

Treatment

- May require hydrocodone, oxycodone, or MS Contin® for pain relief.
- Antimetabolite (dependent on cell type).
- Irradiation therapy depending on sensitivity.
- Frequently requires opiate to control pain.
- May require lumbosacral brace for stabilization and pain control.

Multiple Myeloma

Multiple myeloma (ICD 9 203.0) is a malignant plasma cell tumor of bone marrow associated with bone destruction and pathologic fractures. LBP is the initial symptom in 35% of individuals with multiple myeloma. The clinical course is that of gradual progression of the tumor with mean survival of 5 yr.

Diagnosis

- Pain when lying down.
- Diffuse bone tenderness.
- Monoclonal antibodies.
- Abnormal immunoglobulin production including Bence-Jones protein in the urine.
- Hypercalcemia and increased sedimentation rate.
- Normal alkaline phosphatase in most cases.
- Osteolysis on X-ray.
- Bone marrow aspirate or biopsy shows increased plasma cells.

Treatment

- Melphalan.
- Prednisone or dexamethasone.
- Multiple drug regimen, which may include vincristine, melphalan, cyclophosphamide, or BCNG.
- May require hydrocodone, oxycodone, or MS Contin® for pain relief.

VASCULAR

Abdominal Aortic Aneurysm

Abdominal aortic aneurysm (ICD9 441.3 with rupture or 441.4 without rupture) is a common disorder. Without rupture, abdominal aortic aneurysms are frequently slowly progressive and asymptomatic. Rupture produces epigastric, flank, and LBP, which may begin as a dull ache and progress to a sharp tearing pain. The pain may radiate to the hip or thigh.

Diagnosis

- Pulsatile abdominal mass with or without calcification.
- Mass on abdominal ultrasound or CT.

Treatment

- Surgical excision with graft if aneurysm >5 cm (41% risk of rupture within 5 yr if >5 cm).

PELVIC/RETROPERITONEAL

Endometriosis

Endometriosis (ICD9 617.9) results from functioning endometrial tissue occurring outside the uterine cavity, which undergoes the same monthly cycle of growth and shedding with bleeding. Its prevalence is 3% of females in the 15–50 age group. Endometrial implants in the colon or rectovaginal septum may produce LBP radiating to the thighs. The pain may be intermittent or more constant but usually increases with menses.

Diagnosis

- Uterine or pelvic tenderness on pelvic exam.
- Increase of pain with menses.
- Laparoscopy with biopsy.

Treatment

- Oral contraceptives to regulate menses.
- Danazol (Danocrine®).
- NSAID or acetaminophen.
- Surgery to remove foci of abnormal endometrial implants.

Prostatitis

Prostatitis (ICD9 601.0) is an inflammatory infection of the prostate gland that is associated with pain in the low back and perineum often accompanied by urinary frequency, dysuria, and nocturia.

Diagnosis

- Symptoms described above.
- Tender enlarged prostate.
- Positive urine culture.

Treatment

- Antibiotics, especially trimethoprim-sulfamethoxazole.

Caveat

Antibiotics may be required for 6–12 wk to clear infection.

Pelvic or Retroperitoneal Neoplasms

Pelvic or retroperitoneal neoplasms are a source of LBP.

Leiomyomas produce heaviness in the pelvis and dull aching low back and leg pain. Surgical excision may be required to prevent the pain. Back pain associated with benign ovarian tumors is unusual. When it does occur, it is aching in quality and usually sacral in location. Likewise, malignant ovarian tumors only occasionally are responsible for LBP. When pain does occur, it is usually aching and present in the paraspinous and sacral areas. Transvaginal ultrasound is more sensitive than CT for detecting the presence of malignant ovarian tumors. Primary malignant tumors of the prostate or testes may produce dull or sharp LBP. Testicular carcinoma markers include α-fetoprotein and human chorionic gonadotropin. Renal carcinoma is associated with flank or back pain and hematuria in 41%.

Retroperitoneal Hematoma

Retroperitoneal hematoma (ICD9 568.81) is an uncommon reason for LBP, but must be considered in patients with the acute onset of LBP who are anticoagulated with warfarin. Femoral neuropathy may be associated with the bleed.

Diagnosis

LBP with focal neuropathy from lumbosacral plexus.

Treatment

Discontinue or reduce dosage of anticoagulant.

PSYCHOLOGIC DISORDERS

Psychologic disorders resulting in or resulting from psychologic factors are common in LBP *(46)*. Most individuals with chronic LBP are depressed and will have Minnesota Multiphasic Personality Inventory abnormalities with abnormal depression and hysteria scores. It is not within the scope of this chapter to detail the multiple psychiatric diagnoses associated with back pain. However, the clinician dealing with LBP must differentiate those with factitious, exaggerated pain response, or conversion hysteria problems from the diagnoses described above. That differentiation is not always easy. In addition, the clinician must have a method of dealing with those patients who have chronic pain syndromes. That methodology is also not easy.

Chronic Pain Syndromes

Chronic pain syndromes are defined by the Office of Disabilities of the Social Security Administration as intractable pain of 6 mo or more duration with the following:

1. Marked alteration of behavior with depression or anxiety.
2. Daily activities significantly restricted.
3. Frequent use of medical facilities.
4. Excessive use of medication.
5. No demonstrable relationship with an organic disorder.
6. History of multiple, nonproductive tests, treatments, and surgeries.

Diagnosis

Chronic pain syndrome is more a behavior pattern than a diagnostic term, with known pathophysiology and natural history *(46)*. Seligman's term "learned helplessness" describes in part one of the problems patients and clinicians encounter in meeting and treating this disorder. Etiology and natural history are not well-defined; therefore, treatment is eclectic and frequently empirical. Treatment usually involves a behaviorally oriented program to preclude many of the reinforcers of learned helplessness, including concerns about lack of employment opportunity, reluctance to return to a stressful job situation, fear of losing medical benefits, avoidance of responsibility, protection from rejection, excessive caretaking by family, and "entitlement" to drugs and financial compensation. Many of these secondary gains may be more subconscious than conscious/volitional. All pain medications should be given under a written signed contract, which should include:

1. All medications, particularly opiates, must come from only one physician and one pharmacist.
2. The physician and pharmacist will communicate whether other prescriptions are being used.
3. Frequent patient office follow-ups, not telephone calls for refills, are required.
4. No early refills. If the prescription is lost the patient will bear the consequence of not having the medication until the planned time for refill.
5. A signed agreement regarding medications; violations of the agreement to result in no further prescriptions for the same or similar medications.

Factitious Pain Syndromes

Factitious pain syndromes are conscious/volitional pain prevarications for specific gain, usually involving monetary compensation or personal convenience. Identification of this category requires documentation of:

1. Physical complaints and disabilities during examination that are not observed in outside activities when the individual does not feel he or she is being observed.
2. A distinctly exaggerated pain response to minimal stimulus during examination.
3. Either no physical etiology apparent after comprehensive examination or complaints that are excessively exaggerated in the presence of minimal physical findings.

Treatment of this problem is difficult. Hostile aggressive accusations are usually ineffective. Statements that include the individual in a discussion of why the exaggeration of symptoms is present may be more helpful in resolving the complaints.

Psychogenic Pain Syndrome

Psychogenic pain syndrome is a term that includes hysteria, conversion disorder, functional pain, and somatoform pain disorders. Individuals with this pain syndrome often exhibit the problems characteristic of the mnemonic "MADISON," proposed by Hackett and Bouckoms *(47)*.

*M*ultiplicity of pain (and other) symptoms.
*A*uthenticity, a drive to prove the symptoms are real.
*D*enial of stresses and problems that may produce the symptoms.
*I*nterpersonal variability, symptoms change with the audience.
*S*ingularity, their case is the worst ever.
*O*nly effective medical help is from your intelligent kind treatment.
*N*othing in the past has helped.

Treatment

The treatment of chronic pain disorders involves:

- Behaviorally oriented comprehensive treatment program.
- Informative intercommunication between the patient, the patient's family, and all health professionals involved.
- Appropriate and time-limited use of medications for pain, anxiety, and depression under written signed contract.
- A time-limited treatment plan developed with the patient and family to deal with reduction in secondary gains.

If the above are unsuccessful, consideration should be given to procedural techniques for pain control, which include:

- Implantation of electrical stimulator.
- Implantation of catheters and pumps for intrathecal analgesic administration.

EXERCISE THERAPY FOR LBP

Home exercise programs are important to involve the patient in the treatment process. Those programs reduce pain by restoring normal biomechanics through increasing flexibility, mobilization of soft tissues, and prevention of the complications from immobilization, including loss of strength and bone demineralization *(48)*. Current exercise research suggests the following:

- Exercises for strengthening abdominal and back muscles improve overall fitness and decrease the incidence and duration of recurrent LBP *(49,50)*.
- For acute back pain, McKenzie-type exercises produce earlier return to work and less pain and recurrences over a 1-yr period of follow-up *(22)*.
- In chronic LBP, extensor strengthening can produce decreased pain, fewer sick days, improved strength, improved range of motion, and improved endurance *(48,50)*.

Two exercise programs that are commonly used in the treatment of LBP are William's exercises and McKenzie exercises. William's exercises emphasize flexibility and isometric strengthening of the abdominal and pelvic muscles. Typically patients perform these exercises in a supine position, flexing the hip and knee toward the abdomen, performing a straight leg raise to stretch the hamstrings, or a pelvic tilt held isometrically. Variations of these exercises include single vs double leg lifts. Expansion of the William's program includes abdominal crunches and prone trunk lifts for strengthening.

Although traditionally described as "extension" exercises, the McKenzie exercises are better described as an evaluation and treatment approach. Patients are evaluated with repetitive spine motions that determine positions that aggravate and alleviate pain. Any position that aggravates peripheral or leg pain is avoided. Any position that leads to relief or centralization of the pain from the leg to low back is taught to the patient as a home exercise program. Postural analysis is also a key component to the McKenzie program. Motions that diminish pain in the back or legs are emphasized during the period of acute pain. Subsequent exercises are then used to normalize and return the spine to pain-free lumbar range of motion. Home exercise programs are taught that can be used by the patient if the pain recurs. This provides a program that provides a cost-effective treatment for any recurring pain that occurs. However, if a home program is used, written instructions should include the warning that, if any of the "red flags" identified in the beginning of this chapter occur, then the patient should seek immediate medical attention. Those red flags include loss of bowel or bladder control, weakness in the legs, severe exacerbation of the pain, or aggravation of the pain in the supine position.

A simple concept categorizing the diagnostic etiologies into those affecting the anterior elements of the spine, those affecting the posterior elements, and a soft tissue subset assists in developing appropriate exercise recommendations for LBP.

Anterior Elements of the Spine

Anterior elements of the spine include the vertebral body, the intervertebral disk, and the anterior longitudinal ligament. Diagnoses in which the anterior elements are affected include:

- Osteoporotic compression fractures.
- Traumatic compression fractures.
- Vertebral epiphysitis.
- Annular tears.
- Disk herniations with or without radiculopathy.
- Degenerative disk disease.

In these anterior element disorders:

- Pain is aggravated by flexion exercises, bending, or sitting.
- Avoid stationary bicycle exercises, nordic track ("cross country machines"), stair climbers (which frequently require a forward flexed posture), rowing, and William's flow back flexion exercises.
- Exercises should emphasize extensor strengthening.
- Utilize McKenzie exercises, walking, swimming (crawl), and recumbent stationary bicycles with lumbar support.

Posterior Elements of the Spine

Posterior elements of the spine include the spinal canal, foramen, and facet joints. Diagnoses in which the posterior elements are primarily involved are:

- Spinal stenosis.
- Facet pain syndrome and arthropody.
- Facet arthropody associated with scoliosis.
- Lumbar spondylosis.
- Spondylolisthesis.

In posterior element disorders of the spine:

- Avoid extension exercises.
- Emphasize William's flexion exercises, bicycling, rowing, or nordic track.
- Sacral joint involvement such as in ankylosing spondylitis, traumatic sacroiliitis, and seronegative spondyloarthropathies may respond. However, special care must be taken with ankylosing spondylitis to prevent flexion ankylosis.

Soft Tissue Subset

Soft tissue subset includes musculotendinous strains and sprains, piriformis syndrome, fibromyalgia, and myofascial pain syndromes. Relative rest or avoidance of activities that aggravate the pain with an emphasis on stretching *specific* involved tissues and a graded progression to a home strengthening program is often successful. Encouragement of weight loss and the development of a practical lifetime exercise program is important to prevent reinjury or exacerbations.

For patients with nerve root irritation in any diagnostic subset or those with multilevel disk degeneration and facet degeneration involving both anterior and posterior elements, pool exercises with water temperature of at least 80°F are indicated.

Some patients find any activity painful. Those patients should have a physical therapy evaluation to determine a spinal functional position that allows the patient pain-free motion. This position is then emphasized in a vigorous strengthening program such as dynamic lumbosacral stabilization.

REFERENCES

1. Agency for Health Care Policy and Research. Acute low back problems in adults: assessment and treatment. Quick Reference Guide. Rockville, MD: US Public Health Service, 1994; AHCPR publication No. 95–0643.
2. Koes BW, Bouter LM, van der Heijden GJ. Methodological quality of randomized clinical trials on treatment efficacy in low back pain. Spine 1995; 20: 228–235.
3. Fast A. Low back disorders: conservative management. Arch Phys Med Rehab 1988; 69: 880–891.
4. Shekelle PG, Adams AH, Chassin MR, et al. Spinal manipulation for low back pain. Ann Int Med 1992; 117: 590–598.
5. Borenstein DG. Low back pain: medical diagnosis and comprehensive management, 2nd ed. Philadelphia: Saunders, 1995.
6. Porter RW, Ralston SH. Pharmacologic management of back pain syndromes. Drugs 1994; 48: 189–198.
7. Deyo RA, Diehl AK, Rosenthal M. How many days of bed rest for acute low back pain?: a randomized clinical trial. N Engl J Med 1986; 315: 1064–1070.

8. Wolfe F, Smythe HA, Yanus MB, et al. The Americal College of Rheumatology 1990 criteria for the classification of fibromyalgia. Arthritis Rheum 1990; 33: 160–172.

9. de Girolamo G. Epidemiology and social costs of low back pain and fibromyalgia. Clin J Pain 1991; 7 (Suppl 1): S1–7.

10. Reiffenberger DH, Amundson LH. Fibromyalgia syndrome: a review. Am Family Physician 1996; 53: 1698–1712.

11. Bernard TN Jr, Kirkaldy-Willis WH. Recognizing specific characteristics of non-specific low back pain. Clin Orthop 1987; 217: 266–280.

12. Goldenberg DL. Fibromyalgia, chronic fatigue syndrome, and myofascial pain. Curr Opin Rheumatol 1996; 8: 113–123.

13. Deyo RA, Walsh NE, Martin DC, Schoenfeld LS, Ramamurthy S. A controlled trial of transcutaneous electrical nerve stimulation (TENS) and exercise for chronic low back pain. N Engl J Med 1990; 322: 1627–1634.

14. Calin A. The individual with ankylosing spondylitis: defining disease status and the impact of the illness. Br J Rheumatol 1995; 34: 663–672.

15. Ramos-Remus C, Russell AS. Clinical features and management of ankylosing spondylitis. Current Opinion in Rheumatology 1993; 5: 408–413.

16. Helliwell PS, Zebouri LN, Porter A, Wright V. A clinical and radiological study of back pain in rheumatoid arthritis. Br J Rheumatol 1993; 32: 216–221.

17. Hughes RA, Keat AC. Reiter's syndrome and reactive arthritis. Semin Arthr Rheumatism 1994; 24: 190–210.

18. Linn FV, Peppercorn MA. Drug therapy for inflammatory bowel disease: Part II. Am J Surg 1992; 164: 85–89.

19. Gladman DD. Psoriatic arthritis. Baillieres Clin Rheumatol 1995; 9: 319–329.

20. Mankin HJ. The reaction of articular cartilage to injury and osteoarthritis. N Engl J Med 1974; 291: 1285–1292.

21. Hall S, Bartleson JD, Onofrio BM, et al. Lumbar spinal stenosis: Clinical features, diagnostic procedures, and results of surgical treatment in 68 patients. Ann Int Med 1985; 103: 271–275.

22. Stankovic R, Johnell O. Conservative treatment of acute low-back pain—a prospective randomized trial: McKenzie method of treatment versus patient education in "Mini Back School." Spine 1990; 15: 120–123.

23. Hirsch C, Inglemark BE, Miller M. The anatomical basis for low back pain: studies on the presence of sensory nerve endings in ligamentous, capsular and intervertebral disc structures in the human lumbar spine. Acta Orthop Scand 1963; 33: 1–17.

24. Mooney V, Robertson J. The facet syndrome. Clin Orthop 1976; 115: 149–156.

25. Moran R, O'Connell D, Walsh MG. The diagnostic value of facet joint injections. Spine 1988; 13: 1407–1410.

26. Bell DF, Ehrlich MG, Zaleske DJ. Brace treatment for symptomatic spondylolisthesis. Clin Orthop 1988; 236: 192–198.

27. Kostuik JP, Bentivoglio J. The incidence of low back pain in adult scoliosis. Spine 1981; 6: 268–273.

28. van Dam BE. Nonoperative treatment of adult scoliosis. Orthopaedic Clinics of NA 1988; 19: 347–351.

29. Saal JA, Saal JS. Nonoperative treatment of herniated lumbar intervertebral disc with radiculopathy. An outcome study. Spine 1989; 14: 431–437.

30. White AH, Derby R, Wynne G. Epidural injections for the diagnosis and treatment of low-back pain. Spine 1980; 5: 78–86.

31. Kana S, Wiesel SW. Conservative therapy for spinal stenosis. Semin Spine Surg 1994; 6: 109–115.

32. Moreland LW, Lopez-Mendez A, Alarcon GS. Spinal stenosis: a comprehensive review of the literature. Semin Arthritis Rheum 1989; 19: 127–149.

33. Sinaki M, Lutness MP, Ilstrup DM, et al. Lumbar spondylosis: Retrospective comparison and three-year follow up of two conservative treatment programs. Arch Phys Med Rehabil 1989; 70: 594–598.

34. Alarante H, Hurri H. Compliance and subjective relief by corset treatment in chronic low back pain. Scand J Rehab Med 1988; 20: 133–136.

35. Pace JB, Nagle D. Piriformis syndrome. West J Med 1976; 124: 435–439.

36. Fishman LM, Zybert PA. Electrophysiologic evidence of piriformis syndrome. Arch Phy Med Rehabil 1991; 73: 359–364.

37. Schwartz ST, Spiegel M, Ho G Jr. Bacterial vertebral osteomyelitis and epidural abscess. Semin Spine Surg 1990; 2: 95–100.
38. Riggs BL, Melton LJ III. The prevention and treatment of osteoporosis. N Engl J Med 1992; 327: 620–627.
39. Ayalon J, Simkin A, Leichter I, Ralfmann S. Dynamic bone loading exercises for postmenopausal women: effect on the density of the distal radius. Arch Phys Med Rehabil 1987; 68: 280–283.
40. Sinaki M, Wahner HW, Hodgson SF. Efficacy of nonloading exercises in prevention of vertebral bone loss in postmenopausal women: a controlled trial. Mayo Clin Proc 1989; 64: 762–769.
41. White PA. Osteopenic disorders of the spine. Semin Spine Surg 1995; 7: 187–199.
42. Kaplan FS, Singer FR. Paget's disease of bone: pathophysiology, diagnosis, and management. J Am Acad Orthop Surg 1995; 3: 336–344.
43. Savoia M. An overview of antibiotics in the treatment of bacterial, mycobacterial, and fungal osteomyelitis. Semin Spine Surg 1996; 8: 142–155.
44. Huvos AG. Bone tumors: diagnosis, treatment and prognosis, 2nd ed. Philadelphia: Saunders, 1991.
45. Weinstein JN, McLain RF. Primary tumors of the spine. Spine 1987; 12: 843–851.
46. Covington EC. The psychiatry of chronic back disability. Semin Spine Surg 1994; 6: 269–281.
47. Hackett TP, Bouckoms A. The pain patient: evaluation and treatment. In: Hackett TP, Cassem NH, eds. Massachusetts General Hospital Handbook of General Hospital Psychiatry (2nd ed.), Littleton, MA: PSG Publishing, 1987; pp. 42–68.
48. Hansen FR, Bendix T, Skov P, Jensen CV, et al. Intensive dynamic back-muscle exercises, conventional physiotherapy, or placebo-control treatment of low-back pain. Spine 1993; 18: 98–108.
49. Lahad A, Malter AD, Berg AO, Deyo RA. The effectiveness of four interventions for the prevention of low back pain: a randomized, observer-blind trial JAMA 1994; 272: 1286–1291.
50. Mannishe C, Bentzen L, Hesselsoe G. Christensen I, Lundberg E. Clinical trial of intensive muscle training for chronic low backpain. Lancet 1988; 2 (No. 8626/8627): 1473–1476.

9 PAIN IN THE HIPS AND LOWER EXTREMITIES

JAMES C. LEEK, MD

Key Points

- The differential diagnosis of hip pain can be subdivided into pain in the anterior/inguinal area, lateral hip, and posterior/gluteal area.
- Osteoarthritis is the most common arthritis of the hip. Pain is gradual in onset, relieved by rest, and often accompanied by a limp.
- The femoral head is the most common site of ischemic necrosis. Ischemic necrosis of the femoral head is often bilateral.
- MRI is the most useful diagnostic procedure for ischemic necrosis of the hip or knee. Radiographs are normal or nonspecific early in the course.
- Trochanteric bursitis is the most common cause of lateral hip pain. Underlying hip joint or lumbar spine disease may coexist.
- Meralgia paresthetica (entrapment neuropathy of the lateral femoral cutaneous nerve) causes burning pain in the anterior lateral thigh.
- Osteoarthritis of the knee is one of the most common causes of lower extremity disability. Management is by analgesics, weight loss, modification of activities, physical therapy, and ultimately total knee arthroplasty.
- Patellofemoral pain syndrome is a common cause of anterior knee pain in young adults. Quadriceps strengthening and avoidance of marked knee-flexion activities are important in management.
- Eighty percent of cases of pigmented villonodular synovitis occur in the knee. Brown, serosanguineous synovial fluid is characteristic.
- Achilles tendonitis is commonly caused by athletic overuse or spondyloarthropathies, such as Reiter's syndrome.
- Morton's neuroma causes plantar forefoot pain in the second or third metatarsal interspaces and is usually seen in women.
- Tarsal tunnel syndrome causes poorly localized plantar foot pain.

Table 1
Differential Diagnosis of Hip Pain

Anterior/inguinal pain
  Hip joint
  Groin pull
  Inguinal hernia
  Inguinal adenopathy
  Meralgia paresthetica (anterior/lateral pain)
Lateral hip pain
  Trochanteric bursitis
Posterior hip pain
  Referred lumbosacral pain
  Sacroiliac joint inflammation or infection
  Myofascial pain
  Ischial bursitis
  Hamstring strain

HIP PAIN

• Localization of hip pain determines the differential diagnosis.

Patients typically describe any pain in the general area of the pelvic girdle as "hip" pain. The differential diagnosis varies for pain localizing to the anterior hip or inguinal area, the lateral hip area, or the posterior or gluteal area (Table 1). Hip joint pain is typically referred to the inguinal area or the anterior thigh, although pain referred to the sciatic area or to the knee also occurs. Lateral hip pain usually is due to involvement of periarticular soft tissue and is typically called "trochanteric bursitis."

Hip Joint Pain/Articular Disease

Osteoarthritis of the Hip

Osteoarthritis is the most common articular disease of the hip in adults. Onset is usually gradual with a dull aching pain exacerbated by activities and relieved by rest. Stiffness after activity (morning stiffness or gelling after rest) is usually brief, lasting only a few minutes at most early in the course of disease, and is helpful in distinguishing osteoarthritis from inflammatory arthritis. In inflammatory arthritis, morning stiffness typically lasts 1 h or more. Gradual loss of range of motion is typical of osteoarthritis and should be distinguished from reversible stiffness after inactivity, which, if prolonged, suggests inflammatory arthritis. Symptoms of cracking or crepitation are common. A limp is frequent and often is first apparent to the patient. On examination there is a loss of range of motion, initially limitation of internal rotation, followed by progressive limitation of flexion and extension. Radiographs show asymmetric joint space narrowing and sclerosis of the weight-bearing portion of the joint, in contrast to the diffuse joint space narrowing and lesser degrees of sclerosis seen in inflammatory arthritis. Management is with rest and analgesics with physical therapy for range of motion and muscle

Table 2
Clinical Associations of Osteonecrosis

Trauma
  Femoral neck fracture, hip dislocation
Drugs
  Corticosteroids and cytotoxic drug
Alcohol
Barotrauma/decompression sickness
Rheumatic diseases
  Systemic lupus
  Rheumatoid arthritis
  Systemic vasculitis
  Gout
Hemoglobinopathy
Hyperlipidemias
Pancreatitis

strengthening exercises. Weight loss is important in the obese patient but is difficult due to the limitation of activity. A water exercise program may be helpful. A cane held in the contralateral hand is often of benefit. For more advanced disease, a total hip arthroplasty is highly effective. The most significant limitation of total hip arthroplasty is the limited life-span of the implant *(1,2)*.

Hip involvement is common in inflammatory polyarthritis such as rheumatoid arthritis and the spondyloarthropathies. Management is the underlying management of the inflammatory arthritis with the addition of the physical measures mentioned for osteoarthritis. Hip involvement is rare in gout but relatively common in calcium pyrophosphate deposition arthropathy.

Ischemic Necrosis of the Hip

The femoral head is the most frequent site of osteonecrosis. In the lower extremities, osteonecrosis also occurs at the knee either in the distal femur or the proximal tibia. Conditions associated with osteonecrosis (Table 2) are varied. The most common association is with corticosteroid therapy. Ischemic necrosis of the femoral head is frequently bilateral so that, when this diagnosis is made, early lesions should be sought in the contralateral hip as well as in the knees and shoulders. Management of osteonecrosis is most successful in the early stages. Unfortunately, ischemic necrosis is often asymptomatic in early stages. The first symptom to develop is pain, which may be abrupt in onset and is usually exacerbated by activities. Early in the course, radiographs are normal and gradually develop only nonspecific osteopenia. Eventually, subcortical lucencies or cysts develop, followed by collapse of the subcortical bone forming the so-called crescent sign. Radionuclide bone scan will show avascular areas or increased uptake related to new bone formation and may be useful for screening for ischemic necrosis in multiple sites. The most useful diagnostic procedure is MRI, a sensitive indicator for early stages of ischemic necrosis. Management for early stages of osteonecrosis of the hip consists of limitation of weight bearing, physical therapy, and analgesics. Core decompression of the involved area will decrease pain and frequently slow the progression of the process in early stages. In more advanced cases in which collapse of the femoral head has begun, total hip arthroplasty is the treatment of choice *(3)*.

Bursitis

Trochanteric Bursitis

Trochanteric bursitis is the most common cause of lateral hip pain and is among the most frequent causes of hip pain in middle-aged and older individuals. Pain is prominent at the lateral hip and may radiate somewhat down the lateral thigh. It is often brought on by exercise but may also be noted during sleep, while lying on the trochanteric area. Localized tenderness in the trochanteric area generally somewhat posterior to the trochanteric is characteristic. Trochanteric bursitis frequently coexists with underlying hip joint disease, degenerative disease of the lumbar spine, or radiculopathy so that these entities should be looked for during the examination. Pain of trochanteric bursitis is usually exacerbated by resisted external rotation or abduction of the hip. Treatment consists of modification of activities on a temporary basis and stretching and strengthening exercises for the gluteal muscles, as well as weight loss if appropriate. Nonsteroidal anti-inflammatory drugs are helpful. Corticosteroid injection with local anesthetic into the tender areas is effective. However, recurrences are common *(4)*.

Ischial Bursitis

Ischial bursitis ("Weaver's bottom" or "student's bottom") is usually caused by direct trauma or prolonged sitting and is sometimes seen in cyclists. Pain is in the lower buttock or posterior thigh. Tenderness is present over the ischial tuberosity. Treatment is the avoidance of prolonged sitting or padding the seating surface. Nonsteroidals or a local corticosteroid injection may be helpful.

Meralgia Paraesthetica

Meralgia paresthetica is a syndrome of burning pain, paresthesias, and numbness of the anterior lateral thigh caused by an entrapment neuropathy of the lateral femoral cutaneous nerve at the inguinal ligament. It is most frequently seen in obese patients, in pregnancy, or in diabetes. It may also be precipitated by a constricting corset or belt. Sensation may be limited in the anterior lateral thigh on examination. Palpation of the inguinal ligament at the anterior superior iliac spine may provoke pain. These findings may be absent, and a diagnosis based on symptoms must be made. Treatment is weight reduction, avoidance of constricting garments, or appropriate padding. Occasionally, a corticosteroid injection at the area of compression near the anterior superior iliac spine may be helpful. Surgical decompression is rarely necessary *(5)*.

KNEE PAIN

Arthritis of the Knee

Arthritic involvement of the knee joint is very common, with osteoarthritis of the knee being most common in older adults. Along with osteoarthritis of the hip, that of the knee is one of the most common causes of lower extremity disabilities. Inflammatory arthritides, including rheumatoid arthritis, and the seronegative arthritides, such as Reiter's syndrome and psoriatic arthritis, also frequently affect the knee. Both gout and pseudogout produce acute arthritic episodes within the knee. The differential diagnosis of the inflammatory arthritides is noted in Chapters 4 and 10. As in the hip, osteoarthritis of the knee is characterized by pain provoked by activity and relieved by rest. Acute inflammatory episodes may occur following minor trauma or due to an associated crystalline arthropathy. On examination, crepitus with range of motion is frequent, and flexion contractures occur as disease progresses. Radiographically, joint space loss is usually asymmetrical, involving one compartment more than the others; typically, the medial compartment is the most involved. Disproportionate or isolated involvement of the patellofemoral compartment suggests CPPD arthropathy. As in the hip, management is by weight loss and modification of weight-bearing activities. The use of a cane, usually in the opposite hand, may be helpful. Walking and running exercises can be replaced by a swimming program. Analgesics or nonsteroidal anti-inflammatory drugs, and quadriceps strengthening and range-of-motion exercises are appropriate. Total knee arthroplasty is indicated when conservative treatment fails (6).

Patellofemoral Pain

Anterior Knee Pain or Patellofemoral Pain

Anterior knee pain or patellofemoral pain is very common and often occurs in younger individuals. A variety of abnormalities of patellofemoral architecture may contribute. Symptomatically, the pain may be vaguely described initially, but this is generally anterior in distribution. Clicking and popping are usually noted by the patient, particularly when climbing or descending stairs, which typically increases pain. Prolonged sitting may also exacerbate pain. Crepitus is present on examination by palpating the patella during flexion and extension of the knee. Pain can be elicited by patellar compression against the femur or resistance of patellar contraction during knee extension. Most patients have minimal radiographic changes of the patellofemoral joint. Conservative treatment includes avoidance of activities associated with marked knee flexion, such as deep knee bends. Quadriceps strengthening exercises in extension are important. Nonsteroidal anti-inflammatory drugs or analgesics can be used. A patellar brace or strap may be helpful. Excessive tightness in the quadriceps or hamstring muscles should be corrected during the rehabilitation program. Failure to respond to a conservative rehabilitation program indicates consideration of surgical debridement and/or realignment of the patella (7).

Bursitis and Tendonitis with the Knee Region

Anserine Bursitis

The anserine bursa is located in the medial aspect of the knee, approx 3–4 cm below the joint line between the medial collateral ligament and the tendons of the sartorius, gracilis, and semitendinosus muscles. This is a common cause of medial knee pain in middle aged or older individuals and is often associated with underlying osteoarthritis, obesity, and valgus deformities of the knees. On examination, there is tenderness over the area of the bursa. Management includes activity modification, stretching exercises of the quadriceps and adductor muscles, and nonsteroidal inflammatory agents or corticosteroid injection locally *(8)*.

Prepatellar Bursitis

Prepatellar bursitis causes swelling superficial to the distal half of the patella and is usually due to local trauma such as frequent kneeling. Traumatic bursitis must be distinguished from septic bursitis, which is generally associated with overlying erythema, warmth, and marked tenderness. If infection is suspected, a tap of the bursa should be performed. Staphylococci are the usual organisms. Treatment of traumatic bursitis is by padding of the knee or avoidance of these activities, and analgesic or anti-inflammatory medication.

Patellar Tendonitis

Patellar tendonitis is a cause of anterior patellar pain in athletes and is usually associated with jumping and running activities. There is tenderness on examination over the patellar tendon or insertion in the tibia. Management is by rest, icing, and nonsteroidal therapy. Stretching of the quadriceps muscles and a gradual return to athletic activities with appropriate warm up is important.

Iliotibial Band Syndrome

Lateral knee pain in athletes, particularly runners, may be due to friction from tightness of the ilia tibial band. The ilia tibial band is an extension of the fascia lata, which inserts on the lateral tibia and may produce friction and pain at the lateral femoral condyle. Tenderness is present at the lateral femoral condyle on examination. Treatment is with rest, ice and stretching of the hip abductors *(9)*.

Pigmented Villonodular Synovitis

Pigmented villonodular synovitis is a monoarticular proliferative process of the synovium, considered to be a benign tumor of the synovium. Young adults are most commonly affected and 80% of cases occur in the knee. There is insidious onset of swelling and pain with dark brown or serosanguineous synovial fluid obtained on joint aspiration. Arthroscopy and/or synovial biopsy are diagnostic. Treatment is by total synovectomy. However, recurrences are common. Differential diagnosis of hemorrhagic joint fluid includes trauma, coagulopathies or iatrogenic overanticoagulation, and other tumors *(10)*.

ANKLE AND FOOT PAIN

Ankle Arthritis

Osteoarthritis of the ankle is relatively common in older adults, particularly in the presence of prior trauma, instability, or occupational risk, such as in dancers. Inflammatory arthropathies commonly involve the ankle, including rheumatoid arthritis, the seronegative spondylorthropathies, and crystal-induced arthritis. The ankle is particularly commonly involved in gout. In osteoarthritis, pain is typically exacerbated by

Table 3
Causes of Achilles Tendonitis

Athletic overuse
Trauma
Reiter's syndrome
Ankylosing spondylitis
Psoriatic arthritis
Rheumatoid arthritis
Gout
Calcium pyrophosphate deposition disease
Heel cord contractures

weight-bearing and relieved by rest, and generalized swelling of the ankle is present. Instability should be looked for. Arthrocentesis for synovial analysis and radiographs are useful diagnostically. The ankle is aspirated by the dorsal approach at the joint line medial to the extensor hallucis longus. In addition to appropriate anti-inflammatory therapy, supportive well-cushioned shoes are important. Bracing is useful if instability is present.

Achilles Tendonitis

Pain in the region of the Achilles tendon may be due to a number of causes (Table 3). Running and athletic activities are among the most common causes, generally associated with less local inflammation than tendonitis seen in Reiter's syndrome and the spondyloarthropathies. Fluoroquinilone antibiotics (e.g., norfloxacin) may be associated with the development of Achilles tendonitis or Achilles tendon rupture. Fluoroquinilone antibiotic treatment should be discontinued in any patient who develops Achilles tendon inflammation *(11)*. Calcaneal spurs with new periosteal bone formation and fluffy calcifications may be seen both at the Achilles insertion and at the plantar fascial insertion in Reiter's syndrome. Management consists of nonsteroidal anti-inflammatory drugs, rest, and gradual stretching exercises. Heel lifts are useful. Since the Achilles tendon is subject to rupture, corticosteroid injections are used infrequently *(12)*.

Achilles Tendon Rupture

Achilles tendon rupture may occur during exercise in middle-aged and older individuals. The patient may report a sensation of snapping or an object striking the back of the leg, followed by difficulty in walking or standing on the toes. On examination, local swelling is generally present. A palpable tendon defect may be seen but is not always present. Rupture can be confirmed by ultrasound or MRI. Treatment is by immobilization and/or surgical repair *(13)*.

Plantar Fasciitis (Plantar Heel Pain)

Plantar heel pain is far more commonly caused by mechanical factors than inflammatory arthritis. Plantar fasciitis due to inflammatory arthritis is most common in Reiter's

Table 4
Causes of Metatarsalgia

Hallux valgus
Hallux rigidus
Stress fracture of the metatarsal or sesamoid bones
Rheumatoid arthritis or other inflammatory arthritis of the metatarsophalangeal joints
Prolonged standing or walking
Wearing of high-heeled shoes
Morton's neuroma
Gout (acute episodes)

syndrome and other spondyloarthropathies. Periosteal calcifications or erosions at the insertion of the plantar fascia may be seen in Reiter's syndrome. Inflammation of the plantar fascia due to injury or overuse is common in runners and dancers and is seen in older individuals with less vigorous activities. Pain is present at the plantar aspect of the heel with weight-bearing activity, and localized tenderness is usually present. In older individuals, calcaneal spurs are often present and are usually not directly responsible for symptoms. Obesity and pes planus are additional risk factors. Management includes analgesics or nonsteroidal anti-inflammatory drugs for a short period and the use of a viscoelastic heel pad or a heel cup. Calf and heel cord stretching exercises are very important and probably the most useful long-term measure. Correcting any foot deformities present with appropriate arch supports is useful, as is weight loss in the obese patient *(14)*.

Metatarsalgia

Metatarsalgia or forefoot pain may be caused by a wide variety of conditions, many of which are related to trauma or structural abnormalities of the foot (Table 4). Most of these conditions are associated with gradual onset of pain precipitated by walking or exercise and relieved by rest. Gout is the exception with very acute, inflammatory episodes of pain, typically in the first metatarsophalangeal (MTP) joint with asymptomatic intervals. Rheumatoid arthritis generally involve all of the MTP joints with significant morning stiffness. Symmetrical polyarthritis elsewhere is generally present. However, rheumatoid arthritis may present with a forefoot pain or a bunion pain. A single, diffusely swollen toe (sausage digit) is suggestive of Reiter's syndrome or other spondyloarthropathy. Hallux valgus, the lateral deviation of the first toe at the MTP joint, is among the most common causes of forefoot pain and is often exacerbated by inappropriate shoe wear. Underlying degenerative disease may lead to hallux rigidus. Sesamoiditis or stress fractures of the sesamoid bones are particularly common in dancers.

Appropriate modifications of shoes are crucial to adequate management of forefoot pain. Shoes with correct fit and adequate room in the metatarsal area are important. Unloading the metatarsal region by metatarsal bars added to the sole of the shoe behind the metatarsal heads or padded shoe inserts are helpful. Weight loss in the obese patient, avoidance of high-heeled shoes, and modification of activities are also important. Surgical therapy may be required when conservative measures are unsuccessful *(15)*.

Morton's Neuroma

Morton's neuroma is an entrapment neuropathy of the interdigital nerve and is a frequent cause of metatarsalgia. This syndrome is seen predominantly in women and presents as well-localized pain, usually of gradual onset involving the second and third metatarsal interspaces. Pain may be burning or aching and radiate into the third or fourth toe. It is exacerbated by wearing tight shoes, particularly high heels, or walking on hard surfaces. Pain is relieved by rest and removing the shoes. Plantar palpation of the intermetatarsal spaces reveals tenderness in the involved interspace. This should be distinguished from tenderness at the metatarsophalangeal joint, which is more suggestive of joint involvement. Lateral pressure on the metatarsophalangeal joints while the interspace is palpated will often reproduce the symptoms. Conservative treatment is with a low-heeled shoe of adequate width with a metatarsal pad placed proximally to the tender area. Nonsteroidal anti-inflammatory drugs or a corticosteroid injection into the interspace may be helpful. Surgical excision of the neuroma is indicated when these measures are unsuccessful *(16)*.

Tarsal Tunnel Syndrome

Tarsal tunnel syndrome is a compression neuropathy of the posterior tibial nerve in the tarsal tunnel formed by the distal tibia and the flexor retinaculum behind the medial malleolus. This syndrome may be precipitated by trauma such as a severe ankle sprain or a distal tibial fracture, by tenosynovitis of the flexor tendon, inflammatory synovitis as in rheumatoid arthritis, or space occupying lesions such as ganglions or synovial cysts within the tarsal tunnel. The patient presents with burning pain and paresthesias in the plantar aspect of the foot, which, in distinction from Morton's neuroma, is not well-localized. Symptoms are exacerbated by activity and relieved by rest, although night pain and paresthesia are common, as in carpal tunnel syndrome. Percussion or palpation along the course of the posterior tibial nerve may reproduce symptoms. Sensory nerve loss in the plantar aspect of the foot is often unreliable. Diagnosis is confirmed by nerve conduction study. MRI is useful for imaging the tarsal tunnel, particularly when surgical treatment is being considered. Conservative treatment consists of appropriate footwear or orthotics to correct pronation or a valgus hindfoot deformity. A nonsteroidal anti-inflammatory or local corticosteroid injection into the tarsal tunnel area may be helpful. Surgical decompression of the tarsal tunnel is most successful when a specific lesion can be identified preoperatively *(16)*.

REFERENCES

1. Dieppe P. Management of hip osteoarthritis. Brit Med J 1995; 311(7009): 853–857.
2. Quinet RJ, Winters EG. Total joint replacement of the hip and knee. Med Clin N Amer 1992; 76(5): 1235–1251.
3. Mankin HJ. Non-traumatic necrosis of bone (osteonecrosis). N Engl J Med 1992; 326: 1437–1439.
4. Shbeeb MI, Matteson EL. Trochanteric bursitis. Mayo Clin Proc 1996; 71: 565–569.
5. Wiezer MJ, Franssen H, Rinkel GJ, Wokke JH. Meralgia paraesthetica: differential diagnosis and follow-up. Muscle and Nerve 1996; 19(4): 522–524.
6. Massardo L, Watt I, Cushnaghan J, Dieppe P. Osteoarthritis of the knee joint: an eight year prospective study. Ann Rheum Dis 1989; 48: 833–897.

7. Tria AJ, Palumbo RC, Alicia JA. Conservative care for patellofemoral pain. Orthop Clin N Amer 1992; 23: 545–554.

8. Butcher JD, Salzman KL, Lillegard WA. Lower extremity bursitis. J Am Fam Physic 1996; 53: 2317–2324.

9. Barber FA, Sutker AN. Iliotibial band syndrome. Sports Medicine 1992; 14(2): 144–148.

10. Myers BW, Masi AT, Feigenbaum SL. Pigmented villonodular synovitis and tenosynovitis. Med 1980; 59: 223–238.

11. McGarvey WC, Singh D, Trevino SG. Partial achilles tendon ruptures associated with fluoroquinolone antibiotics: a case report and literature review. Foot and Ankle International 1996; 17(8): 496–498.

12. Hunter SC, Poole RM. The chronically inflamed tendon. Clinics in Sports Medicine 1987; 6: 371–388.

13. Hattrup SJ, Johnson KA. A review of ruptures of the achilles tendon. Foot and Ankle 1985; 6(1): 34–38.

14. Hurwitz SR. Heel pain in the adult. Bull Rheum Dis 1996; 45: 1–3.

15. Gould JS. Metatarsalgia. Ortho Clin N Amer 1989; 20(4): 553–562.

16. Mann RA. Nerve entrapment syndromes. The Foot and Ankle Syndrome, Part II. In: Szabo RM, ed. Nerve Compression Syndrome's Diagnosis and Treatment. Slack, 1989; 293–308.

10 MUSCULOSKELETAL PAIN

RICHARD H. WHITE, MD

Key Points

- The key to diagnosing an articular or periarticular process is the physical examination.
- The symptoms of fibromyalgia may suggest a polyarthritis, but physical examination reveals numerous tender points and no synovitis.
- In patients with a monoarticular arthritis, examination of the joint fluid is critically important, particularly in making a diagnosis of septic arthritis and crystal induced arthritis.
- A positive ANA test or an elevated RF titer often leads to an inappropriate diagnosis of systemic lupus erythematosus or rheumatoid arthritis.
- The diagnosis of polymyalgia rheumatica is based on the history and clinical findings. An elevated ESR only increases the probability that PMR is present.
- Paget's disease is commonly present in asymptomatic individuals who have a markedly elevated serum alkaline phosphatase level.
- The pain of osteomalacia is dull and difficult to localize. The bones most commonly affected are the pelvis and vertebrae in the low back.
- The diagnosis of a vertebral compression fracture should be considered in any postmenopausal woman who presents with sudden onset of mid-back pain, particularly a thin Caucasian woman who is not on replacement estrogen therapy.
- In patients with symptomatic osteoporosis, treatment to enhance bone formation should be started using oral calcium, vitamin D, estrogen replacement in women, and, in selected cases, either nasal calcitonin or oral alendronate.

ARTHRITIS AND PERIARTICULAR PAIN

Overview

If one defines arthritis as inflammation or injury confined to a joint, the number of potential causes and the spectrum of symptoms associated with these processes is extremely large. Mild degenerative arthritis may cause minimal stiffness that improves with motion, without any pain. On the other extreme, an acute septic joint or acute gout may cause excruciating pain with minimal or no motion at all *(1)*.

There is no strict definition of what constitutes a "periarticular disease." The term merely means that the cause of the problem originates in tissues adjacent to a joint. Suffice it to say that these structures, which include ligaments, bursae, tendons, and connective tissue, may be inflamed or injured, causing pain that is felt by the patient to be "in the joint." Examples include acute subacromial bursitis (shoulder pain) and a strained medial collateral ligament of the knee (knee pain).

There are no characteristics of arthritic or periarticular pain *per se* that can allow the clinician to make a prompt, accurate diagnosis in each case! Pain in or around a joint certainly suggests that an articular or periarticular problem may be present, but occasionally the symptoms may be referred from within the joint or from a more distant site. Shoulder pain, for example, may be caused by cholecystitis, a trigger-point process or cervical nerve-root entrapment without any shoulder pathology.

- The key to diagnosing an articular or periarticular process is the physical examination.
- Historical information its certainly very important, but it must always be interpreted in light of physical examination findings.
- Thus, when evaluating a patient complaining of joint pain, it is wise to expeditiously proceed early to an initial examination of the symptomatic region(s).

Such an examination may allow a prompt diagnosis, such as the presence of a trigger finger, or at least allow a more focused approach when completing the history.

Evaluation of the Patient

History

The historical information that is most helpful in making a diagnosis includes the following:

1. The location of the painful joint(s) or periarticular process.
2. The duration and temporal pattern of the pain.
3. The essential demographic information (age, gender, ethnic background).
4. Any history of local injury.
5. The family history.
6. The occupational and sports history.
7. A social history.

The number of causes of arthritis and arthritis-like pain is large, which prohibits extensive discussion of the historical and physical examination characteristic of each disorder. However, it is clear that a history of recent injury increases the likelihood that one is dealing with a traumatic orthopedic problem. Morning stiffness that gradually improves over 30 min to several hours is characteristic of inflammatory arthritis, whereas individuals with osteoarthritis complain of severe pain and stiffness that lasts for just a few moments (gelling phenomenon), followed by low-grade or moderate pain that persists for the remainder of the day. Movement of the joint(s) causing the greatest degree of pain suggests an inflammatory process, as does the gradual increase in the number of affected joints.

Physical Examination

A detailed examination is of paramount importance in making an accurate diagnosis. The key questions that need to be addressed are:

- Is the site of pain confined to the joints, or is it a periarticular process?
- Is there pain in a single joint/region, or is more than one joint/region affected?
- Is inflammation present? Specifically, is there synovitis (tender, palpable synovium, or joint effusion).
- What are the ancillary findings, both locally and systemically?

Unfortunately, some joints are covered by layers of muscle, such as the hip joint and vertebral facet joints, making it impossible to directly palpate these joints. Information can be obtained by assessing range of motion as well as local tenderness.

The following are some examples of how the physical finding can focus the differential diagnosis. A patient may present with pain in the wrist. Careful examination may reveal tenderness confined only to the radial aspect, together with other findings characteristic of tendinitis of the abductor pollicis longus (De Quervain's tenosynovitis). In this particular example, a history of occupational stress, such as playing the harp, strongly suggests a diagnosis of traumatic tenosynovitis, while recent unprotected intercourse with a new partner may suggest gonococcal tenosynovitis.

- Determining if the painful process is focal versus multifocal is extremely important.

For example, the differential diagnosis of a single inflamed ankle is different from an inflamed ankle together with an inflamed knee and proximal interphalangeal joint. Similarly, if symmetrical polyarthritis is detected, the differential diagnosis changes radically. The most common causes of monarticular arthritis and polyarticular arthritis are listed in Tables 1 and 2 (see ref. 2).

- The presence or absence of inflammation is of paramount importance in generating a differential diagnosis.

A painful first metatarsal phalangeal joint with deformity suggests a degenerative bunion, whereas if the same joint is very red, warm and tender, gout is the likely diagnosis.

- Ancillary physical findings are often critically important.

The differential diagnosis of a single, hot, swollen knee may be dramatically narrowed in the presence of other findings, such as erythema nodosum, iritis, tophi, or a local skin infection on the arm. Proximal interphalangeal joint pain with triggering of the finger on flexion makes the diagnosis of stenosing tenosynovitis.

Differential Diagnosis

Space does not permit a discussion of the differential diagnosis of all of the hundreds of causes of arthritis and periarthritis. However, differentiating an articular or periarticular disorder from a nonarticular disorder is very important. The most common causes of pain simulating "arthritis" are listed in Table 3.

Table 1
Differential Diagnosis of Monoarticular Arthritis

Acute (onset over hours)
 Septic Arthritis
  N. gonorrhea
  S. aureus
  Streptococci
  H. Influenzae
  Other: Gram-negative rods
 Gout
 Pseudogout (calcium pyrophosphate deposition disease)
 Reactive arthritis
  Reiter's syndrome
  Inflammatory bowel disease
  Acute sarcoidosis
  Acute rheumatic fever
 Spondylitis (HLA B-27 related)
 Psoriatic arthritis
 Aseptic necrosis
 Other: hemarthrosis, mechanical problem, initial manifestation of a systemic rheumatic disease, metastatic cancer, lymphoma
Subacute or chronic (onset over days)
 Infectious arthritis
  Tuberculosis
  Fungal arthritis
  Lyme arthritis
 Chronic gout
 Chronic pseudogout
 Posttraumatic degenerative arthritis
 Reactive arthritis
 Loose body, mechanical derangement
 Neuropathic arthropathy (Charcot joint)
 Pigmented villonodular synovitis
 Sarcoid arthritis

Myofascial pain syndromes are discussed in other chapters of this book. On examination there is local tenderness in muscle, often with a palpable tight band of muscle. No joint or tendon abnormalities are detected.

In cases of referred pain, examination of the painful region often reveals no local findings. However, examination of other areas of the body may point to the diagnosis. An example is knee pain in the child, which may be caused by arthritis in the hip.

Neuritic pain may be severe and localized to a joint. For example, acute brachial neuritis often feels like shoulder arthritis. Examination of the shoulder is normal, unless muscle weakness has developed.

Table 2
Differential Diagnosis
of Polyarthritis

Common causes
  Acute viral syndrome
  Rheumatoid arthritis
  Systemic lupus erythematosus
  Psoriatic arthritis
Less common causes
  Gout
  Pseudogout
  Gonococcal arthritis
  Acute rheumatic fever
  Sarcoidosis
  Systemic rheumatic diseases
    Primary Sjögren's syndrome
    Polymyositis/dermatomyositis
    Scleroderma/CREST Syndrome
    Still's disease
    Vasculitis
    Polymyalgia rheumatica
  Serum sickness
  Subacute bacterial endocarditis
  Erosive osteoarthritis

Table 3
Disorder-Stimulating Arthritis
or a Periarticular Problem

  Myofascial pain syndrome
  Referred pain
  Neuritic pain
  Fibromyalgia
  Bone pain
  Factitious pain

Fibromyalgia may feel to the patient like total body arthritis. However, physical examination of the joints is normal, and there is widespread symmetrical tenderness over multiple spots on the body.

Bone pain can be either difficult to localize or it may be very focal and mimic arthritis. An example of the latter is metastatic cancer to the acromion or humerus, which may mimic rotator cuff tendinitis. Radiographs or a bone scan may be necessary to make the proper diagnosis.

Table 4
Tests of High Specificity in the Setting of Clinically Evident Arthritis or Periarthritis

Synovial fluid
  Culture positive for bacterial, fungal, or acid-fast organisms
  Characteristic crystals seen for gout and pseudogout
Radiographs
  Osteomyelitis adjacent to septic joint
  Classic erosions of gout
  Changes of a neuropathic process (Charcot joint)
  Sarcoid changes in bone
  Lytic lesion of metastatic cancer
  Sacroiliitis in setting compatible with a spondyloarthropathy
Autoantibodies
  Anti–double-stranded DNA in a setting compatible with systemic lupus erythematosus
  Anti-Smith antibody in a setting compatible with systemic lupus erythematosus
  Anti-Scl 70 (topoisomerase I) in setting compatible with scleroderma
  Antineutrophil cytoplasmic antibody (c-ANCA) in setting compatible with Wegener's
    granulomatosis
  Anticentromere antibody in setting compatible with CREST syndrome

Diagnostic Tests

- For most focal disorders, involving one joint or one periarticular region, the clinical findings alone are often sufficient to make a diagnosis.
- However, in patients with a monoarticular arthritis, examination of the joint fluid is critically important, particularly in making a diagnosis of septic joint (culture, white blood cell count, and Gram stain), or a crystal-induced arthritis.

Radiographs may help if certain classic findings are present, but findings are often nonspecific. A blood chemistry panel, a complete blood count, and a urinalysis are indicated if one suspects any systemic disorder. A myriad of tests are available that may aid in excluding or making a diagnosis of one of the systemic rheumatic diseases, particularly tests for various autoantibodies.

- It must be stressed that, because many immunologic tests are nonspecific (e.g., screening ANA, complement tests, rheumatoid factor, and the erythrocyte sedimentation rate), a positive result by itself does not make a diagnosis.

Tests that do have high specificity and that are useful in making specific diagnoses are listed in Table 4.

Treatment

The treatment of an arthritis or periarthritis depends on the etiology. A simple outline of the most commonly used treatments for osteoarthritis, rheumatoid arthritis, and spondylitis or reactive arthritis is shown in Table 5. An infectious processes is treated with antibiotics, whereas a variety of locally injected or systemic anti-inflammatory

Table 5
Treatment of Osteoarthritis, Rheumatoid Arthritis, and Spondylitis (Reactive Arthritis)

Osteoarthritis	Rheumatoid Arthritis	Spondylitis, Reactive Arthritis
Acetaminophen 3–4 g/d in divided doses, with or without nonsteroidal treatment	Nonsteroidal anti-inflammatory drugs	Nonsteroidal anti-inflammatory drugs, with misoprostol 100 µg tid if at high risk for gastrointestinal bleeding
Nonsteroidal anti-inflammatory drugs, with misoprostol 100 µg tid if at high risk for gastrointestinal bleeding	Disease modifying agents Methotrexate, 7.5–20 mg once weekly Hydroxychloroquine, 400 mg/d Sulfasalazine 2–4 g/d (divided)	Sulfasalazine 2–4 g/d, particularly for peripheral arthritis in patients with Reiter's or psoriasis
Physical therapy, use of cane, and so on	Low-dose prednisone, 5–7.5 mg/d	Physical and occupational therapy, proper posturing, and so on
Orthopedic surgery, joint replacement	Other drugs: Parenteral gold D-penicillamine Cyclosporine, 2.5 mg/kg Oral cyclophosphamide Physical and occupational therapy Orthopedic surgery, joint replacement surgery	

agents are used for most cases of arthritis, and physical therapy with or without surgery is useful in the remaining cases.

FIBROMYALGIA

Definition

Fibromyalgia is a syndrome of unknown etiology that is characterized by:

1. Widespread pain felt by the patient to be in the joints or soft tissues adjacent to joints, usually with associated stiffness and fatigue, with;
2. Widespread tenderness on palpation of soft tissues, with specific areas characteristically affected (see below); and
3. Nonrestorative or nonrefreshing sleep, with pain, fatigue, and stiffness notably present after arising.

American College of Rheumatology criteria for classification of fibromyalgia are listed in Table 6 (3). This syndrome occurs in 2–5% of patients followed by primary care

Table 6
American College of Rheumatology Criteria for Classification of Fibromyalgia

History of widespread pain (present in all of the following sites):
 Right and left sides of the body, including shoulders and buttocks
 Above and below the waist
 In the axial skeleton (cervical spine or anterior chest, thoracic spine or low back)
Pain on digital palpation (performed with about 4 kg of force) in 11 of the following
   18 points (one point on each side):
 Occiput: at suboccipital muscle insertions
 Low cervical: at anterior aspects of intertransverse spaces at C5-C7
 Trapezius: at midpoint of upper borders
 Supraspinatus: at origins, above scapula spine near medial border
 Second rib: at second costochondral junctions, just lateral to junctions on upper surfaces
 Lateral epicondyle: 2 cm distal to epicondyle
 Gluteal: in upper outer quadrants of buttocks in anterior fold of muscle
 Greater trochanter: posterior to trochanteric prominence
 Knee: at medial fat pad proximal to joint line

providers and occurs in up to 20% of referrals to rheumatology and pain clinics. Over 80% of affected individuals are women, and most are between the ages of 30 and 55 yr. The separation of fibromyalgia into "primary" (without associated disease) and "secondary" (if there is an underlying disease) categories is not particularly useful. The clinician must decide if pain and widespread tenderness are disproportionate to the physical findings associated with the underlying disease (such as osteoarthritis).

Because patients rarely, if ever, present with the complaint of, "I think I have fibromyalgia," it behooves any practitioner to become familiar with this syndrome lest patients be inappropriately diagnosed as having a systemic rheumatic disease, like rheumatoid arthritis.

Evaluation of the Patient

History

The severity of fibromyalgia pain spans a wide spectrum, from modest to severe and incapacitating. Minimal efforts, such as walking or doing routine activities, may cause disabling pain that interferes and even prevents completion of simple tasks (4). The pain is most often described as a chronic aching pain that is deep in the tissues and that is invariably made worse by direct palpation. Other major features are fatigue and poor sleep, with considerable pain and fatigue on awakening (see Table 7) (5).

- Although the pain is described as being unrelenting and disabling, patients with fibromyalgia do not appear to be experiencing severe pain during the course of the interview.
- Although they often appear moderately depressed and uncomfortable, there is a striking disparity between the clinically apparent intensity of the pain and the subjective level of the pain.

Table 7
Principal Findings in Patients with Fibromyalgia

Historical

Widespread pain, often attributed to the "joints"

Poor "nonrestorative" sleep; awaken tired and not refreshed

General fatigue, which may be profound

Moderately depressed mood, some are very anxious

Aggravation by cold air, stress, and poor sleep

Nothing seems to help the pain, particularly nonsteroidal anti-inflammatory agents

Description of pain disproportionate to apparent level of pain during the interview

Physical examination

Diffuse, symmetric tender points

Skin-roll tenderness over the trapezius with wincing and withdrawal

Absence of inflamed joints

Absence of a specific trigger-point

Asked to rate the level of pain on a scale of 0–10 points (where 0 is no pain and 10 is the most severe pain the patient has ever experienced in his or her entire life), most patients rate the pain as >5, and many patients rate the pain as high as 9 or 10! Many studies have documented that patients with fibromyalgia have a lower threshold for pain. This has led some researchers in the field to call fibromyalgia a disorder characterized by pain amplification.

Although the intensity of the pain of fibromyalgia appears to be excessive or exaggerated, the symptoms are clearly very real. Not only are descriptions of the pain and associated symptoms remarkably similar between individuals, but even otherwise healthy individuals experience the symptoms of fibromyalgia after sleep deprivation for longer than 24 h, particularly the fatigue, muscle stiffness, and pain in and about the region of the neck, shoulders, and scapular regions. Whereas symptoms abate after sleep in the average individual, patients with fibromyalgia rarely experience dramatic improvement in their symptoms.

- Initially, patients with fibromyalgia tend to localize their pain to:

  1. The lower back region;
  2. The neck and scapular region; or
  3. Multiple joints.

Careful questioning and physical examination disclose that the pain and tenderness are widespread.

- The pain of fibromyalgia is generally worse:

  1. When exposed to cold drafts of air;
  2. During times of more intense emotional stress; and
  3. After a night of poor sleep.

Exercise or stretching may improve or worsen the pain. Nothing uniformly helps all patients with fibromyalgia.

- A majority of patients admit to either feeling depressed, having previous depression, or having excessive anxiety.

However, overt major psychiatric illness is not a typical feature. Whether the depressed affect is a result rather than the cause of the pain remains unanswered.

Physical Examination

The characteristic and necessary physical findings are: diffuse, symmetric tenderness in specific regions of the body (*see* Table 4), together with the absence of any objective evidence for injury or synovitis.

An effort should be made to apply approximately the same amount of pressure to each area in each patient. The tenderness is usually felt in the immediate area that is palpated. This pattern of local pain in many locations stands in contrast to myofascial trigger-point pain, which produces a zone of electric-like radiated pain extending away from a specific single contact point. The local tenderness of fibromyalgia over the body is so striking, and so specific, that a brief physical examination of classically affected areas is recommended during the initial interview in all patients with diffuse joint pains. The presence of characteristic findings of fibromyalgia allow the physician the opportunity to ask certain questions that might not otherwise come to mind, such as the quality of sleep, level of fatigue, presence of psychiatric symptoms, and effect of cold drafty air.

Early criteria for fibromyalgia were proposed by Smythe (Bulletin of Rheumatic Disease 28:928-931, 1977). He found:

- Characteristic local tenderness over the midpoint of the trapezius while rolling the skin. This remains a very useful test.

One gently picks up a 1-in. fold of skin over the upper third of the scapula with both hands and then moves the source (or rolls) the skin-fold cephalad over the trapezius muscle by picking up new skin on the leading edge and leaving skin on the trailing edge of the roll. A normal individual experiences little or no pain, whereas more sensitive patients can have a gradient of responses from: (1) mild discomfort, to (2) irritating pain, to (3) pain leading to wincing, to (4) severe pain and pulling away form the examiner. The latter two responses are commonly noted in patients with fibromyalgia.

Differential Diagnosis

- There are no serious systemic disorders that mimic fibromyalgia.

Nevertheless, symptoms of diffuse joint pain or diffuse bone pain or widespread stiffness are seen in a variety of other disorders, which may arouse the suspicion of fibromyalgia. However, the major feature that distinguishes fibromyalgia from other disorders, namely widespread areas of tenderness, including skin-roll tenderness, is generally lacking in patients with these other disorders. Table 8 lists disorders that may transiently be considered in a patient with widespread pain. It should be stressed that patients with the chronic fatigue syndrome may have fibromyalgia as well.

- Symptoms and objective findings should always be the driving force in making any medical diagnosis, particularly a rheumatic disease.

Table 8
Distinguishing Features of Disorders Associated with Widespread Pain

Polymyalgia rheumatica: principally occurs in individuals over the age of 60; rather precipitous onset of stiffness in the shoulder and pelvic girdle; absence of skin and soft-tissue tenderness

Myofascial pain syndromes: local soft-tissue problems with trigger-point pain; symmetrical involvement very atypical

Diffuse arthritis: joints are warm, swollen, and tender; areas that are characteristically tender in patients with fibromyalgia are unaffected

Bone pain of osteomalacia, multiple myeloma, hyperparathyroidism: aching pain, greater in some bones than others, with absence of local tenderness in soft tissues

In patients meeting criteria for fibromyalgia, screening for rheumatic disease by ordering nonspecific tests, such as a screening ANA, RF, and ESR, should be avoided unless there are signs or symptoms suggesting a rheumatic disease. This is because a false-positive test is much more likely than a true-positive test in a patient with a low probability of having a systemic rheumatic disease. Rheumatologists are deluged with referrals of patients with fibromyalgia who happened to have a low titer ANA or modestly elevated ESR.

- A positive ANA test or an elevated RF titer often leads to the inappropriate diagnosis of systemic lupus erythematosus or rheumatoid arthritis.

Unfortunately, patients frequently latch on these diagnoses, because they "explain their symptoms." It is appropriate to order tests that can be readily interpreted, such as a complete blood count, urinalysis, chemistry panel, and thyroid-stimulating hormone level. Skeletal radiographs may be appropriate when there are signs of osteoarthritis together with fibromyalgia.

Treatment

- There is no known effective medical treatment for fibromyalgia.

Some medications nonspecifically lessen symptoms. Indeed, treatment of this condition with unknown pathogenesis is so ineffective that physicians should avoid assuming the role of taking primary responsibility for controlling the pain and associated symptoms. A better model is one in which the doctor assumes the role of a "coach," leaving the primary responsibility of "working out" or "discovering" the means of reducing symptoms to the patient. As the coach, the physician can support the patient and make suggestions, such as trying different types of physical exercise and trying various methods to reduce stress.

Medications that may help alleviate some of the symptoms nonspecifically downmodulate pain. These include:

- Amitriptyline, which, when given in low doses of 10–50 mg each evening at bedtime, may help 30–40% of patients initially, with diminution of response over time.
- Cyclobenzaprine, 10–30 mg/d.

Nonmedical treatments may be equally or more efficacious compared to analgesic or tricyclic antidepressant treatment. Exercise, particularly cardiovascular fitness training, may be of some benefit. Biofeedback training may also be useful in selected patients.

POLYMYALGIA RHEUMATICA

Definition

Polymyalgia rheumatica (PMR) is a condition characterized by rather abrupt onset of significant stiffness and aching, particularly in the shoulder and hip girdle regions in individuals over the age of 50 yr, and especially over the age of 65 yr *(6)*. In greater than 90% of cases, the Westergren erythrocyte sedimentation rate is elevated above 50 mm in the first hour. It may be a manifestation of giant-cell arteritis, and it shares features with elderly onset rheumatoid arthritis *(7,8)*.

Evaluation of the Patient

History

Patients with PMR give a characteristic history of:

- Rather abrupt onset over several days to weeks of significant muscle aching and stiffness in the shoulder and hip regions.

There is usually no prior history of any previous rheumatic condition. A small proportion of patients recall the onset of symptoms after trauma or vigorous exercise.

- Symptoms of giant-cell arteritis (temporal arteritis) coexist in a significant percentage of cases, and these symptoms should be sought in cases of suspected PMR:

  1. Unilateral headache (either temporal or occipital) with or without scalp tenderness;
  2. Jaw claudication;
  3. Ocular ischemia (transient diminution in vision or frank unilateral blindness); and
  4. Fever.

Some individuals may also complain of peripheral arthritis. PMR is rare in black individuals and more common in Caucasians of Scandinavian descent.

Physical Examination

Overt findings are often not present, and the only finding is moderate pain during examination of the shoulders, neck, hips, and, occasionally, other peripheral joints. If giant-cell arteritis is present, one of the temporal or occipital arteries may have a diminished pulse and be tender. A bruit may be appreciated over a carotid or subclavian artery and, if visual symptoms have developed, the optic disk may show pallor, or the entire retina may show signs of ischemia. Some peripheral joints may show signs of inflammation, particularly the knees.

Differential Diagnosis

Superficially PMR may mimic fibromyalgia, although the onset of PMR is usually more abrupt, and patients with PMR do not have widespread local tenderness. The incidence of fibromyalgia is low in individuals over the age of 65, whereas the incidence of PMR increases with age, being quite common in individuals over the age of 80. If several peripheral joints are inflamed, rheumatoid arthritis is often suspected *(9,10)*. A subset of individuals with elderly onset rheumatoid arthritis present with PMR-like axial stiffness, and most of these patients have a high sedimentation rate without an elevated titer of rheumatoid factor *(8)*.

Diagnostic Tests

- The diagnosis of PMR is based on the history and clinical findings. An elevated ESR merely increases the probability that the diagnosis of PMR is correct.
- Rapid clinical improvement to treatment with a low dose of oral prednisone, 15 mg/d, is also very characteristic.

In approx 15% of individuals with PMR, but without symptoms of giant-cell arteritis, a temporal artery biopsy will reveal arteritis.

- It is not necessary to order a temporal artery biopsy on patients presenting with PMR alone.

A bone scan, which may be very helpful diagnostically, usually shows uptake in joints in the symptomatic regions, such as the glenohumeral joints and the hip joints.

- Frequently there is an associated normochromic, normocytic anemia, with the hematocrit in the range of 27–35%. In addition, the alkaline phosphatase level is often moderately increased.

Treatment

Treatment with low doses of oral prednisone (15 mg/d or less) usually is sufficient. Occasionally higher doses in the range of 30–40 mg are necessary to bring symptoms under control. The dose of prednisone is tapered slowly over the ensuing 6 mo, down to 7.5–5 mg/d if possible. If the patient remains free of symptoms, corticosteroid therapy may be tapered further with complete discontinuation after 12–18 mo of treatment. A flare of the disease occurs in approx 15–20% of cases.

- Physicians should aggressively institute treatment to prevent glucocorticoid-induced osteopenia, using oral calcium, vitamin D, estrogen replacement in women, and, if osteopenia is significant, either nasal calcitonin or oral bisphosphate therapy.

OSTEOMYELITIS

Osteomyelitis is an acute or chronic infection in the bone, which usually affects children and older adults *(11)*. In acute cases there is abrupt onset of systemic toxicity (with fevers and chills) with local symptoms of an abscess developing in the region of the affected bone. More chronic cases present less dramatically with local tenderness and swelling over the involved bone.

- The majority of older individuals with osteomyelitis have longstanding diabetes mellitus with small-vessel disease leading to ischemia of the extremities.

Osteomyelitis also commonly develops in a vertebra of elderly individuals after transient bacteremia. These individuals may present with the insidious onset of malaise, and mild to moderate back pain without any fever. Local tenderness on percussion of the vertebrae should arouse suspicion of possible osteomyelitis.

- A bone scan is usually more sensitive than plain radiographs in detecting osteomyelitis.

Left untreated, a vertebral osteomyelitis can lead to an epidural abscess and even spinal cord compression. The diagnosis is made by needle aspiration and culture.

CANCER

Primary tumors of the bone are rare. More commonly there is metastatic cancer to bone, particularly lung cancer, prostate cancer, sarcomas, gastrointestinal cancer and myeloma in men, and breast cancer and lung cancer in women *(12)*. Other causes of metastatic disease to bone include thyroid cancer, renal cell carcinoma, squamous cell carcinoma of the head and neck, melanoma, and hematologic malignancies.

History

In most cases, the patient with metastatic disease to bone presents with local, progressively worsening pain that is nonmechanical, in that it is not improved with rest. In most cases, the patient is over the age of 50 yr and has a history of a primary malignancy. Systemic signs such as weight loss, fever, and malaise should be sought.

- The history of locally worsening pain, which is not characteristic of myofascial pain, fibromyalgia, or arthritis should prompt an evaluation for a local problem, such as tumor or infection.

Physical Examination

Local tenderness on deep palpation, particularly percussion tenderness, is a common but not invariable finding. The overlying muscles are not exquisitely tender. If nerves or tendons are compressed or entrapped, a variety of findings may be seen. An extreme example is back pain with neurologic findings (such as lower extremity weakness) caused by cauda equina or spinal cord impingement.

Diagnostic Tests

Plain radiographs of the region may be diagnostic. Blood chemistry findings may include hypercalcemia or an elevated alkaline phosphatase. There may be anemia, and the ESR is elevated in a substantial percentage of patients. The ESR is generally not a useful screening test, but it has been shown to be of some use in evaluating patients with back pain who have symptoms suggesting something other than muscle strain or disk pain.

PAGET'S DISEASE

Paget's disease of bone is a disorder associated with locally abnormal bone formation and degradation. It develops in individuals over the age of 40, the incidence rising with age. There are lytic and sclerotic changes in the bone, leading to striking radiographic changes that are diagnostic. Most cases are asymptomatic with only 10% progressing to become clinically overt.

- The most common sign in an asymptomatic individual is elevation in the serum alkaline phosphatase.

The majority of cases of Paget's involve a single long bone, particularly the femur, tibia, and humerus. Widespread disease is unusual and may be associated with a high cardiac output state. Pain is not common, but when it occurs there is a deep ache that is not associated with movement. A common presentation is pathologic fracture of the involved bone. Skeletal bowing may develop in a weight-bearing bone. Skull involvement is not uncommon and may lead to skull enlargement and a variety of neurological complications, including cranial nerve impingement and palsies. When treatment is indicated, calcitonin or bisphosphonates are generally used.

OSTEOMALACIA

- Osteomalacia is a disorder characterized by impaired mineralization of the bone, caused by deficiencies in vitamin D, calcium, or alkaline phosphatase *(13)*.

In children the condition is called rickets, which affects mineralization of the bone and cartilage, leading to abnormal skeletal growth.
Although most affected adults are asymptomatic, bone pain may be present.

- The pain of osteomalacia is dull and difficult to localize. Regions most commonly affected are the pelvis and low back.

In advanced cases there may be local tenderness over the low back, pelvis, and legs. There may also be associated proximal muscle weakness, with muscle atrophy. Pseudofractures are seen on radiographs, particularly in the pelvis and scapulae. True fractures following minimal trauma are also seen in vertebrae and long bones. Hypocalcemia is a common laboratory finding, which by itself may cause problems such as tetany, seizures, diarrhea, and headache.

OSTEOPOROSIS WITH COMPRESSION FRACTURE

Osteoporosis is the most common disorder of bone *(14)*. It is essentially synonymous with osteopenia, which means too little bone, and pathologically there is a decrease in the overall amount of mineralized bone. The disorder is extremely common in the population, particularly in thin, elderly, postmenopausal women, in whom bone loss is accelerated.

- The prevalence of osteoporosis increases with age, and, as bone becomes thinner, the probability of a fracture—particularly vertebral, wrist, and hip fractures—increases.

History

A vertebral compression fracture is the most common presenting sign of osteoporosis, particularly in individuals between the ages of 60 and 70. Pain can be quite severe or mild, depending on the individual's tolerance to pain as well as extent of the fracture. Symptoms gradually decrease over a period of 4–6 wk, as the fracture heals.

Physical Examination

Back pain caused by a compression fracture is usually well-localized between the sixth thoracic vertebrae and the third lumbar vertebrae *(15,16)*. There is usually intense local pain over the vertebral body. Percussion often accentuates the pain, and radiographs show partial collapse of the body of the vertebra.

Diagnostic Tests

- The diagnosis of osteoporosis should be considered in any postmenopausal woman who presents with sudden onset of mid-back pain, particularly thin Caucasian women who are not on replacement estrogen therapy.

The diagnostic tests of choice are plain films or a bone scan.

Treatment

Immediate therapy is limited to analgesic medication.

- Long-term treatment should focus on restoration of bone mass, using:
    1. Estrogen replacement in women;
    2. Oral calcium (1 g of elemental calcium daily) with vitamin D (400 IU/d), and, when bone loss is more advanced;
    3. Nasal calcitonin; or
    4. A bisphosphonate agent (e.g., alendronate, 10 mg/d).

HYPERPARATHYROIDISM

Bone disease due to hyperparathyroidism is becoming a rather rare disorder in the United States, as hypercalcemia and hypophosphatemia are frequently detected on a screening chemistry test leading to a diagnosis at an early stage of the disease, before any bone changes or bone symptoms have developed.

- The diagnosis of hyperparathyroidism is most often made in evaluating symptoms associated with hypercalcemia, particularly muscle weakness and malaise.

Bone disease is more common in the setting of chronic renal failure, when secondary or tertiary hyperparathyroidism frequently develops. There is nothing highly characteristic of the bone pain that may develop in patients with untreated hyperparathyroidism. There is a gradual thinning of the bone, leading to an increase in the chance of fracture.

- The finding of subperiosteal resorption of bone on radiographs, particularly in the phalanges, is characteristic (called osteitis fibrosa cystica).

When fractures do occur, the characteristic bony changes are often noted, or hypercalcemia and hypophosphatemia are detected on a routinely ordered chemistry panel. In very advanced disease, locally destructive cystic lesions called "brown tumors" may develop in the long bones or in the pelvis.

MUSCULOSKELETAL INJURIES

The number of musculoskeletal injuries that can occur is too large to discuss in this brief overview. Essentially every muscle and tendon in the body may be subjected to overuse or injury, leading to local musculoskeletal pain *(17)*. Arthritis, periarticular

Table 9
Common Muscle Injuries

Quadriceps strain
Hamstring strain
Gastrocnemius strain
Hip adductor strain
Lumbar paraspinal muscle strain

pain, and myofascial pain have been discussed in this and other chapters. The most common muscle injuries are listed in Table 9.

Following unaccustomed heavy exercise or work, muscle soreness may develop that can last from 12–24 h. When there is abrupt, excessive stretch on the muscle, injury can result, causing local pain, swelling, and tightness. These strains are also called pulls, tears, or, in the most severe cases, complete ruptures. For the muscle to be injured, there is usually a history of an acute major event. This stands in contrast to tendinitis, which usually develops when there is repeated microtrauma over hours or days. The muscle injury usually occurs near the junction of the muscle belly and the tendon. When injury does occur, there is immediate development of local edema, presaging an inflammatory response. Bleeding is usually not a major feature of a muscle strain, although minor bleeding does occur.

Quadriceps strains develop following a vigorous contraction, such as following a jump or a kick. The tear may be partial or complete. Clinically one sees a bulge in the proximal thigh just above the muscle–tendon junction.

The hamstring muscles in the posterior thigh are prone to strain, particularly in runners and kickers. Any of the three major muscle bellies may be affected, but the biceps femoris is the most commonly affected. In more severe cases one may palpate partial or complete tearing of the muscle just above the muscle–tendon junction.

The medial aspect of the gastrocnemius muscle is commonly injured during sporting activities. There may be the sensation of an acute tear or pop in the calf. Careful examination should exclude the possibility of a tear in the Achilles tendon.

Many sports that involve running may lead to injuries to the groin, particularly the adductor brevis, gracilis, pectineus, and iliopsoas. Hip flexion may be very painful, preventing running or kicking. Complete rupture is rare. Unless the history is straightforward, other causes of groin pain that should be excluded include an inguinal or femoral hernia, epididymitis, urinary tract infection, and (in children) osteitis pubis.

Paraspinal muscles in the back are commonly strained during even routine activities. There is the acute or subacute onset of tightness and pain in the paraspinal muscles or in the ligaments over the sacrum. Pain generally subsides over hours to several days after conservative treatment.

Treatment

Treatment for muscle strains includes acutely icing the injured muscle, resting the involved muscle, initiating nonsteroidal anti-inflammatory drug therapy (followed by gradual stretching) and strengthening of the muscle. A sports trainer or physical therapist should be consulted regarding the timing and extent of a rehabilitation program.

REFERENCES

1. Esterhai J Jr, Gelb I. Adult septic arthritis. Orthop Clin North Am 1991; 22(3): 503–514.
2. Webb J, Nash PT. Polyarthritis. A diagnostic approach. Aust Fam Physician 1990; 19(10): 1533, 1536,1537, 1540–1542.
3. Wolfe F, Smythe HA, Yunus MB, et al. The American College of Rheumatology 1990 Criteria for the Classification of Fibromyalgia. Report of the Multicenter Criteria Committee Arthritis Rheum 1990; 33(2): 160–172.
4. Hawley DJ, Wolfe F, Cathey MA. Pain, functional disability, and psychological status: a 12-month study of severity in fibromyalgia. J Rheumatol 1988; 15(10): 1551–1556.
5. Wolfe F. Fibromyalgia: the clinical syndrome. Rheum Dis Clin North Am 1989; 15(1): 1–18.
6. van Schaardenburg D, Breedveld FC. Elderly-onset rheumatoid arthritis. Semin Arthritis Rheum 1994; 23(6): 367–378.
7. Bacon PA, Farr M. Assessment of rheumatoid arthritis. Curr Opin Rheumatol 1991; 3(3): 421–428.
8. DiBartolomeo AG, Brick JE. Giant cell arteritis and polymyalgia rheumatica. Postgrad Med 1992; 91(2): 107–109, 112.
9. Smith CA, Arnett F Jr. Diagnosing rheumatoid arthritis: current criteria. Am Fam Physician 1991; 44(3): 863–870.
10. Michet C Jr, Evans JM, Fleming KC, O'Duffy JD, Jurisson ML, Hunder GG. Common rheumatologic diseases in elderly patients. Mayo Clin Proc 1995; 70(12):1205–1214.
11. Laughlin RT, Wright DG, Mader JT, Calhoun JH. Osteomyelitis. Curr Opin Rheumatol 1995; 7(4): 315–321.
12. Kanis JA. Bone and cancer: pathophysiology and treatment of metastases. Bone 1995; 17(2 Suppl): 101S–105S.
13. Hutchison FN, Bell NH. Osteomalacia and rickets. Semin Nephrol 1992; 12(2): 127–145.
14. Edwards BJ, Perry HM 3rd. Age-related osteoporosis. Clin Geriatr Med 1994; 10(4): 575–588.
15. Lee YL, Yip KM. The osteoporotic spine. Clin Orthop 1996; 323: 91–97.
16. Lukert BP. Vertebral compression fractures: how to manage pain, avoid disability. Geriatrics 1994; 49(2): 22–26.
17. Pearson AM, Young RB. Diseases and disorders of muscle. Adv Food Nutr Res 1993; 37: 339–423.

11 Comprehensive Pain Management in the Patient with Cancer

Scott Christensen, MD
John Linder, LCSW
John Meyers, PHARMD
Frederick J. Meyers, MD

Key Points

- Pain is a subjective experience that can only be defined and described in terms of the perception of the patient.
- The patient's perception of pain is influenced by psychological, social, and drug factors.
- Pain is often undertreated.
- Appropriate pain relief provides acceptable and even superior quality of life in the terminally ill patient.
- Healing in the absence of cure: psychological, social, and spiritual support for culturally diverse populations through the multidisciplinary team approach.

INTRODUCTION

- Pain is a subjective experience that can only be defined and described in terms of the perception of the patient.
- The perception of pain is influenced by psychological, social, and drug factors.
- The many types of pain may have a clear, in contrast only, a subtle relation to the pathology present.
- Pain is often not accurately assessed and appreciated and, therefore, undertreated.
- Appropriate pain relief provides acceptable and even superior quality of life in the terminally ill patient.

There is a science and art to comprehensive palliative care (Fig. 1). Intractable pain is one of the greatest fears of patients with cancer and their families. Pain management

* The Science

Symptom control - The intensive use of opioids and adjunctive drugs for complete pain relief.

Comprehensive care - The appropriate use of the interdisciplinary team (IDT) to resolve social and emotional issues such as disability and social security payments, family conflict resolution and will and funeral arrangements.

Bereavement and grief.

* The Art

Empathy and effective communication

The creative clinician must cultivate an ability to talk to patients despite   disease progression.

A commitment not to abandon - never say " there is nothing left to do."

Home visits and conversation aimed at validating a person's life efforts.

Fig. 1. Science and art of comprehensive palliative care.

in the setting of terminal illness can be challenging both for practitioner and patient and necessarily includes consideration of medical, psychological, and social factors. The appropriate treatment of pain is a necessary first step before the more existential tasks at the end of life can be addressed by the patient and the family.

Many studies have documented the significant undertreatment of pain in the United States and elsewhere. The barriers to treatment include inadequate physician and staff education, unfounded fear of opioid addiction, patient dissatisfaction with analgesic side effects, and state/federal regulation of opioid analgesic prescription. The American Pain Society recently published guidelines *(1)* aimed at improving pain treatment:

- Recognize and treat pain promptly.
- Chart and display patient's self-report of pain.

- Document outcomes based on data.
- Make information about analgesics readily available to patients and families.
- Provide effective analgesic care.
- Develop systems for outcomes evaluation.
- Develop systems for continuous improvement in pain assessment/management.

The goals of pain management should include complete relief of physical pain, minimizing side effects, and enhancing functional capability whenever possible. Attention must be devoted to patient education regarding analgesic treatments in the psychosocial milieu, and to individual patient goals and tolerances. Involvement of appropriate family and significant others is crucial in developing an effective treatment plan.

APPROACH TO PAIN

- A reproducible, symptom-based plan individualized to patient needs proves most helpful.
- Pain-intensity measurement before and after interventions helps to accurately determine therapeutic efficacy.
- Simpler is often better.
- Reassessment of side effects maximizes attainment of treatment goals.
- Patient satisfaction is enhanced through awareness of individual needs and cultural influences.

Nociception is the activity produced in the central nervous system by tissue-damaging stimuli *(2)*. Pain is the perception of nociception. Thus, pain includes organic and psychological factors. Morphine alters the perception of nociception. The treatment of pain needs to be part of a comprehensive or holistic treatment plan.

Opioids need evaluation in clinical settings where the meaning as well as the intensity of pain is a factor. Laboratory animals and volunteers do not include the complex factors that make pain a combination of nociception and suffering or meaning of pain. For example, postoperative appendectomy pain is not severe not only because of the minimal nociceptive damage, but also because the perception of the patient of risk to life and/or suffering is small, not unlike the soldier who sustains a non–life-threatening injury.

A similar construct is important for the treatment of individual patients. The perception patients have of their pain is the key factor in controlling pain. Narcotics alter perception so that the pain, if still present, does not bother them as much. Similarly, psychological and social factors alter the meaning of pain. Suffering, whether physical or psychological, increases the perception of pain intensity. The orchestration of these factors can contribute to the equanimity of the patient and is discussed later in the context of the interdisciplinary hospice team support for the patient and the family.

Etiology

A thorough, detailed, history is essential to establish the nature and potential etiologies of pain. Important questions include location, nature, severity, episodic or continuous, location, radiation, and precipitating or relieving factors. Physical examination also helps in pain localization and discrimination.

Table 1
Pain vs Characteristics

Pain	Causes
Neuropathic	Local compression, ischemia, infiltration. Radicular; electrical, burning, numbness, tingling, superficial
Somatic	Obstruction, distension; dull, throbbing; poorly localized, referred
Bone pain	Destruction of bone cortex; aching, stabbing, soreness
Wasting	Generalized body pain, myalgias, arthralgias

Table 2
Pain Type vs Treatment

Pain	Treatment
Neuropathic	TCAs, propranolol, opioids, NSAIDs
Somatic	Opioids, NSAIDs
Bone	Opioids; XRT, radioactive calcium (Strontium)
General	Sedatives, opioids
Air Hunger	Opioids, sedative, hypnotics

Many types of pain are recognized (*see* Table 1). Proper recognition of pain etiology is essential in implementing effective therapy. Nonneuropathic pain is called nociceptive and refers to tissue damage to primary afferent neurons. Nociceptive pain responds well to opioids or nonopioid analgesics.

Somatic pain is often poorly localized; is usually described as "achy, dull, or throbbing"; and can be caused by obstruction, distention, or infiltration of an organ or viscus. Bone pain caused by neoplasia eroding cortical bone and periosteum is most frequent in axial, weight-bearing areas. Pathologic fractures can result from loss of bone integrity. Patients describe this pain as "aching, stabbing, or gnawing." Generalized pain is often experienced as myalgias and arthralgias, increasing in prevalence as patients lose weight and become progressively more fatigued.

Neuropathic pain is defined as pain due to injury of sensory nerve fibers by compression, infiltration, ischemia, or treatment-induced injury (i.e., chemotherapy). Neuropathic pain is radicular in distribution and is often associated with cutaneous dysesthesias. Patients frequently describe this pain as "electrical, burning, or tingling."

The importance of distinguishing the different etiologies is that specific treatments do exist for different pains (Table 2). For example, neuropathic pain is often refractory to opioids, but it can respond to one of several drugs that share a common property that can be described as a medical sympathectomy. These include tricyclic antidepressants, anticonvulsants (carbamazepine, phenytoin), and propranolol.

Some symptoms are so distressing as to be called pain of a special type and require treatment. Air hunger is usually observed with pulmonary obstruction secondary to bulky nodal disease or restriction due to infiltrative parenchymal disease rather than hypoxia. Relief of this extreme discomfort is regularly achieved with low-to-moderate doses of morphine.

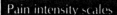

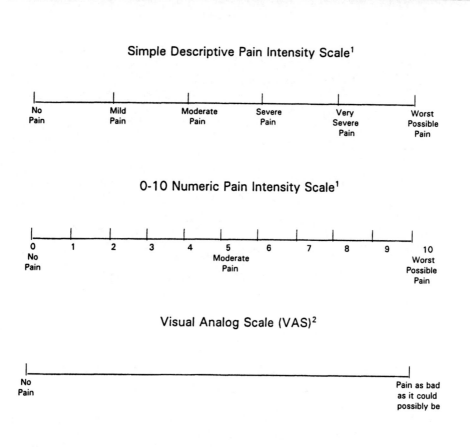

[1]If used as a graphic rating sale, a 10-cm baseline is recommended.
[2]A 10-cm baseline is recommended for VAS scales.

Fig. 2. Quantitative assessments of pain severity.

Two issues deserve emphasis. First is the severity of the pain, the characteristic that defines the selection of the most appropriate level of opioid therapy (Fig. 2). More severe pain is treated with a more potent analgesic, less severe pain with a less potent analgesic. As important as the initial assessment of severity is, re-evaluation to assess the efficacy of the treatment plan also is necessary or critical. Completion of a pain-management scale and the recording of these data at intervals by the patient and the nurse ensures follow-up and evaluation of therapeutic intervention (Fig. 3). This technique of objective evaluation of changes in a regimen should not be overlooked, for it emphasizes to the patient the determination of the interdisciplinary team to relieve suffering. Indirect assessment of pain activity includes recording a patient's mood, activity, enjoyment of hobbies, and interaction with family and friends.

Second, discussion of patient fears, attitudes, and knowledge toward narcotics optimizes therapeutic choices and enhances compliance.

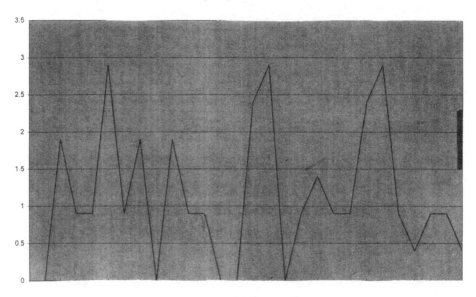

Fig. 3. An example of longitudinal charting of pain severity using a 0–5 scale rather than 0–10.

ANALGESIC INTERVENTIONS CAN BE CLASSIFIED AS SYSTEMIC OR REGIONAL

Systemic treatments include analgesic medications such as opioids and nonopioid analgesics including acetaminophen and nonsteroidal anti-inflammatory drugs (NSAIDs). Adjunctive systemic treatments include sedative-hypnotics and antidepressants of the tricyclic or SSRI classes. Systemic therapies to be tried for the treatment of neuropathic pain include antidepressants, anticonvulsants, and propranolol.

Regional Treatments

Regional treatments include radiotherapy, nerve blockade, and orthopedic fixation. These interventions are most commonly directed at specific disease sites such as spinal cord compression, visceral obstruction, or pathologic fracture and are limited in scope and duration. They can, however, augment systemic interventions and in some cases provide the most effective form of palliation.

SYSTEMIC TREATMENTS

- Narcotic analgesics are most effective for intermediate or severe pain.
- Scheduled dosing is preferred to "prn."
- Combining differing classes of analgesics results in superior pain control.
- Oral analgesic delivery is usually most effective; special circumstances may require alternate methods.

The WHO Analgesic Ladder

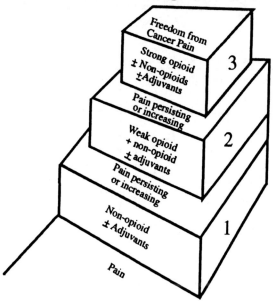

Fig. 4. WHO pain ladder.

Overview

Systemic pharmacologic therapy for cancer pain management is the most common form of pain control. It provides reliable pain relief and allows patients a degree of control. Systemic therapy is both early in the evolution of pain as well as in end-stage care. Too often, however, effective analgesia is not obtained due to unfounded patient or physician fears.

The initial selection of an analgesic should be the least potent necessary to control pain. This concept was strongly reinforced in 1986 by the World Health Organization (WHO). These guidelines provided an "analgesic pain ladder" (Fig. 4) *(3)*.

The ladder is based on the principles of an initial pain assessment followed by reassessment and adjustment of the and potencies and dosing of analgesic interventions. The potency of analgesics is defined as the severity of pain that an opioid able to relieve. The WHO ladder can be "entered" at any point, and "climbed" based on assessment of pain severity. Analgesics can thus be compared for equivalent efficacy, and practitioners should bear this in mind when evaluating new analgesics. Clinical trials of new agents must define pain intensity, and compare new agents to established ones of equal potency. The ladder thus provides an excellent framework for discussion of systemic treatment options.

Pain medications are administered on a scheduled or intermittent basis (Fig. 5). Pain caused by cancer usually is continuous, with periods of intensification or exacerbation. Scheduled analgesic administration is, therefore, preferred and provides a more consistent level of pain relief with fewer unwanted side effects.

The provision of long-acting opioid preparations aims to provide a constant amount of analgesic for baseline pain relief. Breakthrough pain (defined as pain exacerbation

Pharmacokinetic Goals

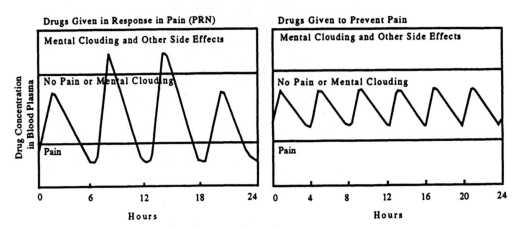

Fig. 5. Intermittent vs scheduled administration of analgesics.

escaping baseline analgesic control) occurs when the patient is on inadequate amounts of long-acting preparations; for example, slow release morphine preparations. The immediate management is for the patient to take short-acting, rapidly absorbed agents added to baseline maintenance therapy.

A common error made in analgesic prescription is to provide inadequate baseline control with excessive intermittent control. The patient experiences a "roller coaster effect," with alternating periods of pain and excessive analgesia. This effect can be avoided by increasing the dose of the slow-release morphine preparation, using methadone on a three- to four-times-a-day schedule or providing morphine or its equivalent by a continuous technique. For example, transdermal fentanyl or continuous intravenous or subcutaneous MS are both effective alternatives.

In general, simple interventions directed at specific complaints, monitored and continually reassessed, tailored to individual patient needs, are the most effective. Costly, complicated, technically difficult plans usually fail. Development of an effective approach to pain is initially time- and resource-intensive, but ultimately should prove both efficacious and cost-effective. Impulses to provide short-term solutions should be curtailed. Drug doses should be maximized before additional agents are added.

Mild Pain

A good beginning point for the treatment of mild pain is found in the nonopioid classes of analgesics, which include acetaminophen and NSAIDs. Aspirin and the various families of NSAIDs control pain by inhibiting prostaglandin synthesis. NSAIDs do not act on the CNS, nor do they affect the perception of pain. Instead, their action is peripheral at the site of tissue injury or inflammation.

Acetaminophen should be regarded as having the same analgesic potency as aspirin. Randomized controlled trials demonstrate the equivalency of acetaminophen to

NSAIDs. A common misconception is that NSAIDs have a selective and superior ability to relieve pain due to bone metastases. The selection of a nonopioid analgesic should thus be based on patient preference, cost, and potential toxicity. For example, many cancer patients can be at increased risk for gastrointestinal bleeding due to thrombocytopenia or concomitant steroid usage. Acetaminophen would then be the nonopioid drug of choice.

Mild pain may not be controlled with NSAIDS alone. Addition of a weak opioid is the most appropriate next step. Codeine and hydrocodone (Vicodin and generics) are the most commonly utilized agents. Both drugs can be obtained without ASA or acetaminophen but are then Schedule-2-controlled substances that require triplicate prescription forms in some states. Thus, they are usually prescribed in combinations that can be ordered on ordinary prescription forms. Acetaminophen is hepatotoxic in large single doses, and NSAIDs have the limitations mentioned above. Dosing of low-potency narcotics should not be increased beyond the amount that gives maximal effect; e.g., 60–90 mg of codeine four to five times a day. Further increases merely increase side effects without substantially affecting greater pain relief *(4)*.

Moderate Pain

A common misconception regarding increasing pain levels is that more of a weaker agent is better. For moderate pain, either an intermediate potency opioid such as oxycodone can be used, or a small amount of a strong opioid such as morphine instituted. Both can be used alone or with previously instituted nonopioid medications.

Oxycodone can be provided with acetaminophen (Roxicet, Tylox, Percocet, Endocet) or with aspirin. The usual caution is to not use more than 8–10 Percocet (40–50 mg) per day because of the fear of hepatic toxicity due to the acetaminophen. Well-done clinical trials confirm that, with oxycodone alone, doses of up to 240 mg/d can be used *(5)*. Even up to these doses, oxycodone is well-tolerated, especially in elderly patients.

The practitioner should also begin to institute appropriate adjunctive measures for control of side effects.

Severe Pain

Treatment of severe pain should begin with a strong opioid via scheduled dosing for baseline pain control. The selection of one of the opioids from this class depends on the preference and knowledge of the practitioner, cost, and important toxicity patterns that are common and predictable.

Intravenous morphine is often used in the acute inpatient setting to establish analgesic dose requirements. Deserving emphasis is that the oral bioavailability of morphine is poor, at most 30%. Thus the conversion to oral preparations requires considerably more than the daily total intravenous dose that provided complete pain relief.

Some patients cannot tolerate morphine for various reasons; in particular, nausea and CNS toxicity as discussed below. Other effective agents include hydromorphone (Dilaudid), methadone (Dolophine), and transdermal fentanyl (Duragesic). Choice among these agents is often dictated by side effects, route of administration, or dosing frequency. No one agent has been demonstrated to be superior. Careful elicitation of patient symptoms, combined with the usage of pain management scales provides guidance toward correct agent choice and analgesic plan development.

Oral Dosing

Oral morphine can be prescribed by using a variety of formulations *(6)* (Fig. 6). One strategy is to begin with oral morphine solution (OMS) concentrate (20 mg/mL). The patient is instructed to start with 5–10 mg (1/4 to 1/2 mL measured by a medicine dropper supplied by the manufacturer) in water, juice, and so on, and to increase the dose until pain relief lasts 4 h. At the time of a regular dosing regimen, conversion to one of the slow-release (SR) preparations may be elected. For example, if a patient is using 30 mg of OMS six times a day, an initial dose of slow-release MS would be 90 mg po b.i.d. The OMS is retained for acute exacerbations; but if the patient uses the OMS concentrate more than occasionally then the fixed dose SR should be increased. Both preparations have very poor absorption in the GI tract, and the patient should be advised that he/she is not using as much MS as the mg dosing would indicate. One way to indicate this is to point out that 90 mg po twice a day is the same as 30 mg iv over 12 h or only 2.5 mg/h.

Hydromorphone (Dilaudid) is available in 2-, 4-, and 8-mg strengths and is very well-absorbed. While a typical dose would be 4–8 mg po every 4–6 h, considerably larger doses of 16 mg are safe when tolerance develops to lower doses. Dilaudid can also be administered iv.

Methadone has a slightly longer half life of other most potent analgesics *(7)*. For emphasis, the once-a-day dosing used to prevent narcotic withdrawal is not the schedule used to provide pain relief. Methadone can be started at 5–10 mg po every 6–8 h and increased every 3–4 d to relief.

Other Routes of Administration

Oral dosing schedules generally are best for most patients. Occasionally, patients may be unable to tolerate oral medications. Alternatives include suppositories, transdermal delivery systems (fentanyl), subcutaneous/intravenous medications, and sublingual preparations. Intramuscular administration (IM) is strongly discouraged. IM dosing is painful, does not provide reliable absorption, and discourages patients from requesting analgesia.

Suppositories

Hydromorphone (Dilaudid) and oxymorphone (Numorphone) are available as suppository preparations. They are particularly useful during the last days of life, when oral administration is compromised by decreased consciousness. Rectal administration of morphine can also be utilized.

Transdermal Administration

While fentanyl is a very short-acting drug when given iv, fentanyl patches (Duragesic) are available as 25, 50, 75, and 100-μg/h patches that last for 72 h. The recommended starting dose is 25 or 50 μg/h with dose escalation every 3 d, when the patches are replaced. The average dose for cancer patients is 200–400 μg/h. A short-acting, rapid-onset supplement such as OMS or hydromorphone must be available to the patient for acute exacerbation. Patients with obstruction of the digestive tract, refractory nausea, or who cannot comply with oral regimens are ideal candidates for transdermal fentanyl.

Recommendations for use of morphine for cancer pain

(1) The optimal route of administration of morphine is by mouth. Ideally, two types of formulation are required: immediate release (for dose titration) and controlled release (for maintenance treatment)
(2) The simplest method of dose titration is with a dose of immediate release morphine given every four hours and the same dose for breakthrough pain. This regular dose may be given as often as required (for example, every hour), and the total daily dose of morphine can be reviewed daily. The regular dose can then be adjusted according to how many rescue doses have been given
(3) If pain returns consistently before the next regular dose is due the regular dose should be increased. In general, immediate release morphine does not need to be given more often than every four hours and controlled release morphine more often than every 12 hours.
(4) Several countries do not have an immediate release formulation of morphine (through such a formulation is necessary for optimal management). A different strategy is needed if treatment is started with controlled release morphine
(5) For patients receiving immediate release morphine every four hours, a double dose at bedtime is a simple and effective way of avoiding being woken by pain
(6) Administration of controlled release morphine every eight hours may be occasionally necessary or preferred
(7) Several controlled release formulations are available. There is no evidence that they are substantially different in their duration of effect and relative analgesic potency
(8) If patients are unable to take drugs orally the preferred alternative routes are rectal and subcutaneous
(9) The bioavilability of morphine by rectal and oral routes is the same, and the duration of analgesia is also the same
(10) The relative potency ratio of oral morphine to rectal morphine is 1:1
(11) Controlled release morphine tablets should not be crushed or used for rectal or vaginal administration
(13) The relative potency ratio of oral morphine to subcutaneous morphine is about 1:2
(14) There is generally no indication for giving morphine intramuscularly for chronic cancer pain because subcutaneous administration is simpler and less painful
(15) Other opioids may be preferred to morphine for parenteral use because of their grater solubility: diamorphine is Britain and hydromorphone elsewhere
(16) Subcutaneous administration of morphine may be practical in patients
      (a) with generalized oedema
      (b) who develop erythema, soreness, or sterile abscesses with subcutaneous administration
      (c) with coagulation disorder
      (d) with very poor peripheral circulation
In these patients, intravenous administration is preferred. Intravenous administration may also be the best parenteral route in patients who, for other reasons, have an indwelling central or peripheral line
(17) The relative potency ratio of oral to intravenous morphine is about 1:3
(18) The above guidelines produce effective control of chronic cancer pain in about 80% of patients. In the remaining 20% other methods of pain control must be considered, including spinal administration of opioid analgesics alone or in combination with local anesthetics or other drugs. There is insufficient evidence to allow recommendation about precise indication for these routes of administration
(19) The buccal, sublingual, and nebulised routes of administration of morphine are not recommended because there is presently no evidence of clinical advantage over conventional routes
(20) Sublingual or transdermal use of other opioids may be an alternative to subcutaneous injection

From Morphine in cancer pain: modes of administration, *British Journal of Medicine*: 312, 825, 30 March 1996

Fig. 6. Recommendations for use of morphine for cancer pain.

Rarely, skin irritation has been reported with transdermal patches, usually an allergic response to the adhesive. Patch removal and appropriate local care resolves the irritation.

Subcutaneous Administration

Subcutaneous administration of morphine has been shown to be both safe and effective *(8)*. This route of administration requires sophisticated pumps and home health support for maintenance, but most patients and/or their care givers can be easily educated in proper usage. Continuous subcutaneous morphine can restore mobility and function and provide increased freedom despite relatively large analgesic doses. Combined with patient controlled anesthesia (PCA) technology, even breakthrough pain can be effectively managed *(9)*. Local irritation or infection can occur at sites of subcutaneous or intravenous needle insertion sites, and thus appropriate monitoring via home health nursing is recommended.

Intravenous morphine or other continuous narcotic infusions require concomitantly greater investments in technology and personnel, and is generally reserved for end-stage care.

Toxicity

Constipation is an invariable side effect of narcotic analgesics to be prevented, not corrected. A detailed patient information sheet describing the daily use of stool softeners and irritant laxatives is encouraged, titrated to patient response. Adequate hydration is essential.

Many patients experience initial clouding of sensorium and even mild confusion when utilizing intermediate/high potency narcotics. These effects are usually transient and minimal once patients are dose-stabilized. The respiratory depression with orally administered narcotics is negligible and is underscored by studies that fail to show impairment of automobile driving skills in patients on oral morphine (10).

Nausea, vomiting, and pruritus commonly seen after beginning oral morphine usually resolve.

CNS stimulation by the metabolites of opioids is frequent (e.g., nightmares) and is underrecognized. Paradoxical pain describes increasing or refractory pain despite increasing doses of a potent analgesic (11). In addition, patients experience a syndrome ranging from anxiety and tremulousness that may progress to hallucinations and seizures. A discussion of the pharmacology provides the reason and the solutions.

The pharmacokinetics and pharmacodynamics of opioids are often altered in chronically ill patients. The older patient and those who have received previous nephrotoxic drugs are particularly susceptible to increased toxicity. Impaired renal function not only prolongs drug effect but also the accumulation of toxic metabolites.

Morphine is metabolized in the liver to 3 morphine glucoronide (3MG) and 6 morphine glucoronide (6MG). The 6MG is the analgesic, but the 3MG is the predominant metabolite. 3MG accumulates in patients with impaired renal function. In many patients, the escalation of iv or oral MS produces only the 3MG. 3MG is not inert but is a CNS stimulant, much like an amphetamine, and produces a characteristic amphetamine-like syndrome of anxiety and tremulousness. The clinician must distinguish the drug effect from the anxiety associated with terminal illness. Most opioids can initiate this toxicity including least potent analgesics such as codeine.

An alternate pathway of metabolism of opioids produces the same effect. The prototype drug is meperidine (12). Meperidine is demethylated to normeperidine, a metabolite that accumulates in patients with azotemia. This frequent toxicity combined with the poor oral absorption of meperidine and its shortest half-life of all the opioids has led to uniform exclusion of meperidine for the treatment of chronic pain. A similar argument could be advanced to reduce its use for acute pain syndromes.

CNS stimulation can be reduced by concomitant use of sedative hypnotics. However, for advanced symptoms of stimulation, the treatment of choice for paradoxical pain is to reduce the daily dose of morphine sulfate to a nontoxic level or even to discontinue completely the MS and to initiate therapy with methadone.

Adjuvant Drugs

Problems occur in pain management when pain is unrelieved (even with very high doses of narcotics), or the type of pain is relatively unresponsive to opioids. The patient's intolerance of side effects can additionally limit maximum opioid dose. Several different classes of agents can be added to narcotics to enhance overall pain relief.

Sedative-hypnotics are most often used to control anxiety or restlessness and to provide sleep. For the many patients who experience nightmares due to opioids, a sedative as bedtime is a very effective adjunct. An important component of pain often overlooked is fear. Benzodiazepines and barbiturates are successful in controlling agitation and add to narcotic analgesic effect.

All sedatives given in sufficiently large amounts can cause paradoxical excitement and an uncontrolled response to painful stimuli. This is due to disinhibition and is frequently an unwanted toxicity. Hepatic function is important in the metabolism of benzodiazepines, barbiturates, and antidepressants. Additionally, benzodiazepines and barbiturates add to the respiratory depressant effects of narcotics and should be added slowly and cautiously.

Antipsychotic tranquilizers also can be helpful in selected patients. Antipsychotics of the phenothiazine group such as chlorpromazine can be combined with a narcotic to give increased sedation without fear of substantially increased respiratory depression. The potentiation of sedation is useful at night but reduces the functional abilities of the patient during the day. As one example, haloperidol (Haldol) is effective when combined with narcotics for evening agitation. Small doses (0.5–1.0 mg) titrated to effect are usually best. For patients with pre-existing psychiatric conditions, antipsychotics may require adjustment, and close psychiatric consultation is recommended. These drugs have a very long half-life and should not be included in fixed combinations with short-acting opioids.

Antidepressants, particularly tricyclics, are helpful with neuropathic pain. Side effects (dry mouth, dizziness, somnolence) can be avoided by beginning with low doses and titrating to maximal analgesic relief. Amitriptyline (Elavil) is commonly employed, although anecdotal efficacy has been reported with imipramine, desipramine, and nortriptyline. The antidepressants exert their effect primarily through sympatholysis. Clinical depression may also augment patients' subjective experience of pain.

CNS stimulants (such as dextroamphetamine) or diet pills (such as Ritalin or phenmetrazine [Prelulin]) can fill an important need by dependably elevating mood and sometimes reducing the lassitude and sedation of opioids. Some caution in prescribing is needed because of side effects such as decreased urinary voiding in men with pre-existing partial outflow obstruction.

Other agents with specific utilities include propranolol (Inderal), which can be very useful for neuropathic pain *(13)*. Anticonvulsants such as phenytoin (Dilantin) and carbamazepine (Tegretol) may mitigate painful neuropathy. Corticosteroids can provide brief relief from cancer pain and improve appetite and sense of well-being *(14)*.

Drugs Not Recommended

Meperidine is not recommended for use as noted above. It has a very poor oral bioavailability, the shortest half-life, and prominent CNS stimulation. Propoxyphene is similarly devoid of analgesic effect but is a prominent CNS stimulant. The opioid agonist–antagonist class of drugs is to be avoided, which includes pentazocine, butorphanolol, and nalbuphine. These agents can precipitate opioid withdrawal in opioid-dependent patients and often produce unpleasant dysphoria, especially in the older patient.

Fixed combinations of opioids and phenothiazines are not recommended because of their disparate half-lives, which leads to cumulative unpleasant sedation.

Barriers to Effective Analgesia

The single greatest barrier to effective analgesia may be the lack of understanding by providers and patients of the difference between tolerance, physical dependence, and "addiction." Tolerance is the need for increasing doses of narcotics to control the same severity of pain. Physical dependence is defined as a withdrawal syndrome evident upon relatively abrupt cessation of the narcotic. The withdrawal syndrome is limited in duration (usually only days), but some symptoms such as insomnia can persist for a month. Rather than addiction, a preferred description of psychological dependence is compulsive abuse. A compulsion is an irrational act repeated over and over again to relieve anxiety; e.g., cigaret smoking, alcoholism, and so on. The euphoria produced by narcotics is dependent on the iv route of administration rather than the oral route. The 4 h of sedation following either route is not the reason for compulsive abuse but rather the explosive relief of anxiety immediately following iv injection or inhalation.

Another important barrier is fear of respiratory depression with narcotic usage. The danger of respiratory depression is less with chronic oral administration of narcotics. Indeed, sedative-hypnotics and barbiturates have a greater effect on medullary respiratory centers than do narcotics. Intravenously administered narcotics can, however, exert a significant respiratory depressant effect and should thus be monitored routinely. Physicians as well as patients should realize that, as tolerance grows, risks from greater dose increments are reduced.

Cooperative group studies have detailed contemporary barriers to effective analgesic therapy *(15,16)*.

Booklets to inform and educate patients and providers are available from the National Cancer Institute *(17)*. Physicians and other providers can obtain this material to be dispensed to patients by calling 1-800-4-CANCER.

REGIONAL TREATMENTS

- Regional therapies are best utilized to address specific, localized problems.
- Radiation therapy is an effective method for palliation.
- Nerve blockade provides effective pain relief.
- Palliative surgical procedures, especially orthopedic fixation of impending weight-baring long bones, provide effective analgesia, eliminate potential complications, and should not be denied to the patient.

Radiation therapy is extremely useful as palliative treatment, and can be provided in many forms. Specific indications for radiotherapy include bone metastases, CNS tumors, and obstructive lymphadenopathy. Electron beam radiotherapy penetrates only a few cell layers and is helpful for disseminated superficial skin disease such as mycosis fungoides or Kaposi's sarcoma. Strontium, a radioisotope analog of calcium, reduces painful osteoblastic bony metastases in 25–35% inpatients on average for 1–3 mo. Patients can experience a transient increase in their pain after initiating strontium and, rarely, external beam radiation. This phenomenon is commonly known as a pain "flare." The usual etiology is local edema and irritation rather than direct injury; the physician must be aware of the potential for flare and adjust analgesics appropriately.

Nerve blockade is another specialized form of regional treatment *(14)*. At times, it is appropriate to block painful neural input as systemic treatment may involve unacceptable toxicity or prove inadequate. Blockade can be accomplished pharmacologically or surgically.

Spinal opioids have become a common, possibly too common, method of providing local pain control. The most common indication is for pain that originates in the lower extremities or pelvis. Most importantly, spinal opioid infusions are ineffective in patients with pain insensitive to systemic opioids. The primary reason to convert to the spinal route is to avoid systemic toxicities of high-dose MS.

Usually accomplished with morphine, the technique relies on implanted catheters or reservoirs to deliver analgesia at local spinal levels. Implantable, continuous infusion morphine pumps are preferable to intermittent reservoir puncture due to decreased infection rates. This intervention is expensive, requiring a surgical procedure and frequent monitoring. Epidural catheters are easier to manage, but are potential sites for infection, decrease freedom of movement, and can be dislodged without careful attention. They are thus poor choices in demented, combative, or incontinent patients. Pump malfunction, while infrequent, is also an important potential complication.

Abdominal visceral pain, while controllable via epidural anesthesia, can also be controlled via nerve blockade outside of the CNS. The most common example is celiac plexus blockade. The plexus can be transected surgically, or infiltrated with a sclerosing agent. Pain due to pancreatic cancer is commonly mitigated in this manner. Reduced gastrointestinal motility can be a complication. Other nerve ganglia can be anesthetized such as in sympathetic blockade, sympathectomy, or spinal nerve root infiltration. All require invasive procedures an may provide only temporary relief. Pain due to head and neck cancers, as well as disseminated meningeal metastases, has been reported to respond to intrathecal morphine (Duramorph). Access devices such as an Ommaya reservoir are required.

Surgical interventions also have specific indications in palliative care. While radiation therapy effectively palliates bone metastases, it does not stabilize bone. Proactive orthopedic fixation may be required to stabilize weight-bearing structures and prevent pathologic fractures. An acceptable indication for fixation is destruction of >50% of bone cortex. Practitioners should aggressively investigate complaints of new or worsening bony pain. Fixation techniques may be unhelpful if bony destruction progresses to the point where remaining "normal" bone is insufficient for anchoring fixation devices. Repeated surgical procedures in the setting of incurable disease, however, are clearly not indicated as morbidity is then outweighed by expected benefit.

UNCONTROLLED PAIN

Clinical situations may arise when pain is inadequately treated, or the patient complains of severe pain. The following "checklist" may be helpful to effectively and efficiently address patient concerns:

- Increasing the dose of the prescribed drug.
- Increasing the potency of the opioid; i.e., stepping up the WHO ladder.
- Considering inpatient hospitalization for continuous intravenous infusion of the most potent opioid to establish dose.

- Considering outpatient continuous intravenous infusion (CIVI) or subcutaneous administration.
- Paradoxical pain: morphine metabolites are out of balance; changing to methadone.
- Orthopedic fixation for advanced long-bone instability.
- Radiation therapy for painful bone metastases.
- Neuropathic pain: central (spinal cord compression) or peripheral; evaluating and adding appropriate nonopioid analgesics.
- Psychosocial issues are overriding. Reassess home, intrapersonal, and interpersonal and financial aspects of illness.

HOSPICE—HEALING IN THE ABSENCE OF CURE

- Hospice addresses medical, psychological, and social concerns.
- Early hospice referral is helpful to establish a constructive, supportive relationship.
- Hospice care is most effective as an extension of the primary physician.
- Hospice referral is generally initiated when curative goals are unable to be met.

Background

The hospice movement has been active in the United States for the past 20 yr. As originally conceived, it offered patients the option of home death rather than hospital-based treatment. The phrase "death with dignity" was coined to reflect prevailing attitudes about appropriateness and invasiveness of terminal care. Importantly, psychological services, such as grief counseling, were provided to both patients and their caregivers (families, significant others, and so on).

Today, hospice programs provide comprehensive medical, psychological, and social support for the terminally ill patient. In general, hospice goals include effective palliation, noninterference with the dying process, and support for patients and their significant others in transition from health, to illness, to death. An underlying value is the belief that death need not be painful, and that patients and their loved ones can resolve important life concerns or issues and achieve mental and/or spiritual peace prior to death.

Cultural and social influences often have profound effects on patient perception of the ability to cope with pain. Language barriers provide challenges to patient education. Educational level provides additional potential challenges. Family dynamics may influence treatment options, particularly regarding opioid usage. Religious convictions may also impact patient ability to accept or comply with proposed treatment. It is incumbent on the entire health care team, including physicians, to become familiar with the major aspects of a patient's sociocultural context to avoid misinterpretations that could negatively affect provision of appropriate analgesia. In culturally diverse populations, it may be necessary to consult with extended family members, religious leaders, or even other community leaders to best meet patient needs *(18)*.

The Role of the Interdisciplinary Team

Fundamental to most hospice programs is the interdisciplinary team. Physicians, nurses, social workers, pharmacists, clergy, and volunteers all participate in providing care for the patient.

The most common psychiatric complaints in the cancer population are depression, anxiety, and delirium, and are more likely to occur in the patient who experiences pain *(19)*. Multimodal treatment involving psychotherapeutic and behavioral interventions, in addition to medical therapies, can enhance pain management.

Each team member participates in identifying problems, developing solutions, and evaluating outcomes. Formal interdisciplinary team meetings are held regularly to coordinate care. Treatment plans are thus adjusted on a continuing basis in response to changing patient needs.

Hospice enrollment benefits patients directly through coordination of medical and psychosocial care. Patients are provided with both nurses and social workers specifically trained in terminal care and end-of-life issues. Every attempt is made to keep the patient comfortable in his/her home environment. Continuous, 24-h, on-call coverage is often provided. In-home continuous infusions, dressing changes, and home pharmaceutical delivery are all appropriate hospice services.

Hospice care by Medicare certified programs is a capitated program of reimbursement that can relieve financial pressures felt by many patients. Medicare and many private insurance programs provide a daily reimbursement to hospice that is used for nursing visits, social work visits, and pharmacy costs. There are many ongoing studies evaluating the cost-effectiveness of palliative care. At this time the barriers to early referral that will fall with further patient and physician education make any conclusion premature.

Many hospices have pharmacies associated with them as well and can provide even more specialized services. New regulations allow the pharmacist to write triplicate prescriptions for patients enrolled in a hospice program. The pharmacist must receive a written order to do so from the physician, but, having done so, this facilitates refills of standing prescriptions. In addition, the pharmacist may partially fill a prescription over 1 mo. Thus, a patient starting a new opioid or who may not survive another month can be given a prescription by the physician for an anticipated 1 mo supply of drug. The pharmacist may dispense a portion; e.g., a 2-wk supply, and then the team can reassess.

Physician management, either through hospice or the patient's primary physician, is enhanced via frequent home visits. Volunteers often provide critical support, particularly to the socially isolated.

The Importance of the Continued Role of the Physician

Referral to hospice programs can be challenging. Often, referral is interpreted by patients as abandonment, or "giving up." Physicians, too, may feel frustration or discomfort at acknowledging the failure of curative-intent treatment. Palliative care is very intensive. A unique opportunity exists at the end of life, when terminal illness will result in death. Physicians and adjunct health providers can reframe the notion that "nothing more can be done." The terminal phase of a disease trajectory is usually most appropriately treated with hospice care. The acknowledged complexity of end-of-life care is indicative of the need for clinical intervention covering the full range of patient distress; medical, interpersonal, intrapsychic, spiritual, instrumental (resource), and posthumous (bereavement).

Hospice joins the strength of a patient's longitudinal relationship with a physician and treatment team to the familiarity and, hopefully, the comforts and convenience of home to promote the use of scarce and waning energy to those activities and pursuits most valuable to the patient. The control that patients can exercise in their home environment is usually greater than in an institutional setting; control and its future or current loss is a central theme at the end of life or in the face of life-threatening illness.

In hospice, the treatment emphasis is the quality of life. Some common concerns include the planning of funerals or memorial services; resolving interpersonal conflicts, particularly those of long standing; providing opportunities for patient and loved ones to discern meaning in the human experience; availability of culturally and denominationally sensitive spiritual care; facilitating the orderly transfer of responsibilities; offering experience-based education on coping at the end of life; instrumental support for the care giving system with volunteers and knowledgeable referral to community resources; and bereavement services for the surviving care giver and loved ones. This list is by no means exhaustive. Advocacy for patient and family often plays an important role; accessing resources and the honoring of treatment decisions often require particular support.

The physician is ill-equipped by standard medical training to participate in the orchestration of end of life *(20)*. Yet patients and families look to the primary physician for leadership and active involvement despite the inexorable progression of cancer.

The physician must be prepared to discuss and participate in the issues above. The physician can provide exposition, noting that cancer or AIDS or other chronic illness are not events, but processes. The astute clinician establishes clear goals based on an assessment of the biology at that point in the process. As the disease changes, the goals change. The transition of the biology must be accompanied by transitions in the knowledge and insight of the patient and the family.

Without such recognition there will be dissonance between the care providers and the patient. But with goal setting and effective transitions come hopefulness, not fear, acceptance of palliative care, and less reliance on unproven methods of treatment.

Finally, there comes an enhanced professional sense of accomplishment as a wholesome and longitudinal relationship develops as physicians follow the patients to the end of their illness, and their families beyond to bereavement *(21)*.

Hospice referral is an important transition, therefore, in the course of the patient's care. Discussion of changing goals, from cure to palliation, can help the patient adjust. Palliative care need not be viewed as "second best," but as important as an active treatment in providing for patient well-being. National guidelines suggest referral to hospice when life expectancy is 6 mo or less. This determination can be difficult to predict, and should be based on objective evaluation of patient condition, trends, and response to active treatment. Practically, hospice referral is appropriate once curative goals are unable to be met and further remission unlikely.

REFERENCES

1. American Pain Society Quality of Care Committee: Quality Improvement Guidelines for the Treatment of Acute Pain and Cancer Pain. JAMA 1995; 274: 1874–2000.
2. Portnoy RK. Cancer pain: pathophysiology and syndromes. Lancet 1992; 339: 1026–1031.
3. Alejandro RJ, Bauman AP. The WHO Analgesic Ladder for Cancer Pain Management. JAMA 1995; 274: 1870–1873.
4. Meyers FJ, Kennedy M, Meyers FH. Pain Management in the Terminally Ill Patient. In: Taylor RS, ed. Difficult Medical Management. WB Saunders, 1991; 478–487.

5. Glare PA, Walsh TD. Dose ranging study of oxycodone for chronic pain in advanced cancer patients. J Clin Oncol 1993; 11: 973–978.
6. Expert Working Group of the European Association for Palliative Care. Morphine in cancer pain: modes of administration. Br Med J 1996; 312: 823–826.
7. Fainsinger R, Schoeller T, Burnern G. Methadone in the management of cancer pain: a review. Pain 1993; 52: 137–147.
8. Shaw HL. Treatment of Cancer Pain by Electronically Controlled Infusion of Analgesic Drugs. Cancer 1993; 72: 3416–3425.
9. Smythe M. Patient-controlled analgesia: a review. Pharmacotherapy 1992; 12: 132–143.
10. Vaini A, Ollila J, Matikainen E, Rosenberg P, Kalso E. Driving ability in cancer patients receiving long term morphine analgesia. Lancet 1995; 346: 667–670.
11. Bowsker D. Paradoxical pain: when the metabolites of morphine are in the wrong ratios. Brit Med J 1993; 306: 473.
12. Kaiko RF, Foley KM, Grabinski PY, Heidrich G, Rogers AG, Inturrisi CE, Reidenberg MM. CNS excitatory effects of meperidine in cancer patients. Ann Neurol 1993; 13: 180–185.
13. Meyers FH, Meyers FJ. Patients with neuropathic pain regularly benefit from treatment with propranolol. Am J Pain Management 1992; 2: 75–78.
14. Marshall K. Managing cancer pain: basic principles and invasive treatments. Mayo Clin Proc 1996; 71: 472–477.
15. Von Roenn JH et al. Physician attitudes and practice in cancer pain management: a survey from the Eastern Cooperative Oncology Group. Ann Int Med 1993; 119: 121–126.
16. Cleeland CS et al. Pain and its treatment in outpatients with metastatic cancer. N Engl J Med 1994; 330: 592–596.
17. Management of Cancer Pain Guideline Panel: Management of cancer pain (Clinical Practice Guideline No. 9; AHCPR publication 94-0592); Management of cancer pain: Adults (Quick reference Guide for Clinicians No. 9; AHCPR Publication 94-0593) Agency for Health Care Policy and Research, US Department of Health and Human Services, 1994 AHCPR Publications Clearing House, PO Box 8547, Silver Springs, MD 20907.
18. Fallowfield L. Psycho-social interventions in cancer. Brit Med J 1995; 311: 1316,1317.
19. Massie MJ, Holland JC. The cancer patient with pain: psychiatric complications and their management. J Pain Symp Management 1992; 7: 99–109.
20. Back AL, Wallace JI, Starks HE, Pearlman RA. Physician Assisted Suicide and Euthanasia in Washington State. Patient requests and physician responses. JAMA 1996; 275: 919–925.
21. Byock IR. Consciously walking the fine line: thoughts on a hospice response to assisted suicide and euthanasia. J Pall Care 1993; 9: 25–28.

12 POSTOPERATIVE PAIN

DENNIS L. FUNG, MD

DEFINING THE PROBLEM

Inadequate Management

- Postoperative pain has a history of being poorly managed. (Large interpatient differences in pharmacokinetics and pharmacodynamics explain the failure of standard doses and intervals to provide adequate analgesia.)
- Successful management of analgesia requires frequent assessment for effectiveness and side effects.
- Complete absence of pain (surgical anesthesia) is usually not the goal of postoperative analgesia.
- Preparation consists of informing the patient of what can or should be done for the anticipated pain, and the method of verbal scoring (0 = no pain and 10 = worst pain imaginable) should be explained.
- Analgesics given prior to experiencing pain have a "pre-emptive" effect, but they should be administered before the surgical procedure begins.
- The types of postoperative pain that seem to benefit the most from epidural analgesia are thoracic and upper abdominal operations that impair chest wall mobility.
- Coagulopathy is an important contraindication to epidural catheter placement.
- In the case of amputations, continuous block of the extremity by epidural for the legs or by brachial plexus block for the arm may reduce the risk of postamputation phantom limb pain.
- Analgesia techniques that are effective in adults are applicable to children.
- A chronic pain patient's requests for additional medication may be mistakenly interpreted as a sign of addiction-based "drug-seeking" behavior instead of legitimate, appropriate requests for adequate analgesia by a patient who had pharmacological tolerance.

Postoperative pain is acute pain. In the absence of postoperative analgesia, pain increases as the effect of anesthesia recedes. At its peak, it may be excruciating (the worst pain the patient has ever experienced). Then over several hours or days, the pain diminishes. Even if untreated, postoperative pain usually disappears with time.

Postoperative pain has a history of being poorly managed. A common practice was to write standard orders that did not take into account variation in patient opiate requirements. Large interpatient differences in pharmacokinetics and pharmacodynamics explain the failure of standard doses and intervals to provide adequate analgesia. In addition to the inflexibility of standardized doses, there was sometimes a deliberate practice of underdosing because addiction or side effects were feared. There also appear to be ethnic biases in the way that analgesia has been prescribed *(1)*.

Sometimes the only noticeable adverse effect of poorly managed pain is patient dissatisfaction. On the other hand, some patients are especially vulnerable to deleterious effects of pain. Patients with coronary artery disease should be spared as much as possible the hypertension, tachycardia, and emotional distress that can accompany postoperative pain. The immobility that pain induces can also be harmful. The price of immobility may come in the form of retained pulmonary secretions, atelectasis, and pneumonia or as pulmonary thromboembolism. Less tangible adverse effects are poor patient cooperation, and increased demands for nursing and medical attention. Potential adverse effects that have also been claimed are hypercoagulability, hypermetabolism, delayed recovery of bowel function, and persistence of pain in the form of a chronic pain syndrome. Ultimately the result can be prolonged recovery, morbidity or mortality, and increased cost of care.

During the past decade there has been increasing recognition of the need to improve postoperative pain management. In 1988 Ready et al. described the Postoperative Pain Management Service at University of Washington *(2)*. In 1992 the Agency for Healthcare Policy and Research (AHCPR) published clinical practice guidelines for acute pain management. *See* Table 1 for a summary of those guidelines.

Planning Postoperative Pain Management

Management of postoperative pain can begin at many points in the course of a patient's surgical experience. It can begin before the operation begins. When alternatives for pain management are discussed with the patient by the person(s) responsible for ordering it, an important aspect of patient education is being performed. The anesthetic selection significantly affects the options and management of postoperative pain. Additionally, the concept of pre-emptive analgesia maintains that events prior to the pain production can modify the experience of pain that follows. Based on this concept, regional anesthesia or the early use of opiate drugs before surgical incision may modify the needs for postoperative analgesia. Intraoperative management, at the least, includes the decision of whether or not to begin the process of analgesia prior to the end of surgery so that the patient arrives in the recovery room with analgesia or partial analgesia. The recovery room nurse plays a key role in the subsequent course of analgesia. Finally, the ward/ICU nursing staff, surgeons, and pain service continue the management of analgesia. It is not always possible to accurately anticipate the magnitude of painful events and all the modifiers of painful experience. Therefore, successful management of analgesia requires continuous assessment of effectiveness. Because of the dangers, assessment for side effects is also necessary.

Table 1
Agency for Healthcare Policy and Research—Clinical Practice Guidelines
for Acute Pain Management

Patients should be informed before their surgery, both verbally and in writing, that effective pain relief is an important part of their treatment, that talking about unrelieved pain is essential, and that the hospital staff should respond quickly to their reports of pain. However, it should also be made clear to patients and their families that the total absence of postoperative discomfort is not normally a realistic goal.

A simple assessment of the intensity of the pain and the pain relief should be recorded on the bedside vital-sign chart or a similar record that encourages easy, regular review by the members of the health care team. The pain assessment should be included in the patient's permanent record. For children, age-appropriate measures should be used.

The institution should determine the pain-intensity and pain-relief levels that will elicit reviewing the current pain therapy, documenting the proposed modifications in treatment, and subsequently reviewing its efficacy.

At regular intervals defined by the clinical unit and the quality-assurance committee, each clinical unit should assess a randomly selected sample of patients in whom surgery has been performed within the last 72 h.

Analgesic drug treatment should comply with several basic principles. Unless contraindicated, every patient should receive an around-the-clock postoperative regimen of an NSAID. For patients unable to take medications by mouth, it may be necessary to use the parenteral or rectal route.

Analgesic orders should allow for the great variation in individual opioid requirements, including a regularly scheduled dose and "rescue" doses for instances in which the usual regimen is insufficient.

Specialized analgesic technologies, including spinal and epidural analgesia and patient-controlled analgesia, should be governed by policies and standard procedure, and managed by physicians who are experts in the administration of these techniques.

Nonpharmacologic interventions are intended to supplement, not replace, pharmacologic interventions. The staff should be able to give patients information about these interventions and support patients in using them.

The procedures for treating pain should be reviewed periodically by using the institutions' quality-assurance procedures.

There is an argument for the earliest possible intervention. Clinical experience suggests it is easier to treat pain early rather than late. It follows that early consideration and intervention of pain management will result in better analgesia. Although postoperative analgesia is one goal, there are other goals in perioperative management besides excellent analgesia. It is conceivable that analgesia that is "too perfect" might interfere with early recognition of postoperative complications, such as compartment syndrome or bowel anastomotic leak. Patient expectations for analgesia may be unreasonable. Complete absence of pain (surgical anesthesia) is usually not the goal of postoperative analgesia.

Assessment of Analgesia Needs and Options

The size and site of surgical incision and the tissues invaded by a surgical procedure are the main determinants of postoperative pain. Incisions in the thoracic and upper

Table 2
Examples of Factors that Determine Analgesic Options

Factor	Analgesic Options
Analgesic needs	Epidural analgesia is not practical for pain above C-5 or for mild pain
Site of postoperative care	PCA is not available for ambulatory patients unless home nursing care is also provided
Likely pain duration	Single-dose intrathecal morphine will not last longer than 12–24 h
Available routes for drug administration	An epidural catheter cannot be safely placed in an anticoagulated patient
Tolerance for side effects	An obese patient with severe pain may not tolerate systemic opiate without ventilation support
Risk acceptance	A patient who fears iatrogenic addiction may refuse systemic opiates
Device availability	Patient control of iv opiates is not advisable without the safeguards of PCA devices
Personnel availability	PCA analgesia is contraindicated in the absence of personnel to monitor for adverse effects and to manage problems

abdominal regions pose the greatest threat to adequate coughing and lung expansion postoperatively. The tissues that give rise to the greatest pain are skin, sensory nerves, and periosteum. Muscle spasm may be a secondary source of pain. The pathology giving rise to pain—ischemia, inflammation, and spontaneous nerve activity—also has implications for treatment decisions.

Patients differ greatly in their ability to tolerate pain. Much depends on the significance of the pain and the patient's attitude toward it. Those who have previously experienced severe pain fear a repetition of that experience, but memory for pain is not entirely accurate. For short procedures, such as colonoscopy and lithotripsy, patients appear to recall memories of pain by the peak pain that was experienced and by the pain toward the end of the experience *(3)*.

Patients also differ in their response to analgesia drugs. Part of the difference is due to pharmacokinetic factors. The rest of the difference in response can be attributed to pharmacodynamic factors, idiosyncratic differences, and predictable changes in response due to tolerance. In patients with chronic pain, the daily amount and the duration of treatment with opiate suggest the presence of tolerance.

The analgesic options available to a patient are determined primarily by whether postoperative care will occur at home or in the hospital. Additional considerations besides analgesic needs that can influence analgesic options are the likely duration of pain, available analgesic routes, ability to tolerate side effects, willingness to accept risks, device availability, and personnel availability. Some examples are given in Table 2. Patients differ in the ease and safety with which the route of analgesic administration can be established. Since surgical patients will have venous access established, intravenous analgesia is an option. On the other hand, extreme obesity or severe spinal osteoarthritis might prevent successful placement of an epidural catheter. Finally, in discussing plans for postoperative analgesia, it will sometimes become clear that a patient has expectations about postoperative pain that seem inappropriate. Such expectations are usually based on prior surgical and analgesia experience or the anticipated effects of surgery.

Patient Preparation

Postoperative pain is something that many patients dread. Its character and magnitude is one of the many unknowns that the preoperative patient faces. Preparation consists of informing the patient of what can or should be done for the anticipated pain. If patient-controlled analgesia (PCA) is one of the options, the operation of patient-controlled infusion pump should be explained The method of verbal scoring (0 = no pain and 10 = worst pain imaginable) should be explained. The patient should be cautioned to use the score as a way of communicating relative degrees of pain, not as a physician or nurse motivator. A patient who describes pain as 11 out of 10 is risking that his or her assessment will not be taken seriously. Patients who have preoperative pain should be allowed to continue their pain medications. While the use of medication prior to arrival in the operating room has become uncommon, there are reasons to suspect that analgesics given prior to experiencing pain have a "pre-emptive" effect.

Pre-Emptive Analgesia

Several laboratory and clinical studies suggest that noxious stimulation can induce central neuronal hyperexcitability and lower the peripheral threshold to noxious stimulation. These changes are prevented by afferent block using local anesthetic, and they are modified by systemic opioids. It is hypothesized that clinical interventions that prevent central transmission of surgical stimulation might result in reduction or delay of postoperative pain. Results from clinical trials are conflicting, however, with some detecting a pre-emptive effect and others failing to. There is evidence that pre-emptive analgesia must be administered before the surgical procedure begins (4). The types of pre-emptive interventions that have been successful in at least one study are listed in Table 3. Although, at present, no consensus has been reached, some clinicians incorporate the concepts of pre-emptive analgesia in their management of postoperative analgesia by instituting early and effective analgesia with local anesthetic blocks and/or systemic opioids.

TECHNIQUES FOR PAIN MANAGEMENT

Wound Infiltration

Skin infiltration with local anesthetic prior to making the incision can provide hours of postoperative analgesia if a long-acting agent such as bupivacaine is used. This method of analgesia qualifies as pre-emptive. Infiltration analgesia is not applicable in areas where cosmetic closure of the skin is intended because of the tissue distortion that can occur. Local anesthetic infiltration is frequently used for small incisions, such as inguinal hernia repairs, arthroscopic procedures, and excision of small lesions.

Table 3
Potentially Effective Pre-Emptive Analgesic Interventions

Interventions	Comments
Epidural or spinal anesthesia	May reduce the incidence of painful phantom sensation if instituted prior to amputation, but it is not known how far in advance of surgery the block is needed in order to be effective
Local anesthetic infiltration	Reduces postoperative analgesic requirements if a local anesthetic is infiltrated before compared to after hernia repair
Nerve block	Reduces postoperative analgesic requirements if a femoral nerve block is performed before compared to after knee surgery
NSAID	Reduces postoperative pain after oral and thoracic surgery, but there is no difference whether the NSAID is given pre- or postoperatively
Opioid	Delays the need for postoperative analgesia if given preoperatively

Oral Analgesia

Oral analgesics are commonly used for mild pain in ambulatory patients and also as hospital discharge medications for patients recovering from more severe postoperative pain. NSAIDs, acetaminophen, and opioids, such as hydrocodone and codeine, are most frequently used. Table 4 lists commonly used drugs and doses and oral bioavailability. When converting from im or iv doses of opioids to oral doses, the first pass effect by the liver has to be accounted for. The magnitude of this effect is a source of variation in the required dose. Generally only about one-half to one-third of an oral dose is systemically available. Meperidine is not recommended for oral postoperative analgesia because the toxic metabolite normeperidine is significantly increased by first-pass metabolism. Potent opiates such as morphine and methadone provide sustained levels of drug and analgesia. Since the onset of analgesia with these drugs is slow, a more rapid-acting drug, such as hydromorphone, can be given as the first analgesic. The most common side effect of opioid analgesia is nausea and vomiting. An anti-emetic, such as metoclopramide 10 mg, droperidol 0.625 mg, or ondansetron 4 mg, will usually have to be given. Selection of a different opioid or substitution of a nonopioid may prevent recurrence.

Intramuscular Analgesia

Intramuscular (im) opioid analgesia was formerly a common way of providing postoperative analgesia. The blood levels following im administration are nearly identical to those following intravenous (iv) administration, except for the slower rise to maximum concentration. Because im administration is periodic with typically a 3- to 4-h period, there is a risk or excessive effect at the beginning of the period and inadequate analgesia at the end. An initial excessive effect can be avoided by using a dose that is barely adequate, but with the disadvantage that the level of analgesia is likely to be

Table 4
Oral Analgesics (Typical Doses for a 70-kg Patient)

Drug	Dose
Opioid	
Codeine (Tylenol 3)	60 mg Q 2 H
Hydrocodone (Lorcet, Lortab, Vicodin)	10 mg Q 3–4 H
Hydromorphone (Dilaudid)	6 mg Q 3–4 H
Methadone (Dolophine)	10 mg Q 6–8 H
Morphine	30 mg Q 3–4 H
Oxycondone (Roxicodone, Percocet, Percodan)	10 mg Q 3–4 H
NSAID	
Aspirin	650–975 mg Q 4 H
Choline magnesium trisalicylate (Trilisate)	1000–1500 mg bid
Ibuprofen (Motrin, Advil, Midol, Pamprin, and so on)	400 mg Q 4–6 H
Indomethacin (Indocin)	25–50 mg Q 8 H
Ketorolac (Toradol)	15–30 mg Q 6 H
Magnesium salicylate	650 mg Q 4 H
Naproxen (Naprosyn)	500 mg loading, 250 mg Q 6–8 H
Other	
Acetaminophen (Tylenol)	650–975 mg Q 4 H Not to exceed 4 g/d

Reprinted with permission from Anesthesiology News.

inadequate for most of the dosing period. Intramuscular injections require the presence of a nurse, and if the order is for "PRN dosing" (as needed), then the patient has to decide that another dose is needed, summon the nurse, wait for the injection, and wait for the effect. Aside from the tendency for being poorly effective, im administration of opioids is painful and can result in abscesses and needle injuries to tissue or nerves. Some patients continue to associate an "im shot" with analgesia and may even prefer it. Usually a trial of PCA is sufficient to convince them of PCA's superiority.

Intravenous Analgesia

Intravenous administration is the most common technique for establishing an initial level of analgesia. Because the latency from iv administration to peak effect is short, titration to effect is more efficiently accomplished. Analgesia from fentanyl or morphine given intraoperatively will persist into the postoperative period. Intravenous administration is continued as needed by the postanesthesia recovery nurse. Orders have to be written with sufficient flexibility so that adequate analgesia is achieved before transferring the patient to the surgical ward. Because of the high nurse-to-patient ratio and the nursing training and experience, PRN orders can be effectively carried out in this setting. In patients unable to take oral analgesics, iv analgesia can be continued by slow iv infusion using a pump. The difficulty with this technique is that over dose or inadequate analgesia must be recognized by the hospital staff and corrected.

$$\text{maximum rate} = \frac{\text{bolus amount} \times 60}{\text{lockout in minutes}} + \text{infusion rate per hour}$$

$$\text{minimum rate} = \text{infusion rate per hour}$$

$$\text{actual rate} = \text{no. boluses per hour} \times \text{bolus amount}$$
$$+ \text{infusion rate per hour}$$

Fig. 1. Calculation of PCA drug administration limits and delivery.

PCA

PCA involves the delivery of iv opioids by a microprocessor-controlled infusion pump. When activated by the patient, the pump delivers a bolus of drug intravenously, and then becomes unresponsive to further requests for drug until the lockout interval (usually 5–10 min) has elapsed. The pump is also able to deliver a constant infusion either alone or in combination with the boluses. The patient has no direct control over the constant infusion. Once the bolus amount and lockout interval have been set, the patient cannot receive drugs at a faster or slower rate than the settings will allow. (*See* Fig. 1 for the calculation of rate limits and actual rate.) The actual amount delivered can be calculated from the PCA record of doses. The use of a basal infusion rate is optional.

With PCA, postoperative pain can be titrated by the patient to his or her needs. All of the variations due to pharmacokinetics, pharmacodynamics, and patient preference are accounted for. PCA is popular with patients because the patient has some control. In addition, PCA makes possible the administration of multiple small doses at short intervals, thus avoiding both excessive dosing and inadequate analgesia. If a patient becomes sedated, additional boluses will not be delivered. The PCA device maintains an internal record of requests for drug by the patient. This record can be compared to the patient's verbal assessment of analgesia when adjusting the PCA parameters. The contraindications to PCA are few. The patient must understand how to use the device for analgesia and must be physically capable of activating the bolus trigger. It is not appropriate for anyone but the patient to activate the bolus injection. Patients who are obese or who have severe pulmonary disease or sleep apnea should be considered for pulse oximetry monitoring in addition to PCA.

PCA orders are usually written on a special order form, and standard drug concentrations are used throughout the hospital. These standardized measures are to avoid confusion and simplify the initiation of PCA bolus injections. Bolus injections are too small and infrequent to be useful in delivering a loading dose, and so loading doses should be administered separately. The loading dose is typically given by bedside iv titration. (*See* Table 5 for typical PCA settings.)

Inadequate analgesia can occur with PCA if the bolus amount is too small or the lockout interval too long. The infusion is used to provide a background level of drug that is added to by the patient's use of the bolus. Although the use of PCA with infusion

Table 5
Typical PCA Settings for a 70-kg Adult^a

Drug	Loading Dose	Dose	Lockout	Infusion
Fentanyl	0.5–1.0 µg/kg	15–75 µg	4–6 min	15–60 µg/h
Hydromorphone	0.01–0.02 mg/kg	0.1–0.5 mg	6–8 min	0.1–0.3 mg/h
Meperidine	0.5–1.0 mg/kg	5–30 mg	6–8 min	5–20 mg/h
Morphine	0.05–0.10 mg/kg	0.5–3.0 mg	6–8 min	0.5–2.0 mg/h

^{a}Lowest doses for extremes of age and ill patients, mid-range for normal adults, highest doses for patients who are inadequately treated by lower doses.
Reprinted with permission from Anesthesiology News.

reduces the risk of inadequate analgesia, it presents some risk of excessive medication. In this respect it has the same drawback as any constant iv infusion. Patients on PCA need to be observed closely (every 1–2 h) while the level of analgesia is being established. Even after PCA use has been stable, patients continue to need periodic observation for signs of oversedation and respiratory depression.

Some problems unique to the PCA device are faulty programming, faulty pump operation, incorrect medication, and bolus activation by someone other than the patient. The iv administration tubing should have an antireflux valve to prevent drug from accumulating retrograde in the iv tubing if the flow is occluded downstream. Without an antireflux valve, it would be possible for the patient to receive an unacceptably large dose when the downstream occlusion is relieved.

Transdermal Opioid

The highly lipid soluble opioid fentanyl can diffuse through intact skin at a rate that is sufficient to provide analgesia. Commercially prepared transdermal patches containing fentanyl are available with transfer rates of 25, 50, 75, and 100 µg/h. The rate of transfer is controlled by the permeability of the patch membrane. Although the patches can deliver a constant rate of fentanyl without cumbersome devices, they are not recommended for acute or postoperative pain. The long delay in reaching a steady level of analgesia makes rapid titration-to-effect impossible.

Epidural Analgesia

Epidural analgesia involves the repeated or continuous administration of analgesic drugs through an epidurally placed catheter. Opioids with or without local anesthetics are the drugs most commonly used. Intermittent epidural injections are usually given by hand. Continuous infusions are administered by an infusion pump. A PCA device can also be used with the epidural route to provide patient control of the epidural doses.

Epidurally administered opioids are thought to act at opiate receptors in the substantia gelatinosa of the dorsal horn. Local anesthetics are thought to act at nerve roots and directly on the spinal cord. The combination of opioid and local anesthetic is synergistic. The concentration of local anesthetic is generally much lower than would be useful if only the local anesthetic were given. Though epidural analgesia may be better in terms of analgesic quality than PCA, it has more restricted applicability. Analgesia is produced only below the upper thoracic area, and is thus not appropriate for some operations. The catheter is usually placed and managed by the anesthesia department, and is thus not as readily instituted as iv analgesia. Patients sometimes prefer the control that PCA gives them over the more passive character of epidural analgesia, and some patients are more comfortable with the concept of iv drugs than with epidurally administered drugs.

The types of postoperative pain that seem to benefit the most from epidural analgesia are thoracic and upper abdominal operations that impair chest wall mobility. The risk of pulmonary complications is reduced. The indications for epidural analgesia can be extended to lower abdominal procedures for patients who have significant pulmonary disease. Other indications are lower extremity orthopedic procedures requiring early ambulation. However, in patients who require a catheter for urinary retention, the presence of the catheter may make ambulation cumbersome. Local anesthetic concentrations sufficient to produce sympathectomy are used in lower extremity vascular surgery to improve blood flow and provide analgesia. It has also been found that epidural local anesthesia reduces the risk of venous thrombosis in orthopedic patients, possibly through an effect on blood coagulability. The use of epidural anesthesia for the prevention of postamputation phantom limb pain has been mentioned in conjunction with pre-emptive analgesia and is further discussed later in the section on continuous regional block.

Epidural analgesia is contraindicated if the patient refuses after discussion of risk, benefits, and alternatives. If the patient has a progressive CNS disease, such as multiple sclerosis, epidural analgesia is contraindicated. While there is no evidence that this form of analgesia would exacerbate CNS disease, new neurologic deficits would be difficult to distinguish from complications due to placement or presence of the epidural catheter. Placement of an epidural catheter is contraindicated in a patient who has either infection near the epidural site or generalized infection, because there is a small risk of inducing an epidural abscess. In all epidural analgesia patients, the epidural site is examined daily for signs of infections, such as erythema, induration, exudate, or tenderness.

Another contraindication to epidural catheter placement is coagulopathy, because an epidural hematoma might result in pressure on neural structures within the confines of the vertebral canal. The degree of abnormality in coagulation tests and platelet count that constitutes "coagulopathy" is not settled. If the patient is fully anticoagulated, an epidural catheter should not be placed. Low-dose heparin for thrombosis prophylaxis is also a contraindication. If anticoagulation is started in a patient who already has an epidural catheter, the catheter should not be removed until coagulation has been restored. Spinal opioid should not cause sensory or motor deficits. If these occur, or if the patient complains of spine pain or spine tenderness, assessment for an abscess or hematoma should begin immediately because the neurologic deficits will become permanent if intraspinal pressure is not relieved within 12 h. If a dural puncture occurs in the process of attempting to place an epidural catheter, an alternative for analgesia should be considered. The presence of a dural puncture may allow entry into the subarachnoid space of enough opioid and/or local anesthetic to produce an intrathecal overdose causing respiratory depression and/or a total spinal block.

If local anesthetic sufficient to cause sensory or motor block is added to epidural opioid analgesia, it will be difficult to decide whether an abscess or hematoma is present.

The concentration of local anesthetic should be reduced to assure that the block is reversible. If local anesthetic sufficient to cause sympathectomy is added, hypotension can occur in a hypovolemic patient. This is prevented by preloading the patient with 500–1000 mL of crystalloid fluid and treated with crystalloid and, depending on the severity, with a vasopressor such as ephedrine 5–10 mg iv. Hypotension can follow induction of epidural analgesia even when no local anesthetic is added. Epidural meperidine has a weak sympatholytic effect. In the case of other opioids, the relief of severe pain is followed by a reduction in sympathetic activity, which may unmask hypovolemia.

The point of entry into the epidural space has important implications in terms of the distribution of analgesia and incidence of side effects. The closer the catheter to the brain, the greater the risk of cephalad migration of opioid and side effects such as pruritus, somnolence, and respiratory depression. Placement of the catheter above the L-2 interspace exposes the patient to risk of spinal cord injury. In the thoracic spine, the epidural space is smaller, and great care must be taken not to puncture the dura. Epidural catheters are marked at 1-cm intervals. The length of catheter inserted is noted at the skin and recorded. The markings are helpful in determining whether that catheter has been withdrawn from its original insertion length.

Two options are available for reducing the cephalad spread of opioid. Placement of the catheter in the lumbar region lengthens the path for cephalad spread. Use of a highly lipid-soluble opioid, such as fentanyl, results in less cephalad spread because the fentanyl is absorbed locally by neural tissue, epidural fat and blood vessels, faster than it spreads to adjacent levels of the spinal cord.

Morphine and fentanyl are currently the most widely used opioids in use for epidural analgesia. Meperidine is useful because it is lipid soluble and analgesic spread is intermediate between that of morphine and fentanyl. Sufentanil is also used and is more lipid-soluble than fentanyl. Lipid solubility is the important physicochemical property that determines the distribution of opioids in the epidural and intrathecal spaces. The relatively poor lipid solubility of morphine explains its predilection to migrate cephalad, causing side effects such as pruritus, sedation, and respiratory depression. It also explains morphine's long duration of effect. The high lipid solubility of fentanyl explains the limited anatomic range of its analgesia and its ready vascular absorption, resulting in clinically significant blood levels. It also explains fentanyl's shorter duration of effect. It has been argued that the high fentanyl blood levels that result from epidural fentanyl infusion account for a significant part of fentanyl's analgesic effect, i.e., that epidural fentanyl infusion is an indirect and costly way of giving iv fentanyl. There is ample evidence however that epidural fentanyl has significant epidural effects apart from any systemic analgesia and that the analgesia is superior to iv fentanyl infusion.

The most common patient complaints related to epidural analgesia are pruritus, urinary incontinence, and inadequate analgesia. Pruritus is attributed to the cephalad spread of local anesthetic. Benadryl is often prescribed, but has unimpressive efficacy. Histamine release is not a characteristic of the pruritus. More consistent relief is obtained from systemic use of opioid antagonists, such as naloxone or nalbuphine. The primary drawback is that analgesia may be impaired. A balance must be determined between the discomfort of pruritus and the discomfort of pain. Intravenous propofol has recently been recommended as an effective antipruritic remedy that does not reverse analgesia. A propofol dose of 10 mg is small enough so that sedation is usually not a problem.

Urinary retention occurs often enough that routine indwelling catheterization is practiced in some institutions. This makes it awkward for patient ambulation and is a reason used to discourage the use of epidural analgesia in patients requiring early ambulation. On the other hand, the superior analgesia and lack of sedation from epidural analgesia promotes early ambulation, and it has been argued that only selected epidural analgesia patients require continuous bladder catheterization.

When inadequate analgesia occurs despite an adequate opioid dose, a cause must be found. The search for an explanation proceeds from the catheter to the infusion pump. If the catheter has been used with local anesthetic, the demonstration of a bilateral sensory block assures that the catheter was placed in the epidural space. If epidural placement is in question, the catheter can be tested with a dose of local anesthetic, after first aspirating to make certain that CSF or blood is not obtained. The catheter site should then be checked for signs of possible dislodgment. If the length of catheter inserted was documented, this can be checked against the markings on the catheter as it is currently positioned. The integrity of the dressing is also a clue to the possible likelihood of catheter dislodgment. The site is also checked for signs of fluid accumulation. A small amount of back-leakage is compatible with adequate analgesia; but if the patient also complains of inadequate analgesia or requires excessively large infusion, an alternative to continued use of the catheter should be considered. If the catheter has been dislodged, the infused solution will frequently follow a path of least resistance back along the catheter. The approximate location of the catheter tip can be estimated from the entry site and the length of catheter inserted. If the tip is not centered at the midpoint of the spinal level corresponding to the surgical dermatomes, part of the incision may be missed by the zone of analgesia. This is verified if the patient states that the lower or upper limit of the incision is painful. When this is the case, an opioid with lower lipid solubility can be tried, or the catheter can be reinserted at a more favorable position. The catheter should be examined for kinks. The connection from the catheter to the infusion pump should be examined for leaks. The pump should be examined for accuracy of the settings. The infusion reservoir should be examined for evidence that the expected amount of solution has actually been delivered by the pump. If sufficient solution hasn't been delivered, either the pump has malfunctioned or the pump has been turned off. Even with a perfectly functioning catheter and infusion system, the patient may have inadequate analgesia if the dose rate is too low, if a sufficient loading dose was not given, or if the patient has tolerance. (*See* Tables 6 and 7 for typical epidural doses and infusion rates.)

The most serious complication of epidural opioid analgesia is respiratory depression. The common causes are rostral spread of an excessive opioid dose, migration of an epidural catheter into the subarachnoid space, and the concomitant administration of a centrally acting sedative or parenteral opioid (*see* Table 8). The earliest sign of rostral spread is progressively increasing sedation. If sedative drugs have been given, it will be difficult to detect rostral spread. Slowing of the respiratory rate and hypoventilation on air resulting in falling pulse oximetry saturation are signs of respiratory depression. Naloxone should be immediately available for reversal of opioid-induced respiratory depression.

Table 6
Typical Epidural Opioid Doses for a 70-kg Adult[a]

Drug	Dose	Onset	Duration
Fentanyl	50–200 µg	5–15 min	2–4 h
Hydromorphone	1.0–1.5 mg	20–30 min	6–18 h
Meperidine	30–100 mg	15–25 min	4–8 h
Morphine	2.5–7.5 mg	30–90 min	6–24 h
Sufentanil	20–50 µg	5–15 min	2–4 h

[a]Lowest doses for extremes of age and ill patients, mid-range for normal adults, highest doses for patients who are inadequately treated by lower doses.
Reprinted with permission from Anesthesiology News.

Table 7
Typical Epidural Opioid Infusion Rates for a 70-kg Adult[a]

Drug	Concentration	Infusion Rate
Fentanyl	2-5 µg/mL	4–8 mL/h
Hydromorphone	0.02 mg/mL	1–6 mL/h
Morphine	0.05–0.10 mg/mL	4–8 mL/h
Sufentanil	1–2 µg/mL	4–8 mL/h

[a]Lowest doses for extremes of age and ill patients, mid-range for normal adults, highest doses for patients who are inadequately treated by lower doses.
Reprinted with permission from Anesthesiology News.

Intrathecal Analgesia

Intrathecal (subarachnoid) injection of opioids can provide hours of analgesia with small doses, with minimal sedation, and without elaborate equipment. Although it is possible to insert a catheter into the subarachnoid space as is done with continuous epidural analgesia, there is possibly a greater risk of neurologic side effects. Intrathecal analgesia is usually accomplished with a single injection of opioid, such as morphine. Since the duration of intrathecal morphine is 8–24 h, significant postoperative pain must be of relatively short duration, or some other form of subsequent analgesia must be planned. One of the most common clinical applications of intrathecal opioid analgesia is for post-Cesarean section pain, as discussed below.

The contraindications to intrathecal opioids are similar to those for epidural opioids. The side effects of intrathecal opioids are also the same as for epidural opioids. Postdural puncture CSF leak and headache can occur with either. It is difficult to compare intrathecal and epidural opioid-induced side effects without first establishing equivalent analgesic doses. For morphine, the ratio of equianalgesic doses is probably 10:1 epidural:intrathecal; i.e., 5 mg given epidurally is approximately equivalent to 0.5 mg given intrathecally (*see* Table 9 for typical doses).

Intra-Articular Analgesia

Both opioids and local anesthetics have been injected intra-articularly after knee surgery. Analgesia by this method suggests a peripheral action of opioids *(5,6)*. The combi-

Table 8
Some Causes of Respiratory Depression from Spinal Opioids

Cause	Comments
Catheter migration from epidural space into an epidural vein	Can occur at any time. Blood is aspirated from the catheter. Rapid respiratory depression after a bolus dose.
Catheter migration from epidural to subarachnoid space	Can occur at any time. CSF is aspirated from the catheter. Rapid respiratory depression after a bolus dose.
Concomitant administration of sedating drug	Standard procedure should be to avoid administration of sedative, tranquilizers, or parenteral opioids.
Incorrect dose or concentration	When unexpected respiratory depression occurs, all syringes and infusion bags should be saved and labeled for later examination.
Incorrect setting on computer-controlled pump	When unexpected respiratory depression occurs, the infusion device should be set aside and labeled for later examination.
Rostral spread	Occurs 6–12 h after a dose. Suggested by progressive sedation. Most commonly seen with low-lipid-solubility drugs like morphine.
Systemic absorption	Occurs within 2 h after a dose.

Table 9
Typical Intrathecal Opioid Doses for a 70-kg Adult[a]

Drug	Dose	Onset	Duration
Morphine	0.2–0.6 mg	15–45 min	8–24 h
Fentanyl	10–25 µg	2–5 min	2–4 h
Sufentanil	5–15 µg	2–5 min	2–4 h

[a]Lowest doses for extremes of age and ill patients, mid-range for normal adults, highest doses for patients who are inadequately treated by lower doses.
Reprinted with permission from Anesthesiology News.

nation of morphine and bupivacaine was found to be superior to either drug alone for postarthroscopy pain *(7)*. Intra-articular opioid has also been effective for anterior cruciate ligament repair *(8)*. However, at least three studies found that, following knee arthroscopy, neither intra-articular morphine nor bupivacaine was an effective analgesic *(9–11)*. Another report found that lumbar plexus block gave better analgesia than intra-articular injection of either bupivacaine or morphine *(12)*. The reason for these discrepancies is unknown. Possibly the technique of injection, the degree of articular inflammation, the type of operative anesthesia, or the use of epinephrine has an influence on the outcome.

Nerve Block

Peripheral nerve blocks, such as digital blocks and penile blocks, are occasionally performed to provide localized anesthesia for minor procedures. If a long-acting agent, such as bupivacaine, is used, the block will slowly regress for several hours after the procedure, allowing time to establish analgesia with oral agents. Although intercostal nerve blocks can provide effective post thoracotomy analgesia, it is usually not practical to repeat the block as often as it will be needed. A technique has been described for placing intercostal catheters for continuous or repeated local anesthetic administration, but this technique does not appear to be widely used. Thoracic paravertebral blocks have also been described for postthoracotomy analgesia with catheter placement. Cryoanalgesia (cryolysis), performed just prior to closing the chest, can provide several days or weeks of analgesia after thoracotomy. Availability of longer acting anesthetic preparations, such as liposomal-encapsulated bupivacaine, may increase the popularity of peripheral nerve blocks for postoperative analgesia.

Continuous Regional Block

Continuous regional block and nerve block are accomplished by the placement of a catheter in close proximity to the innervation of the operative site. Postoperative analgesia by local anesthetic regional blockade has been advocated for amputations and revascularization procedures. In the case of amputations, continuous block of the extremity by epidural for the legs or by brachial plexus block for the arm may reduce the risk of postamputation phantom limb pain. To be effective in preventing painful phantom sensation, it has been recommended that anesthesia be induced preoperatively. When revascularization is desired, the sympathectomy that accompanies regional block may improve blood flow and wound healing.

Continuous brachial plexus blocks, using either axillary or interscalene approach, require the placement of a catheter when the block is first initiated. A loading dose of 0.75% bupivacaine with epinephrine is commonly used to establish anesthesia, and then an infusion of 0.125–0.25% bupivacaine is given at 0.25 mg/kg body wt/h. A continuous technique has also been described for similarly blocking the lumbar plexus to provide unilateral lower extremity analgesia. Although bupivacaine is the longest-acting of the available local anesthetics, there is concern about toxicity from continuous infusion. Cardiotoxicity of bupivacaine is particularly dangerous because of its association with intractable ventricular fibrillation. Phenytoin, a class 1_B antidysrhythmic agent, has been used successfully to reverse bupivacaine-induced dysrhythmias in neonates *(13)*. Other complications from continuous regional block include infection at the catheter site, nerve injury, and injury due to loss of motor control or sensory function.

Interpleural Analgesia

Interpleural analgesia is a technique involving the instillation of local anesthetic into the pleural cavity. The most commonly used agent is 0.5% bupivacaine. Although the procedure has been claimed to be effective for relieving pain from thoracotomy, chole-cystectomy, and renal operations, a number of studies have questioned its efficacy and safety compared to epidural or systemic opioid analgesia. The procedure is only effective for unilateral pain. It requires insertion of a catheter into the pleural space, with attendant risks of pneumothorax and empyema. Absorption of local anesthetic from the pleural cavity is rapid, leading to concern regarding systemic toxicity from bupivacaine. Currently, interpleural analgesia is not a widely practiced technique.

ASSESSMENT OF PAIN AND SIDE EFFECTS

Pain is defined by the International Association for the Study of Pain as an unpleasant sensory and emotional experience that is associated with actual or potential tissue damage, and it is described in terms of such damage. In postsurgical patients, tissue damage is present. The exception might be procedures involving examination only. Amputation (involving nerve, periosteum, and skin), plastic procedures and large incisions (involving skin), and orthopedic procedures (involving periosteum) typically generate significant postoperative pain. There is nothing in the definition of pain about either the appearance or the behavior of a patient who is experiencing pain. There are wide variations in the way that postoperative pain is expressed from unrestrained moaning and screaming to stoic silence. Elevated blood pressure and heart rate are frequently assessed in the recovery room as indications of postoperative pain. These are suggestive but nonspecific signs. Certainly the absence of tachycardia or hypertension does not necessarily correspond to the absence of pain, nor does their presence indicate acute pain.

The most useful information is an estimate by the patient of his/her pain magnitude. This is facilitated by using a numerical score based on a verbally described scale; i.e., zero for no pain and 10 for the worst imaginable pain (verbal numerical rating scale). Similar results are obtained from an unmarked ruler with each end representing the extremes of pain (visual analog scale). This method requires a gesture by the patient and discourages an "off-the-scale" response. Unfortunately pain scores are usually not all "pain." The patient's response may be strongly weighted by emotional factors. Anxiety related to helplessness, fear of complications, or fear of cancer can amplify the score. Measures that recognize and address anxiety will reduce the score. An off-the-scale response, such as "12 out of 10," clearly indicates that the patient is using the score to motivate the nurse or physician rather than to describe a painful experience. Like other clinically generated numbers, the pain score should be part of a more global assessment.

SPECIAL POSTOPERATIVE PAIN PROBLEMS

Patient with Limited Ability to Communicate

Assessment of analgesia requirements is difficult in patients who have limited ability to communicate (see Table 10). Frequently a care giver, such as a parent, nurse or physical therapist, can interpret a patient's responses. If available, a translator or bilingual family member can assist with non–English-speaking patients. An American Sign Language interpreter or written communication can be used with deaf patients. By

Table 10
Patients with Limited Ability
to Communicate

Deaf or mute
Decreased level of consciousness
Intubated or tracheostomy
Non-English speaking
Psychotic
Severe mental retardation
Very young child

observing a patient's responses to pain-producing maneuvers—like position change, coughing, or extremity range of motion—it is usually possible to infer the presence of significant pain.

Ambulatory Surgery and Emergency Room

When patients are going to be discharged to home shortly after surgery, the anticipated pain must be manageable by weak oral analgesics or other techniques that are not associated with significant side effects or risks. Acetaminophen with codeine or hydrocodone usually provides satisfactory analgesia for ambulatory patients. Addition of an NSAID, such as ketorolac, enhances opioid analgesia without simultaneously increasing opioid side effects. Intravenous ketorolac is useful in early recovery before oral intake is established or if postoperative nausea/vomiting is present. Incision infiltration with long-acting local anesthetics, such as bupivacaine, intra-articular instillation of opioid and local anesthetic, and peripheral nerve blocks are also useful ambulatory analgesics. Since peripheral nerve block results in sensory and/or motor block, the patient must be warned of potential injury while the block effects are present.

Post-Cesarean Section Pain

Analgesia following Cesarean section should permit early ambulation and not interfere with the mother's interactions with her newborn child. Cesarean section is a good operation for comparison of postoperative analgesia techniques. The incision is standard and so is the procedure. Many healthy young patients undergo this type of operation. Many clinical studies comparing the postoperative effectiveness of PCA, spinal analgesia, and patient-controlled epidural analgesia have been performed.

In comparisons of PCA, epidural opioid and im opioid for controlling post-Cesarean section pain, PCA caused more sedation but less pruritus than epidural opioid. Both PCA and epidural analgesia provided better analgesia than im opioids *(14,15)*. Is the sedation associated with PCA of clinical significance? In a recent study breast-fed infants whose mothers received epidural bupivacaine for 3 d after Cesarean section gained more weight than infants whose mothers received only diclofenac for analgesia *(16)*. It is not known how PCA would fare in comparison with epidural analgesia in terms of infant weight gain. In a comparison of morphine, meperidine, and oxymorphone PCA, meperidine was associated with fewer maternal side effects, but with lower neonatal neurobehavioral scores, possibly due to high concentrations of normeperidine in breast milk (17,18).

The maternal complications of perinatal spinal opioids do not appear to be different from those encountered in other postoperative situations. There was initially some concern raised about a seemingly high occurrence of herpes simplex reactivation when intrathecal opiates were given for obstetrical analgesia. The natural decline in maternal cell-mediated immunity and the effect of opioids on cell-mediated immunity might explain such an association. At the time of the reports, it was common to use higher intrathecal morphine doses than is currently the practice. Subsequent experience argues against a significant rate of herpes reactivation using current doses and techniques for intrathecal morphine analgesia. Enlargement of epidural veins during pregnancy and thrombocytopenia might increase the risk of epidural hematoma, but this has not been reported despite the wide use of epidural analgesia for labor and epidural anesthesia for Cesarean section. Either morphine PCA or spinal opioid provides safe and adequate analgesia following Cesarean section.

Pediatric Patients

One of the most difficult aspects of providing analgesia to pediatric patients is the difficulty in assessing their response. Children may lack the ability to verbalize their pain. Their response may be to remain unusually quiet. Analgesia techniques that are effective in adults are applicable to children. Techniques that require instruction, such as PCA, may not be practical in very young children. It is generally not acceptable for a parent or nurse to operate the PCA device for a child. Nerve blocks, regional blocks, and spinal opiates have been used successfully in pediatric patients. For example, after major abdominal surgery, epidural morphine is effective with few side effects except that premature children have a high risk of respiratory depression (19). Thoracic epidural fentanyl-bupivacaine has been safely used postthoracotomy in children (20). The technical aspects of analgesia in pediatric patients are more confidently dealt with by those who specialize in pediatric care. Epidural opioid and local anesthetic provide effective analgesia, but there is also a high risk of technical complications (21). Probably the most commonly used method of regional anesthesia and analgesia for young pediatric patients is via the caudal epidural route. The procedure is technically easier and safer in this age group than lumbar or thoracic epidural techniques. Caudal infusions of opioid and/or local anesthetics can be continued postoperatively.

Chronic Pain Patients

Patients who have experienced chronic pain have legitimate fears that their postoperative pain will be inadequately controlled. Tolerance to opioids makes the "usual" opiate doses inadequate. Their request for additional medication may be perceived as addiction-based "drug-seeking" behavior instead of legitimate, appropriate requests for adequate analgesia. A common practice is to involve the pain management specialist in the patient's postoperative analgesic management. Even if regional anesthesia or spinal opioids/local anesthetics are used, it may still be necessary to continue the patient's preoperative pain medications. A reduction in systemic opioid administration might

Table 11
Chronic Pain Medications—Potential Consequences of Abrupt Withdrawal

Drug	Chronic Pain Condition	Potential Consequence
β-Adrenergic blocking drugs; e.g., propranolol, nadolol or metoprolol	Migraine headaches	Hypersensitivity to catecholamines, exacerbation of angina, myocardial infarction, ventricular arrhythmias
Antihypertensive drugs; e.g., clonidine	Postherpetic neuralgia	Rebound hypertension
Antiarrhythmic drugs; e.g., mexiletine		None
Opioid analgesics	Various	Opiate abstinence syndrome
Acetaminophen	Various	None
Salicylates	Arthritis	None
NSAIDs	Various	None
Benzodiazepines; e.g., diazepam or clonazepam	Muscle spasm	Withdrawal syndrome, including grand mal seizures
Tricyclic antidepressants; e.g., amitriptyline	Migraine, diabetic neuropathy, tic douloureux, cancer pain, painful peripheral neuropathy, postherpetic neuralgia, arthritic pain	Withdrawal syndrome (nausea, headache, vertigo, nightmares, malaise)
Anticonvulsants; e.g., phenytoin	Tic douloureux, neuropathic pain	Only a problem for patients who also have seizure disorder
Skeletal muscle relaxants; e.g., baclofen	Muscle spasms	Withdrawal syndrome (hallucinations, seizures)

produce an opiate abstinence syndrome. Also, the postoperative analgesia may not adequately manage the patient's chronic pain. Some pain medications should not be abruptly discontinued (*see* Table 11). Chronic pain patients who are opioid-tolerant will require special precaution. The titration of postoperative pain with large systemic opioid doses entails risks of either overdosing or underdosing. Those who are responsible for assessing the patient's medication response will need to be familiar with the recognition and management of overdose and early abstinence.

Substance Abuse (22)

Patients with a history of substance abuse present a difficult problem for postoperative pain management. The objective is to relieve pain without contributing to addiction. Some of the problems that may have to be addressed are listed in Table 12. Assessment

Table 12
Potential Problems in the Patient
with a Substance Abuse History

Patient reluctance to report drug abuse history
Potential for perioperative relapse
Patient concern about re-exposure to addicting drugs
Pain control in the presence of altered responsiveness (tolerance)
Risk of perioperative access to illicit drugs

includes determining what substances have been abused and which are currently used. The stage of the patient's substance abuse problem should also be ascertained: acutely intoxicated, abstinence syndrome, recovering in a program, or recovered. Finally, the patient's concerns about the use of opioids need to be explored. The widest possible range of options will need to be considered. Nondrug methods—such as TENS, biofeedback, cryotherapy, and cryoanalgesia—may be helpful as adjuncts to reduce the need for opioids. Nonopioid drugs, such as NSAIDs and muscle relaxants, are also likely to reduce the need for opioids. A detailed plan for administration of opioids should be developed for the patient. It will be important to avoid reinforcing analgesic requesting and drug-seeking behavior. Also to be avoided are power struggles and repeated negotiations. Specific opioids, route, prescribing physician, and a plan for tapering should be addressed with the patient. As with chronic pain patients whose tolerance requires that large doses be given, attention to the signs of acute intoxication on one hand and early abstinence syndrome on the other is necessary when opioid tolerance is present. A specialist in the management of addiction may be an appropriate consultant is such cases.

SUGGESTED READINGS

Cousins MJ, Phillips GD, ed. Acute Pain Management. New York: Churchill Livingstone, 1986. Ferrante FE, VadeBoncouer TR, ed. Postoperative Pain Management. New York: Churchill Livingstone, 1993. Macintyre PE, Ready LB. Acute Pain Management. A Practical Guide. London: W. B. Saunders, 1996. Sinatra RS, Hord AH, Ginsberg B, Preble LM, ed. Acute Pain. Mechanisms and Management. St. Louis: Mosby Year Book, 1992.

REFERENCES

1. Ng B, Dimsdale JE, Rollnik JD, Shapiro H. The effect of ethnicity on prescriptions for patient-controlled analgesia for post-operative pain. Pain 1996; 66: 9–12.
2. Ready LB, Oden R, Chadwick HS, Benedetti C, Rooke GA, Caplan R, Wild LM. Development of an anesthesiology-based postoperative pain management service. Anesthesiology 1988; 68: 100–106.
3. Redelmeier DA, Kahneman D. Patients' memories of painful medical treatments: real-time and retrospective evaluations of two minimally invasive procedures. Pain 1996; 66: 3–8.
4. Pasqualucci A, De Angelis V, Contardo R, Colo F, Terrosu G, Donini A, Pasetto A, Bresadola F. Preemptive analgesia: intraperitoneal local anesthetic in laparoscopic cholecystectomy. Anesthesiology 1996; 85: 11–20.

5. Ferreira SH, Nakamura M. II-Prostaglandin hyperalgesia: The peripheral analgesic activity of morphine, enkephalins and opioid antagonists. Prostaglandins 1979; 18: 191–200.

6. Stein C, Comisel K, Haimerl E, Yassouridis A, Lehrgerger K, Herz K, Peter K. Analgesic effect of intraarticular morphine after arthroscopic knee surgery. N Engl J Med 1991; 325: 1123–1126.

7. Allen GC, St Amand MA, Lui ACP, Johnson DH, Lindsay P. Postarthroscopy analgesia with intraarticular bupivacaine/morphine. Anesthesiology 1993; 79: 475–580.

8. Joshi GP, McCarroll SM, McSwiney M, O'Rourke P, Hurson BJ. Effects of intraarticular morphine on analgesic requirements after anterior cruciate ligament repair. Regional Anesthesia 1993; 18: 254–257.

9. Bjornsson A, Gupta A, Vegfors M, Lennmarken C, Sjoberg F. Intraarticular morphine for postoperative analgesia following knee arthroscopy. Regional Anesthesia 1994; 19: 104–108.

10. Raja SN, Dickstein RE, Johnson CA. Comparison of postoperative analgesic effects of intraarticular bupivacaine and morphine following arthroscopic knee surgery. Anesthesiology 1992; 77: 1143.

11. Khoury GF, Chen ACN, Garland DE, Stein C. Intraarticular morphine, bupivacaine, and morphine/bupivacaine for pain control after knee videoarthroscopy. Anesthesiology 1992; 77: 263.

12. De Andres J, Bellver J, Barrera L, Febra E, Bolinches R. A comparative study of analgesia after knee surgery with intraarticular bupivacaine, intraarticular morphine, and lumbar plexus block. Anesthesia Analgesia 1993; 77: 727–730.

13. Maxwell, LG, Martin LD, Yaster M. Bupivacaine-induced cardiac toxicity in neonates: successful treatment with intravenous phenytoin. Anesthesiology 1994; 80: 682–686.

14. Eisenach JC, Grice SC, Dewan DM. Patient-controlled analgesia following Cesarean section: a comparison with epidural and intramuscular narcotics. Anesthesiology 1988; 68: 444–448.

15. Harrison DM, Sinatra R, Morgese L, Chung JH. Epidural narcotic and patient-controlled analgesia for post-Cesarean section pain relief. Anesthesiology 1988; 68: 454–457.

16. Hirsose M, Hara Y, Hosokawa T, Tanaka Y. The effect of postoperative analgesia with continuous epidural bupivacaine after Cesarean section on the amount of breast feeding and infant weight gain. Anesthesia Analgesia 1996; 82: 1166–1169.

17. Sinatra RS, Lodge K, Sibert K, Chung KS, Chung JH, Parker A Jr, Harrison DM. A comparison of morphine, meperidine and oxymorphone as utilized in PCA following cesarean delivery. Anesthesiology 1989; 70: 585–590.

18. Wittles B, Scott DT, Sinatra RS. Exogenous opioids in human breast milk and acute neonatal neurobehaviour: a preliminary study. Anesthesiology 1990; 73: 864–869.

19. Henneberg SW, Hole P{, De Haas M, Jensen PG. Epidural morphine for postoperative pain relief in children. Acta Anaesthesiol Scand 1993; 37: 664–667.

20. Tobias JD, Lowe S, O'Dell N, Holcomb GW III. Thoracic epidural anaesthesia in infants and children. Can J Anaesth 1993; 40: 879–882.

21. Wilson PTJ, Lloyd-Thomas AR. An audit of extradural infusion analgesia in children using bupivacaine and diamorphine. Anaesthesia 1993; 48: 718–723.

22. Williams MJ, Alexander CM. Experiences of recovering substance abuse patients with anesthesia and surgery. Am J Anesthesiol 1995; 23: 14–18.

13 PAIN BY ETIOLOGY

Maurice E. Hamilton, MD

Key Points

Herpes Zoster

- Herpes zoster (shingles) is caused by reactivation of latent varicella-zoster virus (VZV).

- About 15% of patients previously infected with VZV will develop herpes zoster.

- The incidence and severity of herpes zoster increase with age and other causes of impaired cell-mediated immunity, including leukemia, lymphoma, HIV infection, and medications.

- Herpes zoster usually causes severe pain along the affected dermatome for several days prior to the skin eruption; this may be misdiagnosed as cardiac, pulmonary, or abdominal disease.

- Thoracic and lumbar nerves and the ophthalmic branch of the trigeminal nerve are most often affected.

- Involvement of the ophthalmic branch of the trigeminal nerve may cause severe eye disease, including loss of vision; these patients should be referred to an ophthalmologist at once.

- Occasionally, pain from herpes zoster may be present in the absence of skin lesions (zoster sine herpete).

- Disseminated herpes zoster may develop in immunocompromised patients, including patients with lymphoma and graft-vs-host disease.

- Antiviral therapy with valacyclovir, famciclovir, or acyclovir should be initiated without delay as soon as herpes zoster is diagnosed.

- Antiviral agents reduce pain from acute herpes zoster and accelerate the rate of lesion healing. They probably do not decrease the incidence of postherpetic neuralgia, but they do decrease the duration of pain.

- Treatment of pain may include local anesthetic blocks, analgesics, and antidepressants such as nortriptyline or amitriptyline.

- The use of corticosteroids to treat acute herpes zoster has been controversial, but one recent study reported that the addition of prednisone to acyclovir improved the quality of life in relatively healthy patients over age 50.

- Varicella vaccine (Varivax) decreases primary varicella-zoster virus (VZV) infection and restores VZV-specific cell-mediated immunity in older patients, suggesting that it may be possible to reduce the incidence and severity of herpes zoster and its complications in the elderly.

Postherpetic Neuralgia

- Postherpetic neuralgia may be defined as neuropathic pain persisting 1 mo or longer after the onset of herpes zoster.
- Postherpetic neuralgia develops in 10–15% of patients with herpes zoster; the risk increases to about 50% after age 60.
- The primary therapy for postherpetic neuralgia is a tricyclic antidepressant, especially amitriptyline, nortriptyline, or desipramine. Though less effective as analgesics, maprotiline or a selective serotonin reuptake inhibitor may be used for patients unable to tolerate tricyclic antidepressants.
- Other therapeutic options include topical lidocaine or capsaicin, oral opioids, anticonvulsants such as carbamazepine, and transcutaneous electrical nerve stimulation (TENS).
- Patients with pain refractory to these modalities should be considered for referral to a multidisciplinary pain clinic.

Central Pain

- Stroke and spinal cord trauma are the most common causes of central pain, but any lesion in the spinal cord, brainstem, or brain can cause central pain.
- The onset of central pain may be delayed by months or years following the original injury.
- Virtually all patients with central pain have sensory abnormalities, especially to temperature.
- MRI usually identifies the lesion responsible for central pain.
- The therapeutic goal is pain reduction rather than complete pain relief.
- The primary pharmacologic therapy is a tricyclic antidepressant, especially amitriptyline or nortriptyline.
- Other pharmacologic options include anticonvulsants (e.g., carbamazepine), adrenergic agents (e.g., clonidine), and opioid analgesics.
- Psychosocial support is essential in patients with chronic pain to assist with pain coping and to treat depression.
- Physical modalities such as TENS and physiotherapy may provide benefit.
- Therapeutic options for refractory pain include dorsal root entry zone (DREZ), spinal cord, thalamic, and deep brain stimulation.

Psychogenic Pain

- Psychogenic pain represents a pain disorder in which psychological factors play the major role in the onset, severity, exacerbation, or maintenance of the pain.
- Patients with psychogenic pain actually perceive pain.

Table 1
Risk Factors for Herpes Zoster

Age over 50
Cancer (especially lymphoma, leukemia)
HIV infection
Corticosteroids and other immunosuppressants

- Psychogenic pain is poorly localized, does not disturb sleep, and may be relieved by alcohol or psychotropic medication, but seldom by analgesics.

- Weakness of all muscles in a region, superficial tenderness, and occurrence of pain with benign maneuvers suggest psychogenic pain.

- Investigations of possible organic causes of psychogenic pain should be limited.

- Early recognition of psychogenic pain allows prompt referral for psychiatric evaluation and treatment, which may include antidepressants, benzodiazepines, major tranquilizers, behavioral therapy, and psychotherapy.

- Unnecessary medications should be discontinued so they do not reinforce erroneous beliefs regarding the cause of the pain.

HERPES ZOSTER

Varicella-zoster virus (VZV) causes varicella (chickenpox) and establishes a latent infection in sensory ganglia. In Western countries, most varicella infections occur during childhood and are self-limited with little morbidity. However, varicella may cause significant disease in newborns and adults, including pregnant women and immunocompromised patients.

When reactivated, VZV causes acute herpes zoster (shingles), which produces pain and cutaneous lesions in a dermatomal distribution. Immunocompromised hosts may develop disseminated, life-threatening infection. Many patients experience prolonged pain lasting weeks or months following resolution of the cutaneous eruption. This section highlights clinical aspects and treatment of acute herpes zoster. Postherpetic neuralgia is discussed in the following section.

Epidemiology

Cell-mediated immunity (CMI) is the primary host defense against varicella infection and reactivation of the latent virus (1). VZV-specific CMI declines with age, demonstrating marked reduction after age 60. Overall, about 15% of patients who have had varicella will develop herpes zoster, but the incidence and severity increase with age as a consequence of impaired immunity. For individuals aged 50–70 yr, the incidence of herpes zoster is 5–10 cases/1000 persons. By age 80, about one-third of individuals will have experienced herpes zoster (2). Likewise, patients with impaired immunity due to factors such as medications, HIV infection, or neoplasia (especially leukemia or lymphoma) are at increased risk of developing herpes zoster (Table 1). Repeat episodes of herpes zoster are uncommon, presumably due to the vigorous immune response normally triggered by reactivation of VZV.

Table 2
Complications of Herpes Zoster Infection

Cutaneous	Visceral	Ocular	Neurologic
Disseminated lesions	Pneumonitis	Conjunctivitis	Meningoencephalitis
Bacterial superinfection	Pericarditis	Scleritis	Encephalitis
Scarring	Esophagitis	Keratitis	Granulomatous cerebral
Zoster gangrenosum	Gastritis	Iridocyclitis	angiitis
	Hepatitis	Retinitis	Thrombotic cerebral
	Cystitis	Choroiditis	vasculopathy
	Arthritis	Optic neuritis	Optic neuritis
		Ophthalmoplegia	Ophthalmoplegia
			(Cranial nn. 3, 4, 6)
			Ramsey-Hunt syndrome
			Deafness, unilateral
			Transverse myelitis
			Guillain-Barré syndrome
			Peripheral nerve palsies
			Postherpetic neuralgia

Clinical Features

Herpes zoster is characterized by unilateral pain and a vesicular eruption that is usually confined to the dermatome innervated by a single spinal or cranial sensory ganglion *(3)*. Thoracic and lumbar nerves and the first (ophthalmic) division of the trigeminal nerve are most often affected. Herpes zoster infection typically causes sharp, shooting, burning, or aching pain, itching, and paresthesias along the affected dermatome for 2–4 d prior to the appearance of the skin eruption. For many patients, this will represent the most severe pain ever experienced. The pain may be associated with fever and malaise. During this process, the reactivated virus spreads peripherally from the dorsal root or cranial nerve ganglion to afferent neurons along which it propagates to the skin. The cutaneous eruption begins with localized erythema followed by papules that evolve into vesicles, pustules, and crusted lesions. Appropriate precautions must be taken to ensure that persons without previous varicella infection or immunization are not exposed to infectious particles in the cutaneous lesions. The usual duration of these lesions is 7–10 d, but they may last up to 4 wk. Occasionally, pain from acute herpes zoster may occur without skin lesions (zoster sine herpete); in this circumstance, the pain is presumed to be caused by inflammation of neural tissue in the absence of cutaneous infection.

Involvement of cranial nerves may cause serious sequelae (Table 2). When the sensory branch of the 7th cranial nerve is affected, unilateral herpetic lesions may develop on the anterior two-thirds of the tongue and the external ear canal in association with Bell's palsy (Ramsey-Hunt syndrome). Involvement of the 8th cranial nerve may cause unilateral deafness. Zoster affecting the mandibular or maxillary branch of the trigeminal nerve may cause facial and oral lesions.

Herpes zoster ophthalmicus, a potentially devastating complication from involvement of the ophthalmic branch of the trigeminal nerve, has been reported in about 15% of patients with herpes zoster. During the acute phase, headache, fever, chills, and malaise may occur in conjunction with unilateral pain or hypesthesia over the top of the head, forehead, and eye. Within days, characteristic lesions appear along the dermatome. The presence of cutaneous lesions at the tip of the nose indicates involvement of this branch. Conjunctivitis, episcleritis, scleritis, keratitis, iridocyclitis, glaucoma, retinitis, choroiditis, optic neuritis, and extraocular muscle palsies may develop (4). Corneal anesthesia or exposure from lid retraction predisposes to neurotrophic ulcers, which may cause perforation of the eye. Immunologically mediated neovascularization of the cornea may severely impair vision. These patients should be referred immediately to an ophthalmologist.

Prior to or in the absence of skin lesions, herpes zoster may be misdiagnosed as coronary artery disease, pleuritis, cholecystitis, appendicitis, pyelonephritis, kidney stone, intervertebral disk disease, or sciatica. Among elderly or immunocompromised patients with unexplained acute chest or abdominal pain, herpes zoster should rank high in the differential diagnosis. Once the characteristic skin lesions appear, the correct diagnosis is usually obvious. However, both herpes simplex and coxsackievirus infections can cause dermatomal vesicular lesions. If the etiology is uncertain, a Tzanck smear (which can differentiate herpes from other causes) with viral serologic studies or cultures will establish the diagnosis.

Central nervous system (CNS) involvement results when the infection spreads centrally from the ganglion. Even patients without meningeal signs may have cerebrospinal fluid (CSF) pleocytosis and moderate elevation of CSF protein. Symptomatic meningoencephalitis is characterized by fever, headache, photophobia, aseptic meningitis, and vomiting. Other neurologic manifestations include transverse myelitis, cranial or peripheral polyneuritis, and chronic radicular pain. A rare complication is granulomatous angiitis, which may present as contralateral hemiplegia and is diagnosed by cerebral angiography.

Not uncommonly, some vesicles develop at remote sites due to hematogenous dissemination of viral particles. In immunocompetent patients, this process is limited. However, in immunocompromised patients, serious systemic illness may result. Cutaneous disseminated disease develops in about 40% of patients with Hodgkin's and non-Hodgkin's lymphoma, increasing their risk of developing progressive herpes zoster associated with hepatitis, pneumonitis, or meningoencephalitis. Patients who receive bone marrow transplants are at particular risk of developing VZV infection. The development of graft-vs-host disease increases the risk of dissemination and death.

Pathophysiology

The pain from acute herpes zoster results from inflammation and destruction of neural tissue and peripheral tissue, including the skin, as a consequence of viral replication (2). Histologic studies show inflammation with hemorrhagic necrosis and fibrosis in dorsal root ganglia and multinucleated giant cells and epithelial cells with eosinophilic intranuclear inclusions in cutaneous lesions. Inflammation within peripheral nerves may

Table 3
Treatment of Acute Herpes Zoster

Antiviral agent (*see* Table 4)
Analgesic as needed with appropriate precautions
Consider nerve block or topical anesthetic
Consider prednisone in patients over age 50 with mild to severe pain if no contraindication
Consider addition of amitriptyline or another tricyclic antidepressant
Consider carbamazepine if persistent lancinating pain

Table 4
Antiviral Treatment of Herpes Zoster

Agent	Dose	Special Considerations
Acyclovir (Zovirax)	800 mg orally five times daily for 7–10 d; 500 mg/m^2 iv every 8 h for 7 d in immunocompromised patients	Administer intravenously in immunocompromised patients Decrease dose with renal failure
Famciclovir (Famvir)	500 mg orally every 8 h for 7 d	Decrease dose with renal failure
Valacyclovir (Valtrex)	1000 mg orally every 8 h for 7 d	Decrease dose with renal failure

persist for weeks or months and may be associated with demyelination and wallerian degeneration. These processes may lead to scarring of the dorsal root ganglia, peripheral nerves, and skin *(5)*. Permanent morphological changes in the dorsal horn have been described in patients who go on to develop postherpetic neuralgia but not in those with uncomplicated herpes zoster *(6)*.

Treatment

The primary treatment of acute herpes zoster is antiviral therapy, which should be initiated promptly as soon as the diagnosis is made (Table 3). Antiviral agents currently available in the United States for treatment of herpes zoster are acyclovir (Zovirax), famciclovir (Famvir), and valacyclovir (Valtrex) (Table 4). Acyclovir has relatively low bioavailability (15–30%) compared to famciclovir (about 80%) and valacyclovir (55% or higher). Famciclovir and valacyclovir are prodrugs rapidly absorbed from the gastrointestinal tract and metabolized to the nucleoside analogs penciclovir and acyclovir, respectively. These analogs are metabolized by viral enzymes to triphosphate derivatives that inhibit viral DNA replication. Valacyclovir is the least expensive of these agents.

Antiviral agents significantly reduce the pain from acute herpes zoster and accelerate the rate of lesion healing. Whereas antiviral agents probably do not prevent postherpetic neuralgia, famciclovir and valacyclovir have been reported to decrease its duration. In one study, famciclovir reduced the median duration of postherpetic neuralgia from 163 d to 63 d in patients over age 50 *(7)*. In a study comparing valacyclovir to acyclovir in immunocompetent patients over age 50, valacyclovir administered for 7 d reduced the median duration of postherpetic neuralgia to 38 d, compared to 51 d with acyclovir; the percentage of patients with postherpetic neuralgia at 6 mo was 19% with valacyclovir vs 26% with acyclovir (8).

The recommended dose of acyclovir for the treatment of acute herpes zoster is 800 mg (four 200-mg capsules, two 400-mg tablets, one 800-mg tablet, or 20-mL suspension) orally every 4 h five times daily for 7–10 d. For patients with impaired renal function, the dosing interval should be increased to every 8 h for creatinine clearance 10–25 mL/min and every 12 h for creatinine clearance less than 10 mL/min. For immunocompromised patients with normal renal function, acyclovir should be administered intravenously in a dose of 500 mg/m^2 every 8 h for 7 d. Concurrent use of probenecid (Benemid) may decrease renal clearance and increase the plasma concentration of acyclovir.

Famciclovir is administered in a dose of 500 mg orally every 8 h for 7 d. In patients with creatinine clearance 40–59 mL/min, the recommended dose is 500 mg every 12 h. For creatinine clearance under 40 mL/min, this dose should be administered once every 24 h.

The dose of valacyclovir is 1000 mg (two 500-mg caplets) orally every 8 h for 7 d. In patients with renal dysfunction, this dose is reduced to 1000 mg every 12 h for creatinine clearance 30–49 mL/min and every 24 h for creatinine clearance 10–29 mL/min; for creatinine clearance less than 10 mL/min, the dose is 500 mg every 24 h. A thrombotic thrombocytopenic purpura/hemolytic-uremic syndrome has been described in some severely immunocompromised patients treated with high doses of valacyclovir (9). Cimetidine (Tagamet) and probenecid may decrease the renal clearance of acyclovir, the active metabolite of valacyclovir.

Another nucleoside analog, sorivudine, has been reported to be superior to acyclovir for the treatment of localized herpes zoster in patients with HIV infection (10). Administration of sorivudine with 5-fluorouracil (5-FU) or related drugs is contraindicated and has reportedly led to the deaths of 15 people in Japan (11). The Food and Drug Administration recently refused to approve sorivudine for marketing in this country.

For patients experiencing severe pain from acute zoster, local anesthetic nerve blocks may provide dramatic pain relief (2). Some believe that nerve blocks administered early in the course of acute herpes zoster may decrease the incidence of PHN. For trigeminal neuralgia, sympathetic blocks of the stellate ganglion and trigeminal branch blocks may be administered. Nerve blocks are also feasible for zoster in the 2nd through 4th cervical dermatomes. For herpes zoster affecting C5 and lower dermatomes, epidural nerve blocks (sometimes combining local anesthetic with steroids) or peripheral nerve blocks (including intercostal nerve blocks) may be utilized. Although these techniques will generally require the expertise of an anesthesiologist, it is important that the primary physician be aware of these options.

Subcutaneous infiltration of the skin lesions with local anesthetic may also decrease pain from acute herpes zoster (2). Though seldom used, iv administration of lidocaine has been reported to reduce pain from both acute herpes zoster and postherpetic neuralgia.

Many patients require therapy with opioid analgesics, especially if nerve blocks have not been utilized. Depending on the severity of pain, agents such as codeine, hydrocodone, or oxycodone may be prescribed. Antidepressants or anticonvulsants may provide additional analgesic benefit. Use of these drugs is discussed in Chapter 14.

Corticosteroids have been evaluated for their effects on acute herpes zoster and the development of postherpetic neuralgia. One recent study compared the benefit of acyclovir administered orally for 7 vs 21 d, with or without prednisolone (initial dose 40 mg daily, tapered over 3 wk) *(12)*. Administration of corticosteroids was associated with more rapid healing of the rash, and pain reduction was somewhat greater during the acute phase of the disease in patients treated with steroids or acyclovir for 21 d. However, by d 21 there was no difference in the severity of pain between any of the groups, and the duration of pain was the same in all groups. Patients who received steroids reported more adverse effects. Thus, prolonged treatment with acyclovir or the addition of prednisolone produced only limited benefits compared to a 7-d course of acyclovir. Neither additional therapy reduced the incidence of postherpetic neuralgia.

A subsequent study of the effect of acyclovir and prednisone on herpes zoster measured quality-of-life outcomes in addition to duration of pain *(13)*. Participants in the study were generally healthy adults older than 50 yr of age with localized herpes zoster lesions that had been present for less than 72 h. Patients were randomized to receive acyclovir or placebo with or without prednisone. Acyclovir was administered orally in a dose of 800 mg five times daily for 21 d. Prednisone was given in a dose of 60 mg/d on d 1–7, 30 mg/d on d 8–14, and 15 mg/d on d 15–21.

Patients were monitored for lesion healing, resolution of pain, return to usual activity, and return to uninterrupted sleep over a period of 6 mo. The investigators found that the administration of acyclovir plus prednisone did not affect the resolution of pain during the 6 mo after disease onset. However, acute pain was more likely to resolve during the first month after onset of herpes in patients who received prednisone (with or without acyclovir). During the first month after disease onset, prednisone recipients were 1.74 times more likely to return to 100% usual activity than patients who did not receive prednisone, and acyclovir recipients were 1.9 times more like to return to this level of activity than patients who did not receive acyclovir. In addition, prednisone therapy was associated with a shorter duration of interrupted sleep and a shorter period of analgesic use. These data indicate that combination prednisone and antiviral therapy should be considered for patients with herpes zoster who experience moderate or severe pain. However, patients with osteoporosis, diabetes mellitus, and hypertension were excluded from this trial and may not be appropriate candidates for corticosteroid therapy. In addition, the potential benefit of corticosteroids in combination with antiviral agents other than acyclovir is unknown.

Antidepressant therapy initiated at the time of diagnosis of acute herpes zoster in patients over age 60 has been reported to decrease the prevalence of postherpetic neuralgia at 6 mo *(6)*. According to one protocol, all patients over age 60 should be prescribed amitriptyline in a dose of 10 mg at bedtime as soon as acute zoster is diagnosed *(6)*. This dose may be increased to 25 mg after 5–7 d if tolerated. If the pain resolves within 6 wk, the patient is maintained on the same dose for another 6 wk. If the pain persists 6 wk after the onset of shingles, the dose of amitriptyline is increased to 50 mg and subsequently to 75 mg at bedtime if tolerated. One proponent of this strategy has estimated that the combination of antidepressant and antiviral therapy might reduce referrals to pain clinics for postherpetic neuralgia by as much as 90% *(6)*. Nevertheless, this approach has not gained widespread popularity.

Table 5
Varicella Vaccine Precautions[a]

Avoid in immunocompromised states, including congenital immunodeficiency, leukemia, lymphoma, HIV infection, immunosuppressive therapy. (An investigational protocol is available for children and adolescents with acute lymphoblastic leukemia in remission.)

Avoid in patients who have received high-dose steroids within 1–3 mo.

Avoid pregnancy for 1 mo after vaccination.

Avoid if history of anaphylaxis to neomycin.

Do not administer aspirin or salicylates to children for 6 wk after vaccination due to possible risk of Reye's syndrome.

Do not administer vaccine between 3 wk before and 5 mo after transfusion of blood or plasma or receipt of immune globulin preparations, including VZIG, due to reduced efficacy of vaccine. If immunized during this interval, reimmunize or serotest and reimmunize if seronegative.

Vaccine recipients should avoid close contact with susceptible high-risk individuals, including newborns, if they develop an acute rash without other cause within 7–20 d after immunization.

[a]From ref. 16.

Prevention

A significant advance in decreasing morbidity from VZV is the development of varicella vaccine (Varivax), a live attenuated virus strain that induces VZV-specific humoral and cell-mediated immunity in both normal and immunocompromised persons. In one study, a single dose of vaccine protected 95% of children against varicella over a 7-yr period (14). In another trial, during which over 9000 healthy children were followed for periods up to 10 yr after varicella vaccination, the prevalence of herpes zoster was eight cases, similar to that in children after natural infection (15). One case of herpes zoster was also reported during a period averaging 5 yr after vaccination in a group of 1600 adolescents and adults. All nine cases were mild without sequelae. (Cultures from vesicles from one child and one adult among these nine patients revealed wild-type varicella zoster virus, indicating zoster was not caused by the vaccine.)

The current recommendations are to administer a single dose of varicella vaccine to all healthy children between 1 and 12 yr of age with no history of varicella and 2 doses (given 4–8 wk apart) to healthy adolescents and adults with no history of varicella (16). Serotesting of adolescents and adults without a reliable history of prior infection using a sensitive assay such as latex agglutination or ELISA, followed by immunization of only seronegative individuals, may be cost-effective. Special precautions pertaining to administration of this vaccine are listed in Table 5.

At present, it is not known whether the attenuated varicella strain in the vaccine causes herpes zoster, nor is it known whether boosting varicella-specific CMI among the elderly will reduce their risk of developing herpes zoster. A randomized trial is presently underway to determine the incidence of herpes zoster and postherpetic neuralgia following varicella vaccination in individuals over age 60.

Table 6
Pain Definitions[a]

Allodynia	Pain due to a stimulus that does not normally cause pain
Dysesthesia	An unpleasant abnormal sensation
Hyperalgesia	Increased response to a stimulus that is normally painful
Hyperesthesia	Increased sensitivity to stimulation
Hypesthesia (or hypoesthesia)	Decreased sensitivity to stimulation
Hyperpathia	An abnormally painful reaction to a stimulus
Paresthesia	An abnormal sensation

[a]From International Association for the Study of Pain (17).

Conclusion

As the immunity of the adult population declines with advancing age, we can expect an increase in the incidence of herpes zoster over the next few decades unless varicella vaccine proves effective in decreasing reactivation of VZV and the elderly population is immunized. For the present, the appropriate strategy is to decrease morbidity from herpes zoster by early recognition and treatment with antiviral agents and possibly corticosteroids and antidepressants.

POSTHERPETIC NEURALGIA

Postherpetic neuralgia (PHN) may be defined as the persistence of pain for one or more months after the onset of herpes zoster. Rather than a continuation of acute herpes zoster, PHN represents a separate syndrome characterized by pain, allodynia, dysesthesia, and hyperesthesia which may be prolonged and disabling (Table 6) (6).

Epidemiology

Ten to fifteen percent of patients with acute herpes zoster develop postherpetic neuralgia. The risk before age 50 is small but reaches 47% after age 60 and almost 75% after age 70. Additional risk factors include trigeminal nerve involvement, severe initial pain, and sensory loss to thermal stimuli during acute herpes zoster (2,18). Psychosocial factors such as anxiety, depression, life satisfaction, and disease conviction may also be operative (19). The majority of patients with PHN recover, but symptoms persist more than 1 yr in 22% of patients over age 55 and 48% over age 70 (5).

Clinical Features

Patients with PHN experience some combination of three different types of pain: (1) constant, deep burning or aching pain (continuous); (2) brief, spontaneous, recurrent shooting or shocking pain (neuralgic); and (3) sharp, radiating, dysesthetic pain elicited by light touch (allodynic) (2). Neuralgic pain is common, especially during the first year of PHN. Allodynia may persist indefinitely and causes the most disability; gently stroking the skin or wearing clothing may produce severe pain, whereas firm pressure often causes no pain (20). Cold exposure and stress typically exacerbate PHN.

Uncomplicated acute herpes zoster is seldom associated with sensory changes and rarely, if ever, allodynia. In contrast, all patients with postherpetic neuralgia demonstrate loss of tactile and thermal sensation, allodynia, or both in the affected dermatome *(6)*. Continuous pain is typically localized to regions of significant sensory loss, whereas allodynia is generally localized to areas with relatively preserved sensation *(21)*.

The frequency of PHN at various anatomic sites parallels the distribution of acute herpes zoster in most instances. Thus, thoracic dermatomes are affected in about 60% of cases of both herpes zoster and PHN. However, trigeminal herpes zoster, which represents 10–15% of herpes zoster, accounts for about 20% of PHN, whereas lumbar or sacral zoster is less likely to progress to PHN *(2)*. In addition, the proximal portion of the region supplied by a nerve is more likely to be affected than the distal portion. This is obvious when the extremities are involved. It also explains the common involvement of thoracic regions adjacent to the sternum, adjacent to the spine, and midway between the sternum and spine, which represent areas where branches of the intercostal nerves extend from their subcostal location to the skin *(2)*.

Pathophysiology

The observation that infiltration of allodynic skin with dilute lidocaine dramatically reduces pain in many patients suggests that primary afferent nerves, including cutaneous nerve branches, are involved in the pathogenesis of PHN in these individuals *(21)*. Perhaps input from peripheral nociceptive fibers damaged by herpes zoster provides ongoing stimulation of spinal cord neurons, resulting in chronic pain. On the other hand, some patients have severe sensory loss with little or no allodynia and derive little or no pain relief from lidocaine injection, implying that other factors are operative. In these individuals, PHN may represent a disease of the CNS resulting from loss of primary afferent fibers followed by changes in the spinal cord due to deafferentation *(2)*. Permanent morphological changes in the dorsal horn have been described in patients who develop postherpetic neuralgia *(6)*.

Treatment

An important component of therapy for postherpetic neuralgia is a tricyclic antidepressant such as amitriptyline (Elavil), nortriptyline (Pamelor), or desipramine (Norpramin) (Table 7). These agents are most effective when administered early *(22)*. The mechanisms by which antidepressants produce analgesia are presumed to relate to their effects on serotonin and norepinephrine, which have been implicated as neurotransmitters in brainstem to spinal cord nociceptive modulation *(2)*. The analgesic effects of these agents are distinct from their antidepressant effects, as demonstrated by rapid onset of analgesia at doses lower than needed to treat depression. Antidepressants as adjuvant analgesics are discussed in Chapter 14.

All tricyclic antidepressants share certain side effects, including blurred vision, increased intraocular pressure, dryness of the mouth, orthostatic hypotension, cardiac conduction abnormalities, arrhythmias, urinary retention, constipation, sedation, confusion, and seizures. However, desipramine and nortriptyline, the major metabolite of amitriptyline, cause fewer anticholinergic effects, less sedation, and less orthostatic hypotension than amitriptyline *(23)*.

Table 7
Treatment of Postherpetic Neuralgia

Topical therapy[a]	Lidocaine (EMLA or 5% lidocaine gel)
	Capsaicin
Analgesic agent[a]	Codeine
	Hydrocodone
Antidepressant agent	Amitriptyline
	Nortriptyline
	Desipramine
Anticonvulsant agent[b]	Carbamazepine
Somatosensory stimulation	TENS
Pain clinic[c]	Counseling
	Biofeedback
	Relaxation techniques
	Spinal cord stimulation
	Nerve blocks
	Surgical ablative procedures

[a]This therapy is usually administered in conjunction with an antidepressant or anticonvulsant medication.
[b]May be considered with lancinating pain.
[c]If pain is refractory to other modalities.

Many experts recommend that treatment of PHN begin with amitriptyline or nortriptyline in a dose of 10 mg at bedtime in patients over age 65 and 25 mg at bedtime in younger persons (22,23). This dose may be increased every 5–7 d by similar amounts if tolerated until adequate analgesia occurs or a therapeutic serum level is attained. The slow increase in dose is advisable due to the long elimination half-life of these agents, which require 5–7 d to reach a steady-state plasma concentration. A reasonable trial would be a minimum daily dose of 75 mg (the median analgesic dose) or the dose needed to produce a therapeutic serum level for a period of 2 wk. If these agents are not tolerated due to sedation or anticholinergic side effects or provide inadequate analgesia, desipramine may be utilized. The dosing is similar, although desipramine should be administered during the day since it may cause insomnia.

If tricyclic antidepressants are not tolerated, the tetracyclic antidepressant maprotiline (Ludiomil) or a selective serotonin reuptake inhibitor (SSRI)—such as fluoxetine (Prozac), sertraline (Zoloft), or paroxetine (Paxil)—may be administered. However, these drugs tend to be less effective analgesics than tricyclic antidepressants (22), and the incidence of seizures is higher with maprotiline than tricyclics.

Patients should understand that antidepressant medications may relieve pain but seldom abolish it. Whereas some patients note decreased severity of pain, others describe no change in pain, but tolerate it better. Patients must also understand that side effects are likely to occur but may be minimized by using artificial saliva for dryness of the mouth, stool softeners or bowel stimulants if needed for constipation, and "tincture of time" to develop tolerance to sedation.

For patients with lancinating pain or pain unresponsive to antidepressants, physicians may prescribe an anticonvulsant such as carbamazepine (Tegretol) in a starting dose of 100 mg twice daily (*see* Chapter 14). Valproate (Depakene or Depakote), phenytoin (Dilantin), and gabapentin (Neurontin) represent alternative drugs *(5)*. However, anticonvulsants have not been well-studied for treating postherpetic neuralgia, in contrast to antidepressants. Other agents have also been used to treat refractory postherpetic neuralgia. These include the α_2 agonist clonidine (Catapres), neuroleptics such as perphenazine (Trilafon), and antiarrhythmics such as mexiletine (Mexitil).

Oral opioids, such as codeine or hydrocodone, may be administered if needed in conjunction with antidepressant or anticonvulsant therapy. For severe pain, some experts advocate oxycodone or slow-release morphine (after the daily morphine requirement has been determined with immediate-release morphine). End points that can be used for dose titration include analgesia, decreased neurologic abnormalities, and intolerable side effects *(20)*. Problems with addiction have been reported to be uncommon in this population *(22)*. In general, there should be a single prescriber of opioids, and patients with a history of drug abuse should probably be excluded. The reader is referred to the detailed discussion of opioid analgesic agents in the following chapter for additional information.

Most patients are candidates for topical therapy. Benefit has been described with topical capsaicin, topical anesthetics, and topical NSAIDs *(22)*. Capsaicin, derived from the chili pepper, depletes substance P and other neurotransmitters from primary afferent nociceptive fibers by selectively stimulating and then blocking these neurons. These afferents release substance P both peripherally and at their termination in the dorsal horn. Modest (21%) pain relief was reported by 38% of patients with postherpetic neuralgia lasting at least 6 mo in a 6-wk study using 0.075% lotion applied to the affected area seven times daily *(24)*. A more potent preparation containing 0.25% capsaicin is also available. Disadvantages of capsaicin include a burning sensation, which frequently decreases after several days but is intolerable for some patients. The pharmacology of capsaicin is discussed more fully in Chapter 14.

Topical lidocaine preparations have been reported to be effective in PHN and are preferred by some because they do not elicit the burning discomfort associated with capsaicin *(5)*. These include 5% lidocaine gel, 5% lidocaine patch, 5% lidocaine-prilocaine cream (EMLA, a eutectic mixture of local anesthetics), 5% lidocaine with isopropyl alcohol, 9% lidocaine in petrolatum, and 10% lidocaine gel *(2,22)*. In addition, subcutaneous injection of lidocaine into painfully sensitive skin decreases pain associated with PHN, especially in patients with predominantly allodynic pain *(20)*.

Topical NSAIDs such as aspirin in chloroform, ether, or moisturizing lotion have also been utilized. The combination of aspirin 750–1500 mg pulverized and mixed into 20–30 mL of diethyl ether applied topically has been reported to help patients with acute herpes zoster and postherpetic neuralgia *(2)*. The extreme volatility of ether represents a disadvantage of this formulation.

Another therapeutic option is transcutaneous electrical nerve stimulation (TENS), which may provide some benefit in PHN and is generally safe. Presence of a pacemaker represents a contraindication to this modality. Acupuncture has not been demonstrated to be effective in treating postherpetic neuralgia. For patients with PHN affecting dermatomes around the large joints, physical therapy may be utilized to maintain range of motion and muscle strength.

Patients refractory to the modalities discussed above should be referred to a multidisciplinary pain clinic with experience in treating PHN. Potential therapies include intrathecal opioid infusion pumps, spinal cord stimulation, deep brain stimulation, neurolytic nerve blocks, and surgical ablative procedures. Counseling, biofeedback, and relaxation techniques may also provide benefit *(2)*.

Prevention

Is it possible to decrease the risk of developing postherpetic neuralgia? One study reported that administering amitriptyline 25 mg daily for 90 d to patients over age 60 as soon as acute herpes zoster was diagnosed reduced by approx 50% the frequency of pain at 6 mo *(6)*. However, this does not indicate that the incidence of PHN was decreased. Famciclovir and valacyclovir have also been shown to reduce the duration of pain in postherpetic neuralgia, but not the frequency of PHN *(25)*. Nor does administration of corticosteroids during acute herpes zoster appear to decrease the incidence of PHN *(12)*. Thus, no present therapy has been proven to reduce the onset of PHN, although antiviral agents and antidepressants have been reported to shorten the duration of pain.

Conclusion

Prompt administration of antiviral agents during acute herpes zoster decreases the duration of pain but probably not the incidence of postherpetic neuralgia. Antidepressants represent the primary treatment for postherpetic neuralgia, but other modalities are frequently utilized for refractory pain. With effective immunization against varicella, it should be possible to virtually eliminate herpes zoster and its sequelae, including postherpetic neuralgia. Whether the present varicella vaccine produces such benefit is unknown at this time.

CENTRAL PAIN

Central pain is defined as pain that results from injury to the CNS *(17)*. The causative lesion can be located at any level along the neuroaxis from the dorsal horn of the spinal cord to the cerebral cortex. Central pain may be categorized according to anatomic site as pain from spinal cord lesions, pain from brainstem lesions, or pain from cerebral lesions (Table 8).

Causes of Central Pain

Approximately 90% of cases of central pain are caused by strokes *(26)*. The risk of developing central pain following stroke appears to be greatest with thalamic lesions, but central pain may also be produced by cerebrovascular lesions in the brainstem, subcortical white matter, and cortex. Seizures occasionally produce central pain, which may present as abdominal discomfort or pain in an extremity. Central pain from spinal cord lesions is most often associated with trauma or demyelinating disease *(27)*. Almost 50% of patients with multiple sclerosis develop central pain or dysesthesias, usually as a result

Table 8
Causes of Central Pain

Spinal Cord Lesions	Brainstem Lesions	Cerebral Lesions
Trauma	Trauma	Trauma
Hemorrhage	Hemorrhage	Hemorrhage
Infarct	Infarct	Infarct
Arteriovenous malformation	Arteriovenous malformation	Arteriovenous malformation
Infection	Infection	Infection
Neoplasm	Neoplasm	Neoplasm
Multiple sclerosis	Multiple sclerosis	Multiple sclerosis
Syringomyelia	Syringobulbia	Encephalitis
Transverse myelitis		Seizure associated
Herniated disk		

of spinal cord plaques. Hemorrhage, tumors, syringomyelia, syringobulbia, AIDS myelopathy, syphilitic myelitis, and toxic myelopathy may also cause central pain. The development of central pain appears to be idiosyncratic, as not all patients with a given lesion perceive pain.

Clinical Features

The onset of central pain may be delayed for months and occasionally for several years following stroke or spinal cord injury. Patients with central pain experience superficial or deep pain, which is usually constant but may be intermittent. Central pain is most often characterized as burning but may be aching, pricking, or lancinating (28). Pain may increase in response to movement, cold, warmth, emotion, smoking, or other factors. Dysesthesias and paresthesias may be present in association with nonanatomic radiation and poor localization of pain. Temperature sensation is decreased in patients with central pain, and decreased sensitivity to pinprick and deep stimulation is common. Pain may be produced by stimuli that are not normally painful (allodynia), and noxious stimuli may elicit pain that is abnormally intense and prolonged (hyperpathia) (29). In some patients, stimulation of one area may cause pain both in that area and in another part of the body (mitempfindung); or, stimulation on one side of the body may cause pain on the contralateral side (allesthesia) (30).

Central pain following stroke may include all or only a portion of the contralateral hemibody (28). Thalamic pain may tend to be lancinating, whereas pain from brainstem lesions may be burning. Abnormal sensation to pain and temperature is almost always demonstrable in some part of the affected region (26).

Patients with trauma to the spinal cord may experience pain associated with dysesthesias and paresthesias at any level below the injury. The painful regions may be unilateral or bilateral and may fluctuate in size and location. Sensory stimulation above the level of a spinal injury may cause ipsilateral pain below the injury site (synesthesia) (30). Muscle spasms may occur spontaneously or in response to movement or distention

Table 9
Treatment of Central Pain

Pharmacologic treatment	Antidepressant such as amitriptyline or nortriptyline
	Anticonvulsant such as carbamazepine or phenytoin
	Analgesic
	Adrenergic agent such as clonidine
	Other agents such as mexiletine, baclofen
Physical modalities	TENS
	Physiotherapy
Psychiatric intervention	Treatment for depression, pain coping
Invasive modalities	Neurostimulatory techniques
	Ablative procedures

of the bladder or rectum. Lower abdominal or pelvic pain, sometimes acute, may also be triggered by bladder or rectal distention. Multiple sclerosis may be associated with paroxysmal stabbing pain, including trigeminal neuralgia, and Lhermitte's sign, a shock-like pain that radiates down the spine during neck flexion as a result of disease in the dorsal columns of the spinal cord.

Since central pain is often characterized by delayed onset and few objective findings, which may be subtle, physicians and others may doubt the presence or severity of pain *(30)*. Thorough sensory examination is essential for the diagnosis, which can be made on the basis of pain without other cause in combination with abnormal sensation to temperature and pain and a history of previous injury to the CNS. Current MRI techniques identify the responsible CNS lesion in most cases.

Pathophysiology

Three factors have been proposed to be major determinants of central pain *(29)*.

1. Abnormal thalamic function, which may generate the sensation of pain in the absence of input from ascending or descending pathways. If the thalamus is totally ablated, the perception of pain is eliminated *(30)*.
2. Abnormal excitatory and inhibitory activity involving nociceptive or modulatory pathways. Increasing evidence suggests that central pain only occurs in patients who have lesions affecting the spinothalamocortical pathways, which transmit temperature and pain sensation *(31)*.
3. Abnormal receptor function as a consequence of these changes.

Treatment

Therapy of central pain is challenging, because complete relief of pain is seldom attainable. Therefore, a realistic goal for these patients is pain reduction *(30)*. This will frequently include a program that incorporates pharmacologic agents, physiotherapy, transcutaneous electrical nerve stimulation, behavioral therapy, psychotherapy, and possibly neurostimulatory and ablative procedures (Table 9). Coexistent medical disorders associated with pain must also be treated.

Antidepressant therapy represents the primary pharmacologic treatment for patients with central pain *(32)*. Amitriptyline (Elavil), nortriptyline (Pamelor), doxepin (Sinequan), and imipramine (Tofranil) have been used with reported benefit *(30)*. A recommended strategy is to initiate therapy with amitriptyline or nortriptyline (which has fewer side effects) in a dose of 10–25 mg at bedtime, with subsequent dosage increases at 5- to 7-d intervals until pain relief is attained, intolerable side effects develop, or a daily dose of 150 mg (or therapeutic serum level) is reached. Desipramine (Norpramin) has been described as effective for neuropathic pain and may be considered as an alternative agent for treating central pain. Trazodone (Desyrel) may also decrease central pain. Potential side effects of these medications include orthostatic hypotension, sedation, confusion, seizures, increased intraocular pressure, blurred vision, dryness of the mouth, arrhythmias, urinary retention, and constipation; trazodone may also cause priapism.

For patients unable to tolerate these antidepressants, selective serotonin reuptake inhibitors (SSRIs)—such as paroxetine (Paxil) or venlafaxine (Effexor)—may be utilized. Although these agents have fewer side effects than other antidepressants, they appear to be less effective for treating neuropathic pain and have not been well-studied for treatment of central pain.

Anticonvulsants such as carbamazepine (Tegretol) may be effective, especially if the pain has a sharp, stabbing character *(30)*. Therapy with carbamazepine should be initiated in a dose of 100 mg twice daily *(see* Chapter 14). Phenytoin (Dilantin) in a daily dose of 300 mg or more represents an alternative agent. Phenothiazines such as chlorpromazine (Thorazine) and fluphenazine (Prolixin) may be helpful *(27)*.

For patients with persistent pain, analgesics may be prescribed, although central pain may be relatively resistant to these medications. Opioid analgesics are generally administered in a stepwise fashion, starting with those with low potential for abuse *(see* Chapter 14). The objective of analgesic therapy should be to provide continuous pain control such that the pain intensity does not attain a level requiring higher doses of analgesics.

Adrenergic agents such as clonidine (Catapres), β-blockers such as propranolol (Inderal), and calcium channel blockers have also been utilized with reported success in some patients with central pain *(27,30)*. Variable results have been described with mexiletine (Mexitil) and iv lidocaine *(30)*. Baclofen (Lioresal), a γ-aminobutyric acid (GABA) receptor agonist, has been shown to decrease spasm-related pain in patients with spinal cord lesions when administered orally or intrathecally and to decrease dysesthetic pain when infused intrathecally *(33)*.

These modalities may be supplemented with high- (conventional) or low-frequency transcutaneous electrical nerve stimulation (TENS), which is occasionally effective but can also transiently exacerbate the pain *(34)*. Physiotherapy may be utilized to maintain range of motion and strength of affected regions. Psychosocial support should be provided to assist patients with pain coping techniques and to treat depression, which may be associated with suicidal ideation in a significant proportion of these patients *(30)*.

When pain is refractory to these measures, invasive neurostimulatory techniques may be considered. Some patients with central pain originating in the spinal cord benefit from stimulation of the dorsal root entry zone (DREZ) or spinal cord if paresthesias can be

Table 10
Diagnostic Criteria for Pain Disorder (Psychogenic Pain)[a]

1. Pain in one or more regions is of sufficient severity to warrant clinical attention and is the main focus of the clinical presentation.
2. The pain causes significant distress or impairs occupational, social, or other important functional abilities.
3. Psychological factors play a significant role in the onset, severity, exacerbation, or persistence of the pain.
4. The pain is not intentionally produced (as in factitious disorder) or feigned (malingering).
5. The pain is not better explained by a mood, anxiety, or psychotic disorder or dyspareunia.

[a]Adapted from the American Psychiatric Association: Diagnostic and Statistical Manual of Mental Disorders, Fourth Edition, 1994 (35).

elicited at the level of the lesion (30). Spinal cord stimulation should be used before resorting to ablative procedures on the spinal cord. Other therapeutic options in selected patients include stimulation of the thalamus or deep brain. Ablation of brain tissue is not recommended.

Conclusion

Treatment of central pain is challenging, and pain reduction rather than complete pain relief is the usual goal. Antidepressant medications and psychosocial support represent the primary therapy for this disorder. These patients are often candidates for treatment at a multidisciplinary pain clinic and at times may benefit from invasive neurostimulatory procedures.

PSYCHOGENIC PAIN

Psychogenic pain may be defined as pain without organic pathology, although it may also be diagnosed in the presence of organic disease if the complaint of pain greatly exceeds the expected level of pain. Operationally, these criteria have caused confusion—for few patients with chronic pain have no demonstrable organic pathology—and it may be difficult to determine if pain is greater than expected from physical findings.

Diagnostic Criteria

To address concerns such as these, a task force was convened to revise the diagnostic criteria for psychogenic pain. The results are included in the 4th edition of the Diagnostic and Statistical Manual of Mental Disorders (DSM-IV), published by the American Psychiatric Association in 1994. DSM-IV replaced the term "psychogenic pain disorder" (used in DSM-III) with "pain disorder," which is categorized as a somatoform disorder (35). The diagnostic criteria for pain disorder are indicated in Table 10.

Three subtypes of pain disorder are recognized:

1. Pain disorder associated with psychological factors. Psychological factors are judged to have the major role in the onset, severity, exacerbation, or maintenance of the pain. General medical conditions play either no role or a minimal role.

Table 11
Examples of Somatoform Disorders (DSM-IV)[a]

Somatization	Polysymptomatic disorder that begins before age 30, lasts years, characterized by combination of pain, gastrointestinal, sexual, and pseudoneurological symptoms
Conversion disorder	Unexplained symptoms or deficits affecting voluntary motor or sensory function that suggest a general medical condition but are associated with psychological factors
Pain disorder	Pain is the predominant focus of clinical attention and psychological factors have an important role in its onset, severity, exacerbation, or maintenance
Hypochondriasis	Preoccupation with fear that one has or will develop a serious disease based on the misinterpretation of bodily symptoms or functions
Body dysmorphic disorder	Preoccupation with an imagined or exaggerated physical defect

[a]From American Psychiatric Association: Diagnostic and Statistical Manual of Mental Disorders, Fourth Edition, 1994 (35).

2. Pain disorder associated with both psychological factors and a general medical condition. Both psychological factors and a general medical condition are judged to have important roles in the onset, severity, exacerbation, or maintenance of the pain.
3. Pain disorder associated with a general medical condition. Although listed as a subtype of pain disorder in order to defuse the notion that pain associated with psychological factors is less "real" than other pain, this is not considered a mental disorder (36).

Other somatoform disorders include somatization disorder (previously known as hysteria), conversion disorder, hypochondriasis, and body dysmorphic disorder. A discussion of these disorders is beyond the scope of this text, but they are defined in Table 11. The common feature of these disorders is the presence of physical symptoms that suggest a medical disease but cannot be fully explained by a medical condition, the direct effects of drugs, or another mental disorder. To meet criteria for a somatoform disorder, these symptoms must cause clinically significant distress or impairment in function and not be factitious or feigned.

Clinical Features

Patients with pain disorder or psychogenic pain may describe poorly localized pain of vague onset, which occurs in multiple areas that increase in size, varies with mood, does not disturb sleep, and may be relieved by alcohol or psychotropic medication but seldom by analgesics (Table 12). In addition, neurotic symptoms and a personality disorder may be present (37).

Evaluation of the patient suspected of having psychogenic pain should include a thorough neurologic exam, including sensory examination and testing of muscle strength. Weakness in all muscle groups in a particular region, superficial tenderness, and occur-

Table 12
Psychogenic Pain Questions[a]

1. When did the pain first start?
2. Where is the pain felt?
3. Does mood affect the pain?
4. Does the severity of the pain change during the day?
5. What factors make the pain better or worse?
6. Do medications alter the pain?
7. What effect does alcohol have on the pain?

[a]Adapted from ref. *37*.

Table 13
Treatment of Psychogenic Pain

Psychiatric evaluation and treatment	Tricyclic antidepressant
	Benzodiazepine
	Major tranquilizer
	Psychotherapy
Psychological techniques	Behavioral therapy
	Biofeedback
	Self-hypnosis
General	Discontinue unnecessary medications

rence of pain with benign maneuvers support this diagnosis, although the physician must also consider malingering and other psychiatric disorders.

Appropriate tests should be ordered based on findings from the history and physical examination, but the number of diagnostic studies and specialist consultations should be limited. The patient and physician may agree on a "final investigation" *(37)*. This approach discourages the patient from thinking that the physician suspects a serious organic disorder and from focusing on physical symptoms. When the results of these tests are normal, the patient with psychogenic pain may express relief or gratitude (which is associated with a favorable prognosis), or disbelief, anger, or resentment (which is associated with a poor prognosis).

Treatment

Patients should be referred for psychiatric evaluation and treatment as soon as the diagnosis of psychogenic pain is suspected. This referral requires sensitivity, because most patients are certain that they suffer from a physical rather than psychological disorder. One approach may be to advise the patient that factors such as stress and tension may be causing or aggravating the symptoms and that a psychiatrist is the type of physician most knowledgeable in helping patients deal with these factors *(37)*.

Medical treatment of psychogenic pain generally includes tricyclic antidepressants (Table 13). Administration of benzodiazepines as anxiolytic agents and major tranquilizers such as thioridazine (Mellaril), chlorpromazine (Thorazine), or haloperidol (Haldol) may also be appropriate. The potential for fatal overdosage from antidepressants and for abuse of benzodiazepines must be recognized when choosing treatment for an individual patient. A psychiatrist should be involved in this therapy.

Psychological techniques have also been utilized to treat psychogenic pain. These include cognitive behavioral therapy, biofeedback, self-hypnosis, and psychotherapy. Few studies have addressed the efficacy of these modalities for treating psychogenic pain. One study, which compared therapy with amitriptyline to brief outpatient psychotherapy for patients with psychogenic pain, suggested that amitriptyline may be more effective, especially if patients are irritable or depressed *(38)*.

Medications that are not medically indicated should be withdrawn, since they reinforce erroneous beliefs regarding the cause of pain *(37)*. An example would be a cardiac medication for treatment of noncardiogenic chest pain. This process may be difficult, as patients are often psychologically dependent on these medications. Gradual reduction in dose should help convince the patient that these medications are not necessary.

Conclusion

History and physical exam should identify patients with psychogenic pain. The primary physician can optimize patient care by early referral of these patients for psychiatric evaluation and treatment. In addition, unnecessary medications should be withdrawn.

ACKNOWLEDGMENT

The author acknowledges with gratitude the expert assistance of Dr. Vivien C. Abad in the preparation and review of this chapter.

REFERENCES

1. Arvin AM. Aspects of the host response to varicella-zoster virus: a review of recent observations. Neurology 1995; 45: S36–37.
2. Rowbotham M. From mechanisms to clinical syndromes: a comparison of post-herpetic neuralgia and complex regional pain syndromes (RSD and causalgia). Pain symposium. American Academy of Neurology 48th Annual Meeting, San Francisco, March 24, 1996: 1–36.
3. Oxman MN. Immunization to reduce the frequency and severity of herpes zoster and its complications. Neurology 1995; 45: S41–46.
4. Pavan-Langston D. Herpes zoster ophthalmicus. Neurology 1995; 45: S50–51.
5. Kost RG, Straus SE. Postherpetic neuralgia—pathogenesis, treatment, and prevention. N Eng J Med 1996; 335: 32–42.
6. Bowsher D. Pathophysiology of postherpetic neuralgia: towards a rational treatment. Neurology 1995; 45: S56–57.
7. Tyring S, Barbarash RA, Nahlik JE, et al. Famciclovir for the treatment of acute herpes zoster: effects on acute disease and postherpetic neuralgia. Ann Int Med 1995; 123: 89–96.
8. Beutner KR, Friedman DJ, Forszpaniak C, Andersen PL, Wood MJ. Valaciclovir compared with acyclovir for improved therapy for herpes zoster in immunocompetent adults. Antimicrob Agents Chemother 1995; 39: 1546–1553.
9. Valacyclovir. Med Lett Drugs Ther 1996; 38: 3,4.
10. Whitley RJ. Sorivudine: a promising drug for the treatment of varicella-zoster virus infection. Neurology 1995; 45: S73–75.

11. Tyring SK. Early treatment of herpes zoster. Hospital Practice 1996; 31: 137–144.
12. Wood MJ, Johnson RW, McKendrick MW, Taylor J, Mandal BK, Crooks J. A randomized trial of acyclovir for 7 days of 21 days with and without prednisolone for treatment of acute herpes zoster. N Eng J Med 1994; 330: 896–900.
13. Whitley RJ, Weiss H, Gnann JW Jr, Tyring S, Mertz GJ, Pappas PG, et al. Acyclovir with and without prednisone for the treatment of herpes zoster: a randomized, placebo-controlled trial. Ann Int Med 1996; 125: 376–383.
14. Kuter BJ, Weibel RE, Guess HA, et al. Oka/Merck varicella vaccine in healthy children: final report of a 2-year efficacy study and 7-year follow-up studies. Vaccine 1991; 9: 643–647.
15. Varicella vaccine. Med Lett Drugs Ther 1995; 37: 55–57.
16. American Academy of Pediatrics, Committee on Infectious Diseases. Recommendations for the use of live attenuated varicella vaccine. Pediatrics 1995; 95: 791–796.
17. Merskey H, Bogduk N, eds. Classification of chronic pain. 2nd ed. Seattle: IASP, 1994.
18. Bruxelle J. Prospective epidemiologic study of painful and neurologic sequelae induced by herpes zoster in patients treated early with oral acyclovir. Neurology 1995; 45: S78,79.
19. Johnson RW. The future of predictors, prevention, and therapy in postherpetic neuralgia. Neurology 1995; 45: S70–72.
20. Rowbotham MC. Managing post-herpetic neuralgia with opioids and local anesthetics. Ann Neurol 1994; 35: S46–49.
21. Rowbotham MC, Fields HL. Post-herpetic neuralgia: the relation of pain complaint, sensory disturbance, and skin temperature. Pain 1989; 39: 129–144.
22. Watson CPN. The treatment of postherpetic neuralgia. Neurology 1995; 45: S58–S60.
23. Max MB. Treatment of post-herpetic neuralgia: antidepressants. Ann Neurol 1994; 35: S50–53.
24. Watson CPN, Tyler KL, Bickers DR. A randomized vehicle-controlled trial of topical capsaicin in the treatment of postherpetic neuralgia. Clin Ther 1993; 15: 510–526.
25. Boon RJ, Griffin DRJ. Efficacy of famciclovir in the treatment of herpes zoster. Neurology 1995; 45: S76,77.
26. Gonzales GR. Central pain. Sem Neurol 1994; 14: 255–262.
27. Portenoy RK. Neuropathic pain. In: Portenoy RK, Kanner RM, eds. Pain Management: Theory and Practice. Philadelphia: F. A. Davis, 1996; 83–125.
28. Boivie J, Leijon G. Clinical findings in patients with central poststroke pain. In: Casey KL, ed. Pain and central nervous system disease: the central pain syndromes. New York: Raven, 1991; 65–75.
29. Casey KL. Pain and central nervous system disease: a summary and overview. In: Casey KL, ed. Pain and central nervous system disease: the central pain syndromes. New York: Raven, 1991; 1–11.
30. Gonzales GR. Central pain: diagnosis and treatment strategies. Neurology 1995; 45: S11–16.
31. Beric A. Central pain: "new" syndromes and their evaluation. Muscle & Nerve 1993; 16: 1017–1024.
32. Boivie J, Leijon G. Pharmacologic treatment of central pain. In: Casey KL, ed. Pain and central nervous system disease: the central pain syndromes. New York: Raven, 1991; 257–266.
33. Herman RM, D'Luzansky SC, Ippolito R. Intrathecal Baclofen suppresses central pain in patients with spinal lesions. A pilot study. Clin J Pain 1992; 8: 338–345.
34. Leijon G, Boivie J. Central post-stroke pain—the effect of high and low frequency TENS. Pain 1989; 38: 187–191.
35. American Psychiatric Association. Diagnostic and statistical manual of mental disorders, 4th edition. Washington, D.C.: American Psychiatric Association, 1994.
36. King SA. Review: DSM-IV and pain. Clin J Pain 1995; 11: 171–176.
37. Lim LEC. Psychogenic pain. Singapore Med J 1994; 35: 519–522.
38. Pilowsky I, Barrow G. Predictors of outcome in the treatment of chronic "psychogenic" pain with amitriptyline and brief psychotherapy. Clin J Pain 1992; 8: 358–362.

14 TREATMENT OF PAIN

Maurice E. Hamilton, MD
M. Eric Gershwin, MD

Key Points

- Pain represents a complex experience encompassing sensory and emotional components.
- Pain should be treated aggressively during the acute phase, since chronic pain is associated with behavioral and psychological factors that make treatment more difficult.
- Accurate assessment of the severity of pain is essential for appropriate treatment. This is best accomplished by patient self-report using a visual analog or other pain intensity scale.
- Treatment of mild to moderate pain will generally include acetaminophen and, if needed, a nonsteroidal anti-inflammatory drug (NSAID).
- Toradol represents an NSAID available for parenteral administration. It should not be administered to patients taking other NSAIDs.
- Side effects of NSAIDs include peptic ulcer disease, decreased platelet aggregation, renal and hepatic dysfunction, exacerbation of asthma, hyperkalemia, fluid retention, congestive heart failure, hypertension, and CNS symptoms.
- Renal function, potassium, and liver enzymes should be monitored periodically during therapy with NSAIDs.
- Compared to other NSAIDs, nonacetylated salicylates (choline magnesium trisalicylate or salsalate) may be associated with less gastric irritation, platelet inhibition, renal impairment, bronchospasm, and anti-inflammatory activity.
- For more severe pain, opioids are appropriate. These medications are generally administered in a stepwise fashion, starting with "weaker" opioids and progressing to "stronger" opioids if necessary.
- Some opioids may be combined with acetaminophen (e.g., propoxyphene, codeine, hydrocodone, oxycodone). The total daily dose of acetaminophen from all medications should not exceed 4000 mg, owing to the potential for serious hepatotoxicity.

- Opioids may be categorized based on their affinity for the μ-opioid receptor as full agonists, partial agonists, or mixed agonist–antagonists. Partial agonists and mixed agonist–antagonists are favored by some because of a possibly lower incidence of addiction; opioids in these classes may trigger withdrawal in patients receiving opioids.
- The availability of long-acting oral morphine and transdermal fentanyl simplify dosing and may be appropriate for patients with continuous pain requiring opioids. The daily dose of morphine should be established with immediate-release morphine before administering sustained-release morphine.
- Epidural or intrathecal opioids may be utilized in patients unable to tolerate systemic administration due to side effects.
- Patient-controlled analgesia (PCA) permits patients to administer opioids subcutaneously, intravenously, or intraspinally within parameters established by the physician.
- Side effects of opioids include respiratory depression, nausea and vomiting, constipation, increased biliary tract pressure, urinary retention, hypotension, dizziness, dysphoria or euphoria, and altered cognitive function.
- Most opioids are metabolized in the liver and eliminated by the kidneys. They should be administered with caution and generally in lower doses in patients with hepatic or renal disease and in the elderly.
- The metabolites of some opioids have much longer half-lives than the parent compound and may accumulate, especially with renal impairment, leading to drug toxicity. Examples are normeperidine (from meperidine), which may cause tremor and seizures, and norpropoxyphene (from propoxyphene), which may cause cardiac toxicity and seizures.
- Tolerance and physical dependence, which are normal physiologic responses to opioids, must be differentiated from addiction (psychological dependence), which is a behavioral disorder characterized by compulsive securing and use of a drug for nonanalgesic purposes.
- Chronic administration of opioids to patients with cancer is generally accepted, but these patients are often undertreated. Round-the-clock administration of opioids is preferable to as-needed dosing.
- Chronic administration of opioids to patients with chronic nonmalignant pain is less accepted, but some of these patients also require opioids. Adjunctive analgesics and other therapeutic modalities may diminish the need for opioids.
- Physicians should be familiar with laws in their state that may protect them when prescribing opioids for pain relief. These laws may also specify certain requirements for this protection.
- Adjuvant analgesics, such as antidepressants and anticonvulsants, which may be utilized in combination with analgesics or alone, are underutilized by many physicians.
- Topical anesthetics, such as lidocaine and capsaicin, provide additional benefit in some patients.

- Injection of a local anesthetic agent or a neurolytic agent into a localized trigger point, peripheral sensory nerve, or sympathetic nerve plexus may relieve regional pain disorders of benign or malignant etiology.

- Epidural steroids may decrease back pain associated with radicular symptoms, especially if utilized early, but the duration of benefit may be limited.

- The use of marijuana (cannabis saliva) for medicinal purposes is controversial. Marijuana appears to have little, if any, role as an analgesic due to adverse bronchopulmonary and psychotropic effects.

- Acupuncture and transcutaneous electrical nerve stimulation (TENS) are believed to modulate the transmission of nociceptive stimuli. The role of these therapies remains to be defined, but TENS appears to help some patients (either directly or indirectly) and offers the advantage of application by the patient.

- Physical therapy may help patients with muscle pain and spasm through several modalities, including heat (delivered by hot packs, whirlpool, ultrasound), cold, manual therapies, and a therapeutic exercise program.

- Behavioral therapy using operant conditioning, cognitive behavioral therapy, relaxation, biofeedback, or some combination of these, may benefit some patients with chronic pain.

- Patients with pain refractory to usual therapeutic modalities should be considered for referral to a multidisciplinary pain clinic. Some patients, especially those with regional pain, may derive substantial pain relief from nerve blocks or trigger point injections. Patients with pain-related litigation may be advised to resolve the legal issues prior to enrolling.

INTRODUCTION

Treatment of pain is a challenge physicians face each day. Despite the importance of this topic, physicians and other health care providers are often not fully informed regarding recent pharmacologic advances and optimal techniques for managing acute and chronic pain. Since pain is multidimensional, involving "unpleasant sensory and emotional experience associated with actual or potential tissue damage" (*see* ref. *1*), appropriate treatment of pain may require recognition and therapy of cognitive, motivational, behavioral, affective, spiritual, nociceptive, and neuropathic phenomena *(2)*.

This chapter contains practical information regarding selection and administration of analgesic medications, which may be broadly characterized as nonopioid (including acetaminophen and nonsteroidal anti-inflammatory drugs) and opioid analgesics. In addition, adjuvant analgesics (such as antidepressant and anticonvulsant medications) and nonpharmacologic approaches are considered.

GENERAL PRINCIPLES

Acute pain usually results from the perception of a physical stimulus that activates peripheral nociceptive neurons, primarily slow-conducting unmyelinated C fibers and faster-conducting thinly myelinated $A\delta$ fibers, to transmit an electrochemical signal to second-order neurons in the dorsal horn of the spinal cord. These neurons form the spinothalamic and spinoreticular-reticulothalamic tracts to the thalamus, where pain signals are initially processed. Thalamocortical projections terminate in the somatosensory cortex, where pain is consciously localized and characterized, and the cingulate gyrus, a cortical area with many opioid receptors, believed to be involved in the emotional reaction to pain (3). Projections arising in the cortex and hypothalamus descend to the midbrain, reticular formation of medulla, and dorsal horn of the spinal cord, where they inhibit ascending nociceptive impulses by releasing serotonin and norepinephrine.

Substance P and glutamate, present in synaptic vesicles of the C fibers and, to a lesser extent, Aδ fibers, are believed to be the principal neurotransmitters in the pathway from peripheral nociceptors to the spinal cord. Activation of C fibers by nociceptive stimuli leads to release of substance P and other neuropeptides into the surrounding tissue, where they activate mast cells and stimulate the synthesis of inflammatory mediators, including prostaglandins and leukotrienes, to produce neurogenic inflammation (4).

The normal physiologic response to acute painful stimulation includes hyperactivity of the sympathetic nervous system, characterized by findings such as tachycardia, hypertension, pupillary dilatation (mydriasis), and diaphoresis. When pain persists, objective evidence of stimulation of the autonomic nervous system diminishes due to adaptation. With chronic pain, psychosocial forces become operative and often lead to behavioral changes. Especially at this stage, the treatment of pain requires attention not only to the anatomic pathways involved in the sensation of pain, but also to psychological factors. Since treatment of pain is more complex and potentially less successful at this point, pain should be treated aggressively during the acute phase.

In order to treat pain appropriately, accurate assessment of the severity of pain is essential. At times, the physician may be able to infer the intensity of pain from physical findings, such as the presence of acute inflammation. However, since pain is subjective, the mainstay of pain assessment is the patient self-report, which is best accomplished using a pain-intensity scale (5). This may take the form of: a numeric scale (rated from 0 to 10, with 0 representing no pain and 10 representing the worst possible pain); a descriptive scale (no pain or mild, moderate, severe, very severe, or the worst possible pain); a visual analog scale (the patient indicates the severity of pain by marking an "X" on a baseline 10-cm scale with labels ranging from "no pain" to "worst possible pain"); or other graphic scales such as the faces scale (the patient chooses the face with the appropriate degree of grimace). Family members may be able to assist the physician in making this assessment.

Severity of pain and clinical response to therapy will determine the optimal treatment for an individual patient. In general, mild-to-moderate pain should be treated with acetaminophen and, if needed, a nonsteroidal anti-inflammatory drug (NSAID), unless contraindicated (Table 1). Adjuvant agents, such as antidepressant medications, may be added. In addition, electrical stimulation (TENS), acupuncture, behavioral modification, or nerve blocks may be considered. Patients with severe pain should be treated with opioids of sufficient potency and dosage to provide effective analgesia.

Appropriate pain management should improve the patient's physical, social, psychological, vocational, and avocational functioning. Therefore, monitoring these parameters provides crucial information for assessing therapeutic efficacy.

Table 1
Examples of Analgesics for Mild, Moderate, and Severe Pain

Severity of Pain	Analgesic
Mild–moderate	Tylenol
	Nonacetylated salicylate (Disalcid, Trilisate)
	Ibuprofen
Moderate–moderately severe	Propoxyphene with acetaminophen
	Acetaminophen with codeine
	Hydrocodone
	Pentazocine
Severe	Oxycodone
	Morphine
	Hydromorphone
	Levorphanol
	Methadone
	Transdermal fentanyl

NONOPIOID ANALGESICS

Acetaminophen (Tylenol and Others)

For treatment of mild pain, acetaminophen may be sufficient. Maximal analgesic effects are achieved at a dose of 1000 mg. It is usually best to use this maximal dose, which may be repeated every 4–6 h, not to exceed a total of 4000 mg during each 24-h period.

The primary reason that acetaminophen is often preferred over nonsteroidal anti-inflammatory drugs is due to the gastrointestinal toxicity inherent in all presently available NSAIDs. Recognizing this fact, the American College of Rheumatology has recently published guidelines recommending that acetaminophen be considered as first-line medical therapy for osteoarthritis of the hips and knees *(6,7)*. As acetaminophen lacks significant anti-inflammatory properties, it would not be appropriate as primary therapy for an inflammatory process such as rheumatoid arthritis.

Several precautions must be observed. Since acetaminophen may be present in combination with other medications, the total dose from all sources must be reviewed to ascertain that it does not exceed 4000 mg/d. Higher doses may be associated with serious hepatotoxicity. In addition, hepatotoxicity may develop with usual doses of acetaminophen in patients with significant alcohol intake or malnutrition.

If acetaminophen alone is not sufficient for relief of mild to moderate pain, it may be combined with other medications For example, acetaminophen is often used in conjunction with nonsteroidal anti-inflammatory drugs for the treatment of inflammatory arthritis.

Nonsteroidal Anti-Inflammatory Drugs (NSAIDs)

Aspirin and other nonsteroidal anti-inflammatory drugs (NSAIDs) are potent agents that possess both anti-inflammatory and analgesic effects. They may be used to treat mild-to-moderate pain not responsive to acetaminophen alone as well as to treat inflammatory processes such as rheumatoid arthritis. NSAIDs exert their analgesic and anti-inflammatory effects in part by blocking cyclo-oxygenase (COX), an enzyme that converts arachidonic acid to mediators of inflammation such as prostaglandins and oxygen radicals. Some NSAIDs also inhibit lipoxygenase, the enzyme that mediates formation of inflammatory mediators such as leukotrienes from arachidonic acid. Other mechanisms may also contribute to the anti-inflammatory effects of these drugs.

Gastric prostaglandins such as PGI_2 and PGE_2 serve as cytoprotective agents in the gastric mucosa by maintaining blood flow, promoting the secretion of cytoprotective mucus, and decreasing gastric acid secretion. The inhibition of cyclo-oxygenase by NSAIDs decreases levels of these prostaglandins, increasing the potential for peptic ulcer disease. The risk for gastric perforation or major gastrointestinal bleeding has been estimated to be approx 1–4%/yr among patients using NSAIDs. This risk varies somewhat with different NSAIDs and is also dependent on individual risk factors, which include history of peptic ulcer disease, advanced age, concurrent corticosteroid use, disabling arthritis, and possibly smoking and alcohol consumption (6). Although it is recommended that NSAIDs be taken with food, the effect of this approach on the development of peptic ulcer disease is unknown. The incidence of peptic ulcer disease may be reduced in high-risk patients by administering the prostacyclin analog misoprostol (Cytotec) or high-dose (40 mg twice daily) femotidine (Pepcid) (8), and by choosing an NSAID with lower ulcerogenic potential. Nonacetylated salicylates appear to be the safest, although they may have less anti-inflammatory effect. Economic considerations preclude prescribing cytoprotective or H_2 receptor antagonists to all patients receiving NSAIDs.

An exciting recent observation is that cyclo-oxygenase exists as two isoenzymes, termed COX-1 and COX-2. COX-1 is found in blood vessels, the gastrointestinal tract, and the kidneys, whereas COX- 2 is synthesized in response to cytokines and inflammatory mediators. Currently available NSAIDs inhibit both COX-1 and COX-2. Although nabumetone has been reported to preferentially inhibit COX-2, it too may cause gastric ulceration and renal dysfunction. When drugs with selective inhibition of COX- 2 are developed, it may be possible to dissociate gastric and renal toxicity from the analgesic and anti-inflammatory effects of NSAIDs.

NSAIDs are extensively bound to protein, leading to potential displacement and increased activity of other drugs that are protein-bound. Examples include warfarin (Coumadin), digoxin, sulfa drugs, oral hypoglycemic agents, methotrexate, and cyclosporine (5). Certain medications that may interact with NSAIDs are listed in Table 2. Other side effects associated with NSAIDs include decreased platelet function, impaired renal function, hyperkalemia, sodium retention, bronchospasm, hepatic dysfunction, congestive heart failure, hypertension, and central nervous system (CNS) symptoms, such as headache, dizziness, and depression (Table 3) (9). These agents should be used cautiously, if at all, in patients with impaired hepatic or renal function. In general, NSAIDs should be avoided in patients with asthma, although nonacetylated salicylates may be administered cautiously to patients who have not experienced a major reaction to aspirin or other NSAIDs. Monitoring of patients receiving NSAIDs should include

Table 2
Drug Interactions with NSAIDs

Drug or Drug Category	Potential Effect from NSAID
Antihypertensive agents	Decreased hypotensive effect
Digoxin	Increased digoxin levels with aspirin, ibuprofen
Lithium	Increased lithium levels
Methotrexate	Increased methotrexate levels with salicylates and others
NSAIDs	Decreased NSAID levels with salicylates
Phenytoin	Increased phenytoin levels
Probenecid	Decreased uricosuric effect with salicylates (low dose)
Sulfonyurea hypoglycemic agents	Increased hypoglycemic effect
Warfarin	Increased anticoagulant effect[a]

[a]NSAIDs should be used with considerable caution if at all in patients who are anticoagulated; nonacetylated salicylates are generally safest in this circumstance.

Table 3
Side Effects of NSAIDs

Gastrointestinal intolerance and ulceration
Impaired platelet aggregation
Decreased renal function
Hyperkalemia
Peripheral edema
Elevated liver enzymes
Bronchospasm
CNS symptoms
Hypersensitivity reactions
Bone marrow suppression

periodic assessment of electrolytes, creatinine, and liver enzymes. Although uncommon, hyperkalemia or renal failure may occur within days of starting an NSAID.

Many patients respond better to one NSAID than another, but there is no way to predict in advance the response of an individual patient to a particular NSAID. When prescribing an NSAID, the physician should allow sufficient time for the serum concentration to reach a steady-state level and for the drug to exert its effects before switching to another NSAID. This generally means that a particular drug should be administered for at least 2–3 wk, unless side effects preclude such treatment. Since NSAIDs include drugs from different chemical groups (Table 4), there is a theoretical reason to consider changing to an NSAID from another group if a patient does not respond satisfactorily to a particular agent. In practice, however, this classification does not always seem relevant.

NSAIDs available in the United States at this time are described below in chronologic order by group and in Table 5.

Table 4
A Classification of NSAIDs

Alkanones	Nabumetone (Relafen)
Arylacetic acids	Tolmetin (Tolectin)
	Diclofenac (Voltaren, Cataflam)
	Ketorolac (Toradol)
	Bromfenac (Duract)
Fenamates	Meclofenamic acid (Meclomen)
	Mefenamic acid (Ponstel)
Indole and indene acetic acids	Indomethacin (Indocin)
	Sulindac (Clinoril)
	Etodolac (Lodine)
Oxicams	Piroxicam (Feldene)
Propionic acids	Ibuprofen (Motrin, Rufen, Advil, Nuprin)
	Naproxen (Naprosyn)
	Naproxen sodium (Anaprox, Aleve, Naprelan)
	Fenoprofen (Nalfon)
	Ketoprofen (Orudis, Oruvail)
	Flurbiprofen (Ansaid)
	Oxaprozin (Daypro)
Pyrazolidinediones	Phenylbutazone (Butazolidin)
Salicylates	Acetylsalicylic acid (aspirin)
	Choline magnesium trisalicylate (Trilisate)
	Salsalate (Disalcid)
	Diflunisal (Dolobid)

Salicylates

Aspirin (acetylsalicylic acid) and its active metabolite, salicylate, were synthesized In the 19th century. Salicylsalicylic acid or salsalate (Disalcid) and choline magnesium trisalicylate (Trilisate) represent nonacetylated salicylates available in the United States. In contrast to regular or buffered aspirin, enteric-coated aspirin (Ecotrin, Easprin) and the nonacetylated salicylates are preferentially absorbed in the neutral pH environment of the small intestine. Accordingly, they are associated with a lower incidence of gastric irritation than regular aspirin and most other NSAIDs. However, concurrent administration of antacids or H2 receptor antagonists may increase absorption of these preparations through the gastric mucosa.

Salicylates in low doses (serum levels of 5–15 mg/dL) exert analgesic and antipyretic effects. To achieve anti-inflammatory effects, a serum salicylate level of 20–25 mg/dL is generally necessary. Due to considerable individual variation in absorption of salicylates from the gastrointestinal tract, the dose required to achieve a given salicylate level is not predictable. For analgesic effects, therapy with aspirin may be initiated in doses as low as 500 mg twice daily, whereas anti-inflammatory effects may require doses as high as 2000 mg three times daily. Serum salicylate levels are widely available and permit optimal dosing, even though this testing adds to the cost of administering these agents. Diflunisal (Dolobid) is not metabolized to salicylic acid, so salicylate levels are

Table 5
NSAID Doses and Half-Lives

Generic (Brand) Name	Oral Strengths	Half-Life,[a] h	Usual Dose[b]
Aspirin (Various)	81,[g] 325,[g] 500,[g] 975 mg	4–16	500 mg bid[c]- 2000 mg tid[d]
Bromfenac (Duract)	25 mg	1–4	25 mg tid-qid
Choline magnesium salicylate (Trilisate)	500, 750, 1000 mg	4–16	750-1500 mg bid[d]
Diclofenac (Voltaren)	25, 50, 75 mg	1–2	50–75 mg bid
Diclofenac (Voltaren XR)	100 mg	See text[f]	100 mg qd
Diclofenac (Cataflam)	50 mg	1–2	50 mg bid-tid
Diflunisal (Dolobid)	250, 500 mg	8–12	250 mg bid- 500 mg tid[e]
Etodolac (Lodine)	200, 300, 400 mg	7	200–400 mg tid (300 mg qid)
Etodolac (Lodine XL)	400, 600 mg	See text[f]	400–1000 mg qd
Fenoprofen (Nalfon)	200, 300, 600 mg	3	200–600 mg tid-qid
Flurbiprofen (Ansaid)	50, 100 mg	5–6	100 mg bid-tid
Ibuprofen (Advil, Nuprin, Motrin, Motrin IB, Rufen)	200,[g] 400, 600, 800 mg	2	400–800 mg tid (600 mg qid)
Indomethacin (Indocin)	25, 50 mg	4–5	25–50 mg tid
Indomethacin (Indocin SR)	75 mg	4–5[f]	75 mg qd-bid
Ketoprofen (Actron, Orudis KT, Orudis)	12.5,[g] 25, 50, 75 mg	2	50–75 mg tid-qid
Ketoprofen (Oruvail)	100, 150, 200 mg	5–6[f]	150–200 mg qd
Ketorolac (Toradol)	10 mg; also im, iv	4–6	Not to exceed 40 mg orally or 120 mg iv or im/d
Meclofenamate (Meclomen)	50, 100 mg	2–4	50–100 mg tid-qid
Nabumetone (Relafen)	500, 750 mg	24	1000–2000 mg qd
Naproxen (Naprosyn, EC-Naprosyn)	250, 375, 500 mg	14	250-500 mg bid
Naproxen sodium (Aleve, Anaprox, Anaprox DS)	220,[g] 275, 550 mg (equivalent: to 200, 250, and 500 mg naproxen)	14	275–550 mg bid
Naproxen sodium (Naprelan)	Equivalent to 375 and 500 mg naproxen	See text[f]	750–1000 mg qd
Oxaprozin (Daypro)	600 mg	40–60	600–1200 mg qd
Piroxicam (Feldene)	10, 20 mg	50	20 mg qd
Salsalate (Disalcid)	500, 750 mg	4–16	750–1500 mg bid[d]
Sulindac (Clinoril)	150, 200 mg	18	150–200 mg bid
Tolmetin (Tolectin, Tolectin DS)	200, 400, 600 mg	5	200–600 mg tid

[a]Approximately five half-lives are required to approach steady-state plasma concentrations.
[b]These are usual but not necessarily maximal doses for anti-inflammatory effects; analgesic doses may be less. NSAIDs other than bromfenac should be taken with food.
[c]Abbreviations: qd, once daily; bid, twice daily; tid, three times daily; qid, four times daily.
[d]Determined by serum salicylate level for anti-inflammatory doses.
[e]Salicylate levels are not useful for monitoring diflunisal therapy.
[f]Delayed absorption with sustained-release preparation increases effective half-life.
[g]Over-the-counter strength.

not helpful in monitoring this agent. The usual dose of diflunisal ranges from 250 mg twice daily to 500 mg three times daily.

Manifestations of salicylate toxicity often include tinnitus and, especially in the elderly, reversible hearing loss or confusion, which may be the only clue to salicylism. At very high salicylate levels, seizures or coma may develop.

Although all NSAIDs decrease platelet aggregation through inhibition of platelet cyclo-oxygenase, aspirin differs from other agents in that it irreversibly acetylates cyclo-oxygenase, interfering with platelet function for the lifetime of the platelet. In contrast, the nonacetylated salicylates, which are weak inhibitors of cyclo-oxygenase, exert the least effect on platelet function among the NSAIDs and should be considered in patients with bleeding diatheses who require anti-inflammatory agents. Other NSAIDs reversibly block platelet cyclo-oxygenase; platelet function will return to normal 2–3 d after the NSAID is discontinued.

Inhibition of prostaglandin synthesis by aspirin and other NSAIDs may decrease renal blood flow, leading to impaired renal function. This effect, usually reversible, is more common in hypovolemic patients or those with pre-existing renal disease. Nonacetylated salicylates appear less likely to decrease renal function than other NSAIDs. Aspirin and other salicylates may also increase liver enzymes. This has been noted in particular among patients with juvenile rheumatoid arthritis, systemic lupus erythematosus, decreased renal function, and the elderly.

All NSAIDs have the potential to trigger or exacerbate bronchospasm in patients with asthma. It is hypothesized that this is owing at least in part to inhibition of cyclo-oxygenase, leading to increased metabolism of arachidonic acid via the lipoxygenase pathway to leukotrienes (including leukotrienes C4, D4, E4, formerly known as SRS-A or slow releasing factor of anaphylaxis) and other inflammatory mediators. The nonacetylated salicylates, noted above to be weak inhibitors of cyclo-oxygenase, represent the safest nonsteroidal anti-inflammatory agents for use in patients with asthma (although at times they too may worsen bronchospasm).

Special consideration should be given to administering salicylates to patients with gout. Since low-dose salicylates inhibit tubular secretion of uric acid, thereby increasing the serum uric acid level, they are not usually administered to patients with gout (unless antiplatelet effect is desired). Although high-dose salicylate therapy is uricosuric and may lower the serum uric acid level, other NSAIDs are considered more efficacious for treating gouty arthritis.

Pyrazolidinediones

Phenylbutazone (Butazolidin) is mentioned primarily for historical reasons. Introduced in the late 1940s, phenylbutazone is considered the most potent nonsteroidal anti-inflammatory drug. However, other NSAIDs have supplanted this agent due to its potential for serious side effects, including aplastic anemia, peptic ulcer disease, and others. It may be indicated occasionally to treat refractory cases of ankylosing spondylitis but is no longer available in the United States.

Indole and Indene Acetic Acids

Indomethacin (Indocin), a potent cyclo-oxygenase inhibitor, represents a highly effective agent for treating acute inflammatory processes, such as gout. Immediate-release

(25 mg, 50 mg), sustained-release (75 mg), oral suspension (25 mg/5 mL), suppository (50 mg), and intravenous preparations are available. The plasma half-life is variable, perhaps due to extensive enterohepatic circulation, but averages about 4–5 h; the effective half-life of sustained-release indomethacin is longer due to delayed absorption. The usual dose is 75–150 mg/d. Potential side effects include headaches, dizziness, depression, peptic ulcer disease, peripheral edema, hyperkalemia, renal dysfunction, and bone marrow suppression. Because these side effects are more common with indomethacin than most other NSAIDs, alternative agents are generally preferred for long-term use.

Sulindac (Clinoril), a prodrug developed as a less toxic congener of indomethacin, has been represented as possibly having less renal toxicity than most other NSAIDs. It may cause CNS side effects similar to, but generally less severe than, indomethacin. Sulindac and its sulfone and sulfide metabolites undergo extensive enterohepatic circulation, which may increase their gastrointestinal toxicity. The half-life of sulindac is about 7 h, but the active sulfide metabolite has a half-life of up to 18 h. The usual dose is 150–200 mg twice daily. Renal stones composed of sulindac metabolites have been described, and aseptic meningitis has been reported in some patients with connective tissue diseases.

Etodolac (Lodine), an indoleacetic acid approved by the Food and Drug Administration (FDA) for treatment of osteoarthritis, rheumatoid arthritis, and pain, inhibits cyclooxygenase but not lipoxygenase. Maximal analgesia occurs within 1–2 h after a single dose; the half-life is about 7 h, with analgesic effects lasting 4–6 h. The recommended dose is 200–400 mg every 6–8 h, not to exceed 1200 mg/d. An extended-release preparation (Lodine XL) is also available; the recommended dose is 400–1000 mg once daily. Gastrointestinal and renal side effects from etodolac are similar to other NSAIDs.

Propionic Acids

Ibuprofen (Motrin and others) is rapidly absorbed after oral administration but has a short plasma half-life of about 2 h. The usual dose for anti-inflammatory effects is 1200–2400 mg/d (maximal 3200 mg/d); therapy may be initiated at a lower dose for analgesic effects. Although frequent dosing (three to four times daily) represents a disadvantage and may decrease compliance, ibuprofen is relatively well-tolerated and inexpensive. NSAID-associated aseptic meningitis is an uncommon side effect described most often with this drug, primarily in patients with lupus or other connective tissue diseases.

Fenoprofen (Nalfon) also has a short half-life (about 3 h) but is more expensive than ibuprofen and offers no apparent advantage for most patients. The usual analgesic dose is 200 mg every 4–6 h; the anti-inflammatory dose ranges from 300 to 600 mg administered three to four times daily. The total daily dose should not exceed 3200 mg. Fenoprofen has been associated with more cases of acute interstitial nephritis and nephrotic syndrome than other NSAIDs.

Naproxen (Naprosyn, EC-Naprosyn [enteric-coated]) achieves peak plasma concentrations within 2–4 h following administration, whereas naproxen sodium (Anaprox, Aleve, Naprelan) reaches peak concentrations within 1–2 h. Although this difference may be significant for short-term analgesia, it is irrelevant for long-term therapy. The usual daily dose of naproxen is 500–1000 mg (corresponding to 550–1100 mg naproxen sodium). The daily dose should not exceed 1500 mg, which may be given for a limited time if clinically indicated. Plasma half-life is about 14 h (longer in the elderly), permitting twice-daily dosing with Naprosyn and Anaprox. Naprelan, available in strengths equivalent to naproxen 375 and 500 mg, is a controlled-release tablet designed for once-daily administration. Physicians should be aware of the sodium content when prescribing naproxen sodium to patients with hypertension or congestive heart failure.

Ketoprofen is available as Orudis capsules, which release the drug in the stomach, and Oruvail capsules, which contain pellets that are designed to release the drug at a controlled rate in the small intestine. Also approved are Orudis KT and Actron, over-the-counter preparations containing ketoprofen 12.5 mg. Peak plasma levels occur within 1–2 h with Orudis and 6–7 h with Oruvail. Orudis has a half-life of about 2 h, necessitating administration three to four times daily. Because the slow absorption of Oruvail prolongs its elimination half-life, it can be administered only once each day. The recommended dose of ketoprofen is 25–50 mg every 6–8 h for analgesia and 150–200 mg/d for anti-inflammatory effects.

Flurbiprofen (Ansaid) represents another NSAID with a longer half-life (about 6 h) than ibuprofen. The usual adult dose is 100 mg two to three times daily.

Oxaprozin (Daypro) can be administered once daily owing to its long half-life of 40–60 h (which increases with age). This provides convenient dosing and may improve compliance, but when adverse effects occur, they may persist longer. The recommended dose is 600–1200 mg once daily.

Arylacetic Acids

Tolmetin (Tolectin), a heteroarylacetic acid, is structurally similar to zomepirac, an analgesic withdrawn from the market due to anaphylactic reactions. The half-life is about 5 h, necessitating dosing three to four times daily. The usual total daily dose is 600–1800 mg. Tolmetin is one of the few NSAIDs (the others being aspirin, ibuprofen, and naproxen) approved by the FDA for treatment of juvenile rheumatoid arthritis. Anaphylaxis, though uncommon, has been associated with tolmetin more than other currently available NSAIDs; this seems most likely to occur when the drug is resumed after a hiatus. Tolmetin may cause CNS side effects similar to indomethacin. Aseptic meningitis associated with tolmetin has been described in patients with lupus and other connective tissue diseases.

Diclofenac (Voltaren, Cataflam) is a phenylacetic acid derivative available as a delayed-release (enteric-coated) preparation designed to dissolve in the duodenum (Voltaren) and as an immediate-release preparation that dissolves in the stomach (Cataflam). An extended-release preparation designed for once-daily administration (Voltaren XR) is also available. The plasma half-life of diclofenac is short (1–2 h), but the slow absorption of Voltaren prolongs its elimination half-life. The usual total daily dose is 100–150 mg. Elevated hepatic aminotransferase levels are detected in about 15% of persons treated with diclofenac. Liver enzymes should be monitored within the first 8 wk of therapy and periodically thereafter.

Ketorolac (Toradol), one of the few NSAIDs approved for parenteral administration, has moderate anti-inflammatory but potent analgesic properties. Maximal plasma levels occur within 30–50 min following oral or intramuscular administration; the elimination half-life is 4–6 h. The usual im or iv dose for patients under age 65 is a single injection of 60 mg or multiple injections of 30 mg every 6 h, not to exceed 120 mg/24-h period. The recommended oral dose for patients under age 65 is two 10-mg tablets followed by 10 mg every 4–6 h, not to exceed 40 mg/24-h period. This dose should be reduced in the elderly and in patients with renal impairment. Use with caution in patients with hepatic disease. Ketorolac should not be administered with other NSAIDs. Because it may adversely affect fetal circulation and inhibit uterine contractions, ketorolac is contraindicated during labor and delivery.

Bromfenac sodium (Duract) is a newly released NSAID indicated for the short-term (generally <10 d) treatment of pain. It has the advantage of rapid onset and 25 mg brofenac is equivalent to two Percocet tablets. Analgesic effects occur within 30 min and peak at 2–3 h. The recommended dose is 25 mg every 6–8 h, except when taken with high-fat food (which impairs absorption), in which case a 50-mg dose may be used. The total daily dose should not exceed 150 mg.

Fenamates

Meclofenamate (Meclomen) is an anti-inflammatory agent occasionally used for treating inflammatory arthritides. The usual dose is 50–100 mg three to four times daily. Due to a relatively high incidence of gastrointestinal side effects (including abdominal cramps and diarrhea) and rash, meclofenamate is not recommended as initial therapy. Mefenamic acid (Ponstel), indicated only for short-term analgesia and relief of primary dysmenorrhea, is seldom used due to toxicity and the availability of other agents. Plasma half-life is 2–4 h for both meclofenamate and mefenamic acid.

Oxicams

Piroxicam (Feldene) has an average plasma half-life of 50 h and was the first once-daily NSAID available in the United States. This represents an advantage from the standpoint of convenience and compliance and may also explain, at least in part, the relatively high incidence of peptic ulcer disease reported with this medication. The usual dose is 20 mg once daily; higher doses cause significantly greater side effects without concomitant clinical benefit and are not recommended.

Alkanones

Nabumetone (Relafen) is a nonacidic prodrug converted in the liver to one or more active metabolites, mainly 6-methoxy-2-naphthylacetic acid, a potent inhibitor of cyclooxygenase, especially COX-2. This metabolite is eliminated with a half-life of about 24 h, allowing nabumetone to be administered once daily. The recommended dose is 1000–2000 mg/d. The incidence of endoscopically detected gastric lesions has been reported to be less with nabumetone than indomethacin, piroxicam, or ibuprofen.

OPIOID ANALGESICS

Opiates are drugs derived from opium. These include morphine, which is the principal and most active alkaloid of opium, in addition to codeine and various semisynthetic congeners. Opioids refer to all drugs with morphine-like activity, including endogenous peptides known as enkephalins, endorphins, and dynorphins.

Table 6
Classification of Opioids

Full Agonists	Partial Agonists	Mixed Agonist–Antagonists	Other
Codeine	Buprenorphine	Butorphanol	Tramadol
Fentanyl		Dezocine	
Hydrocodone		Nalbuphine	
Hydromorphone		Pentazocine	
Levorphanol			
Meperidine			
Methadone			
Morphine			
Oxycodone			
Oxymorphone			
Propoxyphene			

The CNS contains at least three major classes of opioid receptors, known as μ, κ, and δ receptors. Although individual drugs interact with different groups of receptors, explaining differences in analgesia and side effects, most opioid drugs produce analgesia by activation of μ receptors. μ receptors are found in high concentration in specific areas of the CNS, including the hypothalamus, thalamus, and some cortical areas. Interaction of opioids with these receptors appears to activate descending pathways that inhibit pain sensation. In the spinal cord, opioid receptors are present on terminal axons of primary afferent nociceptive fibers in the dorsal horn. Activation of these receptors may block transmission of nociceptive stimuli to the second-order neurons that comprise the spinothalamic and spinoreticular tracts *(10)*.

Classification

Opioid drugs are classified as full (morphine-like) agonists, partial agonists, or mixed agonist-antagonists, depending on the receptors to which they bind and their activity at these receptors (Table 6) *(5)*. Full agonists—which include codeine, oxycodone, hydrocodone, morphine, hydromorphone, levorphanol, and fentanyl—do not antagonize or reverse the effects of other full agonists given simultaneously. Weaker opioid agonists such as codeine and hydrocodone exhibit an "analgesic ceiling," whereby increasing doses cause greater side effects without significantly greater analgesia *(11)*. On the other hand, the more potent opioid agonists display no analgesic ceiling; the dosage of these agents is limited only by side effects. Partial agonists, such as buprenorphine, are subject to a dose-related ceiling effect and represent less potent analgesics. Mixed agonist–antagonists, including butorphanol, dezocine, nalbuphine, and pentazocine, activate one type of opioid receptor while blocking another type. Due to this antagonism, they may precipitate a withdrawal syndrome in patients receiving an opioid agonist and are contraindicated in such individuals. The analgesic effectiveness of these mixed agents is also limited by a ceiling effect, and they are usually not recommended for treatment of cancer pain.

Table 7
Principles of Opioid Use[a]

1. Choose the appropriate drug and route of administration.
2. Start with a low dose.
3. Titrate the dose until adequate analgesia is achieved or intolerable side effects develop.
4. Learn equianalgesic doses for different opioids and routes of administration.
5. When changing from one opioid to another in an opioid-tolerant patient, begin with 50–75% of the equianalgesic dose. For methadone, begin with 40–50% of the equianalgesic dose. In the elderly, reduce the equianalgesic dose by another 25%.

[a]From refs. *14* and *19*.

Choice of Drug

A stepwise approach is generally recommended, beginning with "weak" opioids and progressing to "strong" opioids, if needed, in conjunction with nonopioid analgesic and adjuvant agents (Tables 1 and 7). Propoxyphene or codeine, often in combination with acetaminophen, is appropriate for treatment of moderate pain. For treatment of more severe pain, hydrocodone or oxycodone, each of which is available in combination with aspirin or acetaminophen, is commonly used. Noncombination opioids are utilized for pain unrelieved by these or similar agents. Physicians should be familiar with analgesic doses and pharmacokinetics of several opioids for pain of varying severity (Tables 8 and 9).

Route of Administration

Opioid drugs may be administered by various routes, and differences in absorption, distribution, metabolism, and elimination affect the dose, dosing interval, and drug toxicity. Oral administration is usually preferred for reasons of convenience and cost *(5)*. Opioids administered by this route are metabolized to varying degrees by the liver following absorption from the gastrointestinal tract (first-pass metabolism), resulting in bioavailability ranging from about 20 to 90% of the administered drug, depending on the compound. Patients unable to take oral medications may be treated by the transdermal, intranasal, or rectal route. The transdermal route is not appropriate for rapid-dose titration.

Severe pain, rapidly increasing pain, intolerable side effects, or inability to tolerate oral or transdermal drugs may warrant parenteral administration of opioids *(12)*. Any opioid formulated for parenteral use may be administered intravenously or subcutaneously, but morphine, hydromorphone, and fentanyl are the opioids most often delivered by these routes (Table 10). Intravenous administration of opioids provides the most rapid onset of analgesia, but the duration of action is shorter than with other routes. Peripheral venous access is usually chosen for short-term therapy and central venous access for long-term analgesia. When intravenous administration is not practical, subcutaneous infusion may be appropriate. The intramuscular route should generally be avoided due to unreliable absorption and pain. Segmental analgesia may be achieved with epidural or intrathecal (subarachnoid) administration of opioids, which enter the cerebrospinal fluid and bind to opioid receptors in the dorsal horn *(see below)*.

Table 8
Equianalgesic Doses and Pharmacokinetics of Opioids

Drug	Equianalgesic Dose[a]	Half-life, h	Duration of Analgesia, h
Buprenorphine	0.4 mg im or iv[b]	1–7	4–6
Butorphanol	2 mg im or iv	3	3–4
	2 mg intranasal	3	4–5
Codeine	200 mg orally	3	4–6
	130 mg im or iv	3	4–6
Fentanyl	Transdermal patch	*See text*	72
	0.1 mg im or iv	3–4	0.5–2
Hydrocodone	30 mg orally	3–4	4–5
Hydromorphone	7.5 mg orally	2–3	4–6
	1.5 mg im or iv	2–3	4–5
Levorphanol	4 mg orally	12–16	4–7
	2 mg im or iv	12–16	4–6
Meperidine	300 mg orally	3–4[c]	4–6
	75 mg im or iv	3–4	4–5
Methadone	20 mg orally	15–30+	Variable
	10 mg im or iv	15–30+	4–6
Morphine	20-60 mg orally	2–3	4–7
	10 mg im or iv	2–3	4–6
Nalbuphine	10 mg im or iv	2–3	4–6
Oxycodone	30 mg orally	2–3	3–5
Oxymorphone	5–10 mg per rectum	2–3	3–6
	1 mg im or iv	2–3	3–6
Pentazocine	180 mg orally	2–3	4–7
	30–60 mg im or iv	2–3	4–6
Propoxyphene	200–300 mg orally	6–12[d]	4–6

[a]These doses represent approximate equianalgesic doses but not necessarily the appropriate therapeutic dose; *see* Table 9.
[b]im, intramuscular; iv, intravenous.
[c]Half-life of meperidine; the half-life of the active metabolite normeperidine is 12–16 h.
[d]Half-life of propoxyphene; the half-life of the active metabolite norpropoxyphene is 30–36 h.

Molecular size and shape, degree of ionization, and lipid solubility determine the effectiveness of absorption through a given route. For example, lipophilic agents diffuse more rapidly through the skin, nasal mucosa, and blood–brain barrier.

Spinal Analgesia

Opioids may be administered into the epidural or intrathecal compartment of the spine for treatment of acute pain, cancer pain, and chronic nonmalignant pain in selected patients with conditions such as lumbar arachnoiditis, vertebral compression fracture, postherpetic neuralgia (PHN), and reflex sympathetic dystrophy *(13)*. This approach is

Table 9
Opioid Analgesic Doses for Moderate to Severe Pain in Opioid-Naive Adults

Generic Name (Brand Name)	Oral Strengths	Oral Dose	Parenteral Dose
Butorphanol (Stadol, Stadol NS[a])	None	Not available	1 mg every 3–6 h
Codeine (Various)[b]	15, 30, 60 mg	15–60 mg every 3–6 h	50–75 mg every 3–6 h
Fentanyl (Oralet, Sublimaze, Duragesic[c])	Oralet for premedication	Analgesic role of Oralet is not determined	25–100 µg/h every 72 h[c] (see text)
Hydrocodone (Lortab, Vicodin)[b]	2.5, 5, 7.5, 10 mg	5–10 mg every 3–6 h	Not available
Hydromorphone (Dilaudid)[d]	2, 4, 8 mg	2–6 mg every 3–6 h	0.75–1.5 mg every 3–6 h
Levorphanol (Levo-Dromoran)	2 mg	2–4 mg every 4–8 h	1–2 mg every 4–8 h
Meperidine (Demerol)	50, 100 mg	50–150 mg every 3–6 h	50–100 mg every 3–4 h
Methadone (Dolophine)	5, 10 mg	2.5–10 mg every 3–8 h	2.5–10 mg every 4–8 h
Morphine (Various)[d]	15, 30 mg	10–30 mg every 3–6 h	5–10 mg every 3–6 h
Morphine, sustained release (MS Contin, Oramorph SR)	15, 30, 60, 100 mg	30–120 mg every 12 h	Not available
Oxycodone (Roxicodone, Percocet, Tylox, Percodan)[b]	5 mg	5–10 mg every 3–6 h	Not available
Oxymorphone (Numorphan)[d]	None	Not available	0.5–1 mg every 3–6 h
Pentazocine (Talwin)	12.5, 25, 50 mg	12.5–50 mg every 3–6 h	30 mg every 3–6 h
Propoxyphene (Darvon N, Darvocet N)[b]	50, 100 mg[e]	50–100 mg every 4–6 h	Not available

[a]Stadol NS nasal spray; see text.
[b]May be administered as combination drug with acetaminophen or aspirin.
[c]Duragesic transdermal patch; see text.
[d]Also available as suppository; see text.
[e]Darvon N is only available as 100 mg strength.

generally reserved for pain that cannot be controlled with systemic opioids due to side effects. If necessary, bupivacaine or another local anesthetic may be added to opioids delivered by the epidural route.

Following epidural injection, opioids cross the dura at a rate dependent on factors such as size and lipid solubility. Those with poor lipid solubility, such as morphine, are

Table 10
Dosage Guidelines for Continuous Subcutaneous
or Intravenous Infusion of Opioids[a]

Drug	Loading Dose[b]	Hourly Infusion Dose[b]
Morphine	0.05–0.20 mg/kg	0.01–0.075 mg/kg
Hydromorphone	0.01–0.03 mg/kg	0.0015–0.02 mg/kg
Fentanyl	0.5–3.0 µg/kg	0.2–2.0 µg/kg

[a]Adapted from ref. 12.
[b]For "opioid-naive" patients; higher doses may be required in patients already receiving opioids. The loading dose may be administered during the initial 30 min of the infusion rather than as a bolus.

absorbed slowly but remain in the dural space longer and spread over more dermatomes than medications with greater lipid solubility, such as fentanyl. Epidurally administered opioids bind to opioid receptors in the substantia gelatinosa of the dorsal horn. They are also absorbed systemically and diffuse within cerebrospinal fluid to the medullary and brain opioid receptors, providing additional analgesia but also contributing to side effects. Nevertheless, this route is associated with greater analgesia at considerably lower doses than required if given systemically. Opioids may also be administered intrathecally, which hastens the onset of action since they do not need to diffuse across the dura. The duration of analgesia following intrathecal injection is prolonged compared to the epidural route. The intrathecal analgesic dose for morphine is about one-tenth the epidural dose, which is about one-tenth the intravenous dose. Fentanyl doses barely change between these routes.

The most potentially serious complication of spinal opiates is respiratory depression, which may occur early (1–2 h) or late (6–24 h) following administration. The early respiratory depression is believed to occur as a result of vascular absorption of the drug, whereas the delayed reaction is attributed to rostral migration of the opioid in the cerebrospinal fluid to the respiratory center in the pons. The incidence of delayed respiratory depression is greater with spinal morphine compared to fentanyl, since morphine demonstrates greater spread. Epidural administration offers the advantage of a lower incidence of respiratory depression, headache, and CNS infection compared to the intrathecal route. As with other routes of administration, urinary retention, nausea, vomiting, sedation, constipation, and pruritus may occur with spinal opioids.

Contraindications to spinal administration of drugs include bleeding diathesis, septicemia, and local infection. Over long periods, fibrosis may develop around epidural catheters, leading to variable CSF opioid concentrations and decreased analgesic efficacy. For treatment longer than 6 mo, intrathecal administration using a totally implanted programmable pump may be considered (13).

Dosing

The appropriate dose of opioid is the amount that provides adequate analgesia with the fewest side effects. This dose will be determined both by the extent of injury or other cause of pain and the ability of the patient to tolerate pain. The clinician should avoid the tendency to prescribe an inadequate dose of opioid and then consider with suspicion requests by the patient for more medication. The need for increased doses of analgesic medication often reflects progression of the disease, especially in patients with cancer. As patients develop tolerance to opioids, they require more frequent dosing. When the dose of opioid is changed, it may be increased or decreased by one-fourth to one-half of the previous dose *(5)*. Although higher doses of opioids are needed for oral than parenteral administration, they are similar for subcutaneous, intramuscular, and intravenous routes.

When one opioid is exchanged for another in an opioid-tolerant patient, the equianalgesic dose (Table 8) should be reduced by approx 50% for initial administration since crosstolerance *(see below)* between narcotics may be incomplete. When converting to methadone, the equianalgesic dose should be decreased by 50–60%, as crosstolerance may be particularly limited between methadone and other strong opioids. For opioid-naive adults, the starting doses listed in Table 9 are appropriate.

When opioids are needed for treatment of chronic nonmalignant pain, intermittent dosing may be appropriate for patients with episodic severe pain, but most patients do better with continuous around-the-clock therapy. Analgesic medication for treatment of acute or cancer pain should be administered on a regular schedule rather than an as-needed (prn) basis. "Rescue" medication to treat breakthrough pain should usually be provided. An appropriate dose is generally 5–10% of the total daily opioid dosage, which may be made available to the patient every 1–2 h if necessary. The number and amount of the rescue doses should be recorded and used as the basis for determining the subsequent 24-h opioid dosage. Treating pain before it becomes severe not only provides greater patient comfort but also reduces total analgesic dosage, since higher doses are needed to treat pain than prevent it.

Patient-Controlled Analgesia (PCA)

In some circumstances, administration of analgesics on a regular schedule can be accomplished most effectively with patient-controlled analgesia (PCA), whereby the patient controls the dosing of analgesic medication administered by continuous subcutaneous, intravenous, or epidural infusion within parameters established by the physician. A loading dose is delivered to achieve a serum level that provides baseline analgesia. Thereafter, the patient pushes a hand-held button to deliver the demand dose. A lockout time ranging from 5 to 15 min follows administration of the demand dose to allow for the full effect before further doses can be given. In addition, the amount of drug administered over a given time period can be limited. General dosing guidelines are indicated in Table 10.

Opioid Use for Chronic Nonmalignant Pain

Although long-term opioid therapy for patients with cancer pain is accepted, use of opioids to treat patients with chronic nonmalignant pain is controversial. Nevertheless, some of these patients fail to achieve adequate analgesia with other modalities. Patients with chronic pain syndromes may be considered for treatment with opioids after other reasonable attempts at analgesia, including adjuvant analgesics and possibly nonpharmacologic modalities, have failed. A history of drug abuse represents a relative contraindication.

Patients should be informed of the small risk of psychological dependence (addiction) and the potential for cognitive impairment with the opioid drug alone or in combination with sedatives or similar agents *(15)*.

For patients with unremitting nonmalignant pain, opioids should be administered on a regular schedule. Long-acting oral agents, such as sustained-release morphine, levorphanol, methadone, or transdermal fentanyl, offer the advantage of prolonged pain relief with less variation in peak and trough serum levels than shorter-acting drugs. The patient should agree on several weeks as the period of initial dose titration, during which time pain reduction as well as possible functional improvement are the goals. If relatively low initial doses of analgesic fail to provide at least partial pain relief for patients not tolerant to opioids, the patient may not be a candidate for this approach. In addition to the analgesic requirement initially determined, the dose may be transiently increased on days of increased pain. One technique is to instruct the patient that one or two extra doses may be taken if needed for pain exacerbation, but this must be followed by an equal reduction of dose on subsequent days *(15)*.

In order to minimize the potential for abuse, only one physician should prescribe analgesic medications for the patient. Patients should be evaluated on a regular basis for effectiveness of treatment, medication side effects, and evidence of drug abuse. Acquisition of opioids from other physicians, uncontrolled dose escalation, or other aberrant behaviors should be followed by tapering and discontinuation of opioid medications *(15)*.

Side effects may occasionally limit the effectiveness of oral opioid therapy. In selected patients with chronic nonmalignant pain, these agents may be administered by the epidural or intrathecal route *(see above) (13)*.

Metabolism

Following absorption, most opioids undergo extensive metabolism in the liver, usually by conjugation. These metabolites may possess analgesic activity, sometimes with half-lives much longer than the parent compound. In such instances, impaired renal function may lead to accumulation of active metabolites and associated side effects. For example, repeated dosing with meperidine in patients with renal dysfunction may lead to accumulation of the metabolite normeperidine with resultant tremor and seizures. Similarly, accumulation of norpropoxyphene from overdosing with propoxyphene may cause cardiac toxicity and seizures. All opioids should be administered with caution and generally in lower doses to patients with hepatic or renal disease.

Special Considerations in the Elderly

Doses of morphine and other opioids administered to elderly patients should generally be decreased due to impaired renal function in addition to a smaller volume of distribution. Appropriate starting doses for analgesics are often lower than the minimum recommended doses. Opioids associated with CNS side effects such as confusion or disequilibrium or with prolonged half-lives (which may be age-dependent) should be used with extreme caution, if at all, in the elderly. Examples of such medications are transdermal fentanyl (Duragesic), levorphanol (Levo-Dromoran), meperidine (Demerol),

Table 11
Side Effects of Opioids

Respiratory depression
Hypotension with or without bradycardia
Sedation
Altered mood and cognitive function
Pruritus
Dry mouth
Nausea and vomiting
Constipation
Urinary retention
Sexual dysfunction
Increased biliary tract pressure
Myoclonus
Inappropriate secretion of antidiuretic hormone (SIADH)

methadone (Dolophine), propoxyphene (Darvon), all of which are associated with long duration of action of the parent compound or metabolite, and pentazocine (Talwin), which may cause delirium and other CNS symptoms.

Side Effects

Opioids are associated with characteristic side effects, including respiratory depression due to impaired responsiveness of the brainstem respiratory centers to carbon dioxide. This is of particular concern in patients with impaired respiratory function, including patients with COPD, in whom sensitivity to carbon dioxide is often depressed. Carbon dioxide retention may also be dangerous for patients with head trauma due to increased intracranial pressure associated with acidosis. Moreover, administration of opioids to these patients may interfere with the ability to monitor their neurologic status (sensorium and pupil size). The depressant effects of opioids may be increased by the concomitant administration of phenothiazines, tricyclic antidepressants, and monoamine oxidase (MAO) inhibitors.

Other typical side effects of opioids include pruritus, dizziness, dysphoria, euphoria, altered cognitive function, sleep disturbances, miosis, dry mouth, hypotension (with or without bradycardia), nausea and vomiting, constipation, increased biliary tract pressure, urinary retention, sexual dysfunction, inappropriate secretion of antidiuretic hormone (SIADH), and myoclonus (Table 11). Morphine and other opioids directly release histamine from basophils and mast cells. For this reason, these agents should generally be avoided in patients with urticaria pigmentosa and systemic mastocytosis, conditions associated with excess numbers of histamine-containing cells.

An expected result of chronic opioid drug use is the development of tolerance and physical dependence. The distinction between these characteristics and addiction is often misunderstood and is discussed later in this chapter. Tolerance and physical dependence are related phenomena that represent normal physiological responses to opioids and neither indicate nor predict the development of drug abuse or addiction. Too frequently, unwarranted fears that addiction may develop result in undertreatment of chronic pain, especially in patients with cancer.

Most side effects from opioids are manageable. Tolerance to respiratory depression usually develops rapidly. Stimulating the patient with sound or light may reverse a mild degree of respiratory depression until tolerance develops. Sedation may be decreased by reducing the dose and increasing the frequency of opioid administration. Tolerance to sedation usually develops within days. If tolerance is incomplete, a CNS stimulant such as caffeine, methylphenidate hydrochloride (Ritalin), or dextroamphetamine (Dexedrine and others) can be used. These agents should be used cautiously in patients with cardiac arrhythmia, coronary artery disease, hypertension, or a history of psychosis *(14)*.

Constipation may be countered by increasing fluid intake, eating foods high in fiber, ingesting fiber supplements such as psyllium (Metamucil), and using stool softeners such as docusate sodium (Colace) or a mild laxative such as a combination of sennosides and docusate (e.g., one Senokot-S tablet per 15–30 mg of sustained-release morphine) *(10)*. Nausea that is constant without exacerbation by eating or movement may be treated with phenothiazines. Nausea aggravated by eating may respond best to metoclopramide (Reglan), whereas nausea precipitated by changes in position or head movement may be treated with transdermally administered scopolamine (Transderm Scop) or meclizine (Antivert) *(14)*.

Should patients receive excess opioid dosage, the medication should be withheld until the symptoms resolve and then resumed with a 25% dosage reduction. In cases of more severe opioid overdosage, aggressive treatment is mandatory.

Opioid Overdose

The combination of coma, depressed respiration, and pinpoint pupils indicates opioid toxicity until proven otherwise. Severe hypoxia may lead to dilated pupils. Treatment requires that an airway be rapidly established and that the patient be ventilated. An opioid antagonist, preferably naloxone (Narcan), should then be administered. Naloxone reverses the respiratory depression, sedation, and hypotension associated with overdose of opioids, including natural and synthetic narcotics, such as propoxyphene, methadone, and diphenoxylate (an ingredient in Lomotil), and narcotic-antagonist analgesics, such as butorphanol, nalbuphine, and pentazocine. In order to avoid precipitating narcotic withdrawal in patients physically dependent on opioids, the standard naloxone dose (0.4 mg) may be diluted in 10–50 mL of normal saline or 5% dextrose solution and administered by slow intravenous infusion. If necessary, additional doses may be given. If no response has been observed after the administration of 2 mg of naloxone, the diagnosis of opioid toxicity should be questioned. Noncardiogenic pulmonary edema may occur with opioid toxicity; treatment of this complication may include positive-pressure respiration. The duration of action of narcotic antagonists is shorter than that of many opioids. For example, the effects of methadone may last as long as 24–72 h. Consequently, patients must be monitored carefully and may require repeated doses of naloxone before the opioid has been eliminated.

Specific opioid agents, grouped according to structure, are discussed *below*.

Morphine and Other Opioid Agonists

Morphine

Morphine represents the standard against which other opioids are measured. It may be administered by the oral, rectal, subcutaneous, intramuscular, intravenous, epidural, or intrathecal route. Oral morphine sulfate is available as immediate-release (MSIR tablets, capsules, or solution; Roxanol solution) or sustained-release (MS Contin, Oramorph SR) preparations. Significant first-pass metabolism by the liver reduces bioavailability of orally administered morphine to about 25–35% of the dose given. Consequently, an equipotent oral dose may be three to four times greater than the parenteral dose. However, as considerable individual variation exists in the degree of first-pass metabolism, the dose must be individualized.

The usual adult dose of immediate-release oral morphine is 10–30 mg every 4 h as needed. For patients with chronic, severe pain (as from cancer), the drug should be administered on a regular basis every 4 h in the lowest dose that provides effective analgesia. Sustained-release oral morphine should only be used in patients who have received immediate-release morphine and require continuous opioid analgesia for more than several days. The dose of sustained-release morphine is based on the daily requirement for immediate-release morphine. The same daily dose of sustained-release morphine can then be administered using either an every 8- or every 12-h schedule. Sustained-release tablets must be swallowed whole and not crushed or chewed. Since the release of morphine from sustained-release preparations is not uniform, use of these formulations will lead to higher peak and lower trough levels than an immediate-release preparation administered every 4 h. Morphine sulfate given as a rectal suppository (RMS and MS/S suppositories) generally produces slightly stronger or equianalgesic effects to morphine administered orally. The usual starting dose is 10–30 mg per rectum every 4 h as needed; analgesic effects occur within 20–60 min.

Morphine administered subcutaneously or intramuscularly at a dose of 10 mg/70 kg of body weight relieves moderate to severe pain in most patients, although some patients require higher doses. For severe pain, morphine may be given intravenously: the initial dose is 2–10 mg/70 kg of body weight. In the postoperative period, patient-controlled analgesia (PCA) has been shown to improve pain control without increasing total analgesic dose.

Morphine may also be delivered epidurally or intrathecally for postoperative or chronic pain relief (generally in patients with cancer). Epidurally administered morphine is rapidly absorbed into the systemic circulation with kinetics similar to morphine given intravenously or intramuscularly. Maximal plasma concentration is achieved within 10–15 min following administration of morphine by any of these routes. Peak cerebrospinal fluid level occurs 60–90 min after epidural administration. Biphasic cerebrospinal fluid elimination kinetics are reported, with an early half-life of about 90 min and a late phase half-life of about 6 h. Intrathecal administration of morphine offers the advantage of bypassing the meningeal barrier (which morphine crosses poorly) and providing a long duration of analgesia. However, the epidural route is usually preferred due to a lower risk of adverse effects, including headache and infection.

Duramorph and Astramorph are preservative-free solutions of morphine sulfate available for intravenous, epidural, or intrathecal administration. Infumorph, also a preservative-free solution of morphine sulfate, is available for use in continuous microinfusion devices for epidural or intrathecal analgesia. Pharmacists and others must be aware that the concentration of morphine in Infumorph (10 or 25 mg/mL) is significantly higher than in Astramorph or Duramorph (0.5 or 1 mg/mL).

Morphine is metabolized in the liver into active (morphine-6-glucuronide) and inactive (morphine-3-glucuronide) metabolites, which are excreted by the kidneys. When morphine is given repeatedly to the elderly or in the presence of renal dysfunction, morphine-6-glucuronide may accumulate, leading to opioid toxicity. As with other opioids, hepatic or renal disease may require dose reduction.

Respiratory depression may occur up to 24 h following either epidural or intrathecal administration of morphine. Other side effects of morphine include somnolence, euphoria, dysphoria, psychosis, dizziness, nausea, vomiting, pruritus, sweating, urinary retention, and hypotension. High doses of morphine may stimulate the cardiovascular system or cause seizures. Morphine should be used with great caution, if at all, in patients with head injury, as it obscures the clinical status of these patients and may increase intracranial pressure.

Hydromorphone

Hydromorphone (Dilaudid), a morphine congener, is approx five times more potent than morphine. Oral bioavailability is low, ranging from 25 to 40% of the administered dose. Analgesia occurs within 30 min following oral administration and within 15 min after parenteral administration and persists for 4–6 h. The short half-life of hydromorphone (2–3 h) makes this drug an alternative agent for patients (including those with renal dysfunction) who derive inadequate analgesia or develop intolerable side effects from morphine *(14)*.

The usual oral dose is 2 mg every 4–6 h. Hydromorphone rectal suppositories (3 mg every 6–8 h) are also available. Parenteral hydromorphone, which may be used for subcutaneous, intramuscular, intravenous, or epidural administration, is available in lower potency preparations (1, 2, or 4 mg/mL) and a high potency (Dilaudid-HP) preparation (10 mg/mL). The usual subcutaneous or intramuscular dose is 1–2 mg every 4–6 h. If administered intravenously, hydromorphone should be infused slowly over at least 2–3 min.

Levorphanol

Levorphanol (Levo-Dromoran), a synthetic congener of morphine, is approximately five times more potent than morphine but may produce less nausea and vomiting. The d-isomer of the codeine analog of levorphanol is dextromethorphan, an antitussive without analgesic effects available in various over-the-counter preparations. The half-life of levorphanol is 12–16 h with duration of analgesia for 6–8 h. The average dose is 2 mg administered either orally or subcutaneously every 4–6 h. Caution should be exercised with repetitive dosing of this drug due to its long half-life (which is greater than the duration of analgesia) and when prescribing this agent for patients with renal failure or elderly patients, in whom the drug and its metabolites may accumulate.

Oxymorphone

Oxymorphone (Numorphan), another morphine congener, is available for parenteral or rectal administration. Administered parenterally, 1 mg of oxymorphone is approximately equianalgesic to 10 mg of morphine; administered rectally, oxymorphone is equianalgesic to morphine on a weight basis. The usual parenteral dose is 0.5–1.5 mg sc or im or 0.5 mg iv every 4–6 h as needed. Analgesic effects are usually noted within 5–10 min of parenteral administration with duration of action approx 3–6 h. The dose per rectum is 5 mg every 4–6 h as needed.

Codeine

Codeine, an alkaloid obtained from opium or prepared from morphine by methylation, is appropriate for the treatment of moderate to moderately severe pain. The analgesic effects of codeine are due to demethylation of a small proportion (about 10%) of the administered dose to morphine. In contrast, the antitussive properties of codeine appear to be related to receptors that bind codeine. Codeine administered orally in a dose of 30 mg is approximately equianalgesic to 325–500 mg of aspirin. Following absorption, codeine is metabolized by the liver, and these compounds are excreted in the urine. The plasma half-life of codeine is 2–4 h.

The usual adult dose of codeine is 15–60 mg every 4 h as needed for pain, not to exceed 360 mg/d. For children, the usual dose of codeine is 0.5 mg/kg. Doses of codeine greater than 60 mg do not significantly increase analgesia but are associated with increased side effects.

Since codeine is often administered in combination with acetaminophen or aspirin, dosing guidelines for the supplemental medication must also be followed (e.g., maximal 24-h dose of acetaminophen is 4000 mg). Acetaminophen 300 mg is available in combination with codeine 15 mg (Tylenol with codeine no. 2), codeine 30 mg (Tylenol with codeine no. 3), and codeine 60 mg (Tylenol with codeine no. 4). The analgesic effects attained with a given dose of codeine may be enhanced by increasing the dose of acetaminophen. For example, administration of two Tylenol with codeine no. 2 tablets provides twice as much acetaminophen but the same amount of codeine as one Tylenol with Codeine no. 3 tablet.

For patients unable to swallow tablets, an oral solution of acetaminophen and codeine (Tylenol with codeine elixir) containing 120 mg of acetaminophen and 12 mg of codeine/5 mL is available. The recommended dosage is 5 mL (1 teaspoon) three to four times daily for 3- to 6-yr-old children, and 10 mL (2 teaspoons) three to four times daily for 7- to 12-yr-old children. Codeine may also be administered by injection.

Overdose with codeine is characterized by respiratory depression, somnolence (which may progress to coma), skeletal muscle flaccidity, cold and clammy skin, and sometimes bradycardia and hypotension. Cardiovascular collapse and apnea may develop. Treatment is with naloxone as previously described.

Dihydrocodeine

Dihydrocodeine (in DHCplus, Synalgos-DC), a semisynthetic analgesic related to codeine, is available in combination with acetaminophen (356.4 mg) and caffeine (30 mg) for treatment of moderate to moderately severe pain. The usual adult dose is 32 mg (2 capsules) every 4 h as needed. Because of the presence of caffeine, this analgesic is more appropriate for treating acute rather than chronic pain.

Hydrocodone

Hydrocodone (in Anexsia, Lortab, Vicodin, and others), a semisynthetic analgesic with actions similar to codeine, is available for oral administration in combination with acetaminophen (2.5, 5, 7.5, or 10 mg hydrocodone with 500–750 mg acetaminophen) or aspirin (5 mg hydrocodone with 500 mg aspirin) for treatment of moderately severe pain. Oral administration of 5 mg is approximately equivalent to 40 mg codeine. The usual adult dose is 5–10 mg every 3–6 h as needed. The plasma half-life is 3–4 h.

Oxycodone

Oxycodone (Roxicodone; in Percodan, Percocet, Tylox), another semisynthetic analgesic related to codeine, is available alone (oxycodone 5 mg as Roxicodone) or in combination with aspirin (4.33 mg oxycodone with 325 mg aspirin as Percodan or 2.17 mg oxycodone with 325 mg aspirin as Percodan-Demi) or acetaminophen (5 mg oxycodone with 325 mg acetaminophen as Percocet or 5 mg oxycodone with 500 mg acetaminophen as Tylox). Oxycodone may produce less sedation and fewer hallucinatory effects than morphine *(16)*.

The usual adult oral dose is 5–10 mg every 3–6 h as needed for moderate to severe pain, although the dose must be adjusted for the individual patient on the basis of severity of pain and patient response. For control of severe, chronic pain (such as cancer pain), oxycodone should be administered every 4 h in the lowest dosage that provides adequate analgesia. When using combination drugs, the usual precautions apply concerning dosing of aspirin and acetaminophen.

Meperidine

Meperidine (Demerol), a phenylpiperidine, exerts pharmacologic effects similar to morphine in equianalgesic dosage, although meperidine appears less likely to cause constipation, urinary retention, or elevation in biliary tract pressure than morphine. Unlike morphine and its congeners, it is not used to treat cough or diarrhea. Meperidine in a dose of 60–80 mg administered parenterally is approximately equivalent in analgesic efficacy to 10 mg of morphine. Meperidine is considerably less effective orally than parenterally due to low (about 50%) oral bioavailability.

The usual dose in adults is 50–150 mg orally, subcutaneously, or intramuscularly every 3–4 h as necessary for moderate to severe pain. Maximal analgesic effects are noted approx 2 h after oral administration and 1 h following parenteral administration. The rate of absorption after intramuscular injection is unpredictable. Local tissue irritation and induration may develop following subcutaneous or intramuscular injection.

Meperidine is metabolized primarily in the liver, where it is converted to meperidinic acid and the active metabolite normeperidine. Although the plasma half-life of meperidine is only 3 h, that of normeperidine varies from about 12 to 16 h. The half-lives of meperidine and normeperidine are prolonged in patients with hepatic disease, and that of normeperidine is also prolonged in patients with renal disease.

Repeated dosing of meperidine may lead to accumulation of normeperidine, which can produce CNS excitability manifested by mydriasis, mood changes, hallucinations, tremor, multifocal myoclonus, encephalopathy, or seizures. The development of myoclonus may necessitate treatment with clonazepam (Klonopin) and a change of opioid. Naloxone may not reverse the CNS effects from normeperidine, although it is indicated to treat respiratory depression from meperidine overdosage. However, administration of naloxone may reverse the suppressant effects of meperidine on the CNS, thereby unmasking the convulsant activity of normeperidine and inducing status epilepticus *(14)*. Meperidine should not be administered to patients receiving MAO inhibitors *(16)*.

Due to the short duration of action and potential side effects from normeperidine, meperidine is not recommended for long-term treatment of cancer pain or other chronic pain requiring repetitive dosing *(14)*.

Congeners of meperidine include diphenoxylate (available only in combination with atropine to prevent abuse as Lomotil and others) and loperamide (Imodium), both of which are used to treat diarrhea.

Fentanyl

Fentanyl, a synthetic congener of meperidine, is available for transdermal (Duragesic), oral transmucosal (Oralet), and intramuscular, intravenous, epidural, or intrathecal (fentanyl citrate as Sublimaze) administration. The fentanyl lollipop may be used for premedication prior to surgery in children; its role as an analgesic agent is not established. Fentanyl citrate is used for anesthesia and postoperative pain and would generally be administered by an anesthesiologist. A dose of 100 µg of fentanyl citrate is approximately equivalent in analgesic activity to 10 mg of morphine or 75 mg of meperidine. Side effects of fentanyl include respiratory depression, which may persist longer than the analgesic effects; fentanyl citrate may also cause muscle rigidity, particularly involving the muscles of respiration.

The Duragesic transdermal system is indicated for the treatment of chronic pain (such as cancer pain) that requires continuous opioid therapy by virtue of inadequate control with nonopioid or intermittently administered opioid analgesics. Fentanyl may be useful in patients with histamine-like reactions to other opioids *(10)*. Duragesic is available as patches that deliver approx 25, 50, 75, or 100 µg/h. Doses higher than 25 µg/h should only be used for patients who are already receiving and are tolerant to opioids.

The Duragesic patch delivers the drug continuously for 72 h, at which time it should be removed and replaced with a new patch at a different site if continued analgesia is required. Analgesic serum levels are achieved in 8–16 h and a steady state is reached in 24 h. Patients should be cautioned to avoid application of heat to the transdermal patch, as this may enhance release of fentanyl. In addition, during transdermal administration of fentanyl, a drug reservoir develops in the cutaneous tissue, which leads to continued drug activity for 17 h or more after the patch is removed. Since this may cause sedation and life-threatening hypoventilation, transdermal fentanyl is contraindicated in the management of acute or postoperative pain.

Methadone

Methadone (Dolophine) is a synthetic opioid appropriate for treatment of severe pain and detoxification or temporary maintenance in patients addicted to heroin or other morphine-like drugs. It has a longer half-life (15–40 h) than any other currently available opioid, which may predispose to delayed toxicity as steady state is approached following initiation of therapy or dosage increase. Analgesic effects occur within 30–60 min (maximal within 4 h) after oral administration and 10–20 min (maximal within 2 h) following subcutaneous or intramuscular injection. Intravenous, epidural, and intrathecal routes of administration are also available. Methadone administered orally is about one-half as potent as when given parenterally. Despite the prolonged duration of many of its side effects, the duration of analgesic activity is variable. Initiation of methadone on an as-needed basis may be prudent to determine the duration of analgesia in an individual patient and reduce the risk of drug accumulation.

The usual adult dose for severe acute pain is 2.5–10 mg orally every 3–6 h as needed. For patient-controlled analgesia, a typical loading dose is 2.5–10 mg administered intravenously over 15–30 min, followed by an initial demand dose of 1 mg. Due to the long half-life of methadone, which is considerably longer than its analgesic effects, caution must be used with repeated dosing, especially in patients with renal failure and the elderly. However, evidence that methadone and its metabolites may be excreted in the feces suggests that drug accumulation in patients with renal dysfunction may be limited (14).

When converting to methadone from another strong opioid in an opioid-tolerant patient, crosstolerance is often incomplete. The methadone dose should be decreased by 50–60% from the calculated equianalgesic dose and then titrated to achieve analgesia. MSIR or hydromorphone may be used if needed for "rescue" analgesia.

Use of methadone for treating narcotic addiction is restricted to the oral form dispensed through hospital or community pharmacies and maintenance programs approved by the FDA and state authorities. When used only to prevent narcotic withdrawal, methadone may be dispensed as infrequently as every 72 h. The methadone abstinence syndrome differs from morphine withdrawal in that the onset is slower and the symptoms are less severe.

Patients addicted to heroin or receiving maintenance doses of methadone may experience withdrawal symptoms when given pentazocine (Talwin) or other opioid agonist-antagonist drugs. Rifampin and phenytoin (Dilantin) may increase the metabolism of methadone and lead to withdrawal symptoms.

Propoxyphene

Propoxyphene (Darvon-N; in Darvocet-N) is an oral analgesic structurally related to methadone. It binds primarily to μ-opioid receptors and produces analgesia and other effects similar to those of morphine. With potency from two-thirds to equal that of codeine, propoxyphene is used for the treatment of moderate pain. It is usually prescribed as propoxyphene napsylate (Darvon-N 100, 100 mg) or propoxyphene napsylate with acetaminophen (Darvocet-N 50 or Darvocet-N 100 containing 50 mg propoxyphene napsylate and 325 mg acetaminophen, or 100 mg propoxyphene and 650 mg acetaminophen, respectively). Propoxyphene hydrochloride (Darvon, 65 mg) and propoxyphene hydrochloride with aspirin and caffeine (Darvon Compound-65 containing 65 mg propoxyphene, 389 mg aspirin, and 32.4 mg caffeine) are also available. An advantage of propoxyphene napsylate is greater stability compared to propoxyphene hydrochloride.

The usual dose of propoxyphene napsylate is 50–100 mg every 4 h as needed for pain; the total daily dose should not exceed 600 mg. The recommended dose of propoxyphene hydrochloride is 65 mg every 4 h as needed with a maximal daily dose of 390 mg. As noted previously, the total daily dose of acetaminophen should not exceed 4000 mg due to potential hepatotoxicity.

Propoxyphene is metabolized in the liver to norpropoxyphene, which has a much longer half-life (30–36 h) than propoxyphene (6–12 h). Norpropoxyphene is believed to cause or contribute to some of the toxic effects that may follow administration of propoxyphene, including respiratory and CNS depression. Hallucinations, seizures, pulmonary edema, and cardiotoxicity, including arrhythmias and conduction disturbances, have been described with high doses. Naloxone antagonizes the respiratory and CNS depression. Depression of the respiratory or CNS is aggravated by the concurrent use of alcohol or other sedating medications. Severe neurologic disease, including coma, has occurred with concurrent use of carbamazepine (Tegretol). Propoxyphene should be administered with caution to patients with hepatic or renal disease, including the elderly, since excretion of the drug and its metabolites may be impaired.

Tramadol

Tramadol (Ultram), a synthetic analgesic with a dual mechanism of action, binds to μ-opioid receptors and inhibits reuptake of norepinephrine and serotonin. Tramadol is converted in the liver by the cytochrome P-450 system to the active M1 metabolite and excreted as unaltered drug and metabolites in the urine. The opioid activity of this drug results from low-affinity binding of the parent compound and high-affinity binding of the M1 metabolite to μ-opioid receptors.

Tramadol administered in a single dose of 50 mg is about equianalgesic to 60 mg codeine for treatment of postoperative pain, although at considerably greater cost *(17)*. Analgesia develops within 1 h following administration and peaks in 2–3 h, corresponding to the maximal plasma concentration. The half-life of tramadol and the M1 metabolite is 6–7 h but may be prolonged in patients with hepatic or renal dysfunction.

The usual dose is 50–100 mg every 4–6 h as needed for moderate to moderately severe pain, not to exceed 400 mg per day. For patients over age 75, the maximum recommended daily dose is 300 mg. If creatinine clearance is less than 30 mL/min, the dose should be reduced to 50–100 mg every 12 h. Metabolism of tramadol is decreased in patients with severe hepatic disease, leading to higher levels of tramadol and decreased levels of the M1 metabolite. Likewise, concurrent administration of quinidine, which blocks the P-450 isoenzyme that converts tramadol to M1, increases serum tramadol levels and reduces serum M1 levels.

Tramadol can produce drug dependence by binding to the μ-opioid receptor, analogous to codeine and other opioids. Although tramadol produces less respiratory depression than morphine, caution should be exercised when administering this drug to patients with pulmonary disease. Other potential side effects include dizziness, nausea, constipation, headache, and somnolence. Seizures have been reported with excessive doses and with coadministration of antidepressants. Naloxone only partially antagonizes tramadol-induced analgesia and other effects.

Opioids with Partial Agonist Effects

Buprenorphine

Buprenorphine (Buprenex), a semisynthetic derivative of thebaine, exhibits partial agonist activity at μ-opioid receptors in the CNS. It is available for intramuscular or intravenous administration for the relief of moderate to severe pain. In analgesic and respiratory depressant effects, 0.4 mg buprenorphine is approximately equivalent to 10 mg morphine.

Analgesia occurs as early as 15 min following intramuscular injection and may persist for 6 h or longer. Maximal effects are observed at about 1 h. When given intravenously, these times are shorter. Plasma half-life averages about 2 h but ranges up to approx 7 h.

The usual dosage for patients 13 yr of age and older is 0.3 mg (1 mL Buprenex), given by intramuscular or slow (over at least 2 min) intravenous injection. This dose may be repeated once, if necessary, 30–60 min after the initial dose and subsequently only as needed at intervals up to 6–8 h. The dose of buprenorphine should be reduced by approximately one-half in the elderly and in patients with respiratory, hepatic, or renal disease.

Side effects are similar to other opioids and include sedation, nausea, vomiting, sweating, headache, dizziness, respiratory depression, and hypotension. Respiratory and cardiovascular collapse have been described in patients who received therapeutic doses of diazepam (Valium) with buprenorphine.

Like other partial agonists, buprenorphine possesses limited activity at μ-opioid receptors, despite strong binding to these sites which may displace more active opioids. This narcotic antagonist activity may cause withdrawal symptoms in persons physically dependent on opioids. The strong binding to μ-receptors also results in a slow rate of dissociation of buprenorphine from these receptors, which is hypothesized to explain its long duration of action and the unpredictable reversal of its effects by opioid antagonists such as naloxone.

For drug overdose, oxygen, intravenous fluids, vasopressors, and other supportive measures should be utilized as appropriate. Although naloxone should be administered, it may not be effective in reversing respiratory depression and other effects of buprenorphine. Doxapram (Dopram), a respiratory stimulant, may be used. Adequate ventilation, using mechanical means if necessary, is essential.

Opioids with Mixed Agonist–Antagonist Effects

Pentazocine

Pentazocine (Talwin) is a synthetic opioid with analgesic properties related to κ-opioid receptor stimulation. This drug also possesses weak antagonist activity at the μ-opioid receptor, deliberately produced in an effort to decrease its potential for drug abuse. Patients receiving opioids, including methadone for treatment of drug addiction, may experience withdrawal symptoms after receiving pentazocine. Pentazocine is the only mixed agonist–antagonist available for oral use.

Pentazocine is available in several forms: (1) 12.5 mg base pentazocine hydrochloride in combination with 325 mg aspirin (Talwin Compound); (2) 25 mg pentazocine hydrochloride base in combination with 650 mg acetaminophen (Talacen); (3) 50 mg pentazocine hydrochloride base in combination with naloxone 0.5 mg hydrochloride base

(Talwin NX), all for oral administration; and (4) pentazocine lactate (Talwin) for subcutaneous, intramuscular, or intravenous injection. Naloxone is added to Talwin NX to reduce the potential for drug abuse. Administered orally, 0.5 mg naloxone is rapidly inactivated by the liver and has no pharmacologic activity, but administered parenterally, naloxone is an effective antagonist to pentazocine and other opioids and may precipitate narcotic withdrawal symptoms.

Pentazocine is indicated for the treatment of moderate to severe pain. Given orally, it is about equianalgesic to codeine on a weight basis. Administered parenterally, 30 mg pentazocine is approximately equivalent to 10 mg morphine. Pentazocine is absorbed well from the gastrointestinal tract and from subcutaneous and intramuscular sites. Due to extensive first-pass metabolism in the liver, the bioavailability of orally administered pentazocine is only about 20%. Pentazocine is metabolized in the liver and excreted primarily by the kidneys. Consequently, as with other opioids, caution should be exercised in administering this agent to patients with hepatic or renal disease.

The usual initial adult dose of Talwin NX is 1 tablet every 3–4 h. This may be increased to 2 tablets every 3–4 h if needed, but the total daily dosage should not exceed 12 tablets. For Talwin compound, the recommended dose is also 1–2 tablets every 3–4 h as needed, not to exceed 12 tablets per day, whereas for Talacen the recommended dose is 1 tablet every 4 hours as needed, not to exceed 6 tablets per day. Onset of analgesia usually occurs within 15–30 min after oral administration (maximal at 1–3 h). Plasma half-life is 2–3 h, and duration of action is usually 3 h or longer.

The recommended parenteral dose is 30 mg by subcutaneous, intramuscular, or intravenous route. This may be repeated every 3–4 h. The sc or im dose may be increased to 60 mg if needed; total daily dose should not exceed 360 mg. Analgesia usually occurs within 15–20 min after intramuscular or subcutaneous injection (maximal at 15–60 min) and within 2–3 min after intravenous injection.

Side effects of pentazocine include sedation, dizziness, nausea, vomiting, and euphoria. Some patients receiving therapeutic doses of pentazocine have developed transient hallucinations (usually visual), disorientation, and confusion.

In contrast to morphine and most μ-opioid receptor agonists, intravenous administration of pentazocine increases systemic vascular resistance and systemic and pulmonary arterial pressure in patients with acute myocardial infarction. Pentazocine produces less elevation of biliary tract pressure than morphine. Following repeated injections of pentazocine lactate, some patients develop fibrosis of the skin, subcutaneous tissue, and muscle at the administration sites, producing a "woody" consistency in the tissues.

Butorphanol

Butorphanol (Stadol) is a synthetic analgesic available for parenteral or nasal administration. Butorphanol and its major metabolites are agonists at κ-opioid receptors and mixed agonist–antagonists at μ-opioid receptors. Indications for this medication include severe (especially acute) pain, preoperative sedation, and balanced anesthesia. Butorphanol is not recommended for use in patients dependent on narcotics due to its opioid antagonist effects; these patients should have a period of opioid withdrawal prior to starting butorphanol.

Butorphanol in a dose of 2–3 mg administered parenterally produces analgesia and respiratory depression similar to 10 mg of morphine. As with pentazocine and other drugs with activity directed primarily toward κ-opioid receptors, the degree of respiratory depression with butorphanol is not proportionately increased with higher doses. Nasal butorphanol (Stadol NS) in doses of 1 and 2 mg produces a similar level of analgesia as morphine in doses of 5 and 10 mg, respectively.

Onset of analgesia occurs within several minutes following intravenous administration of butorphanol, within 10–15 min following intramuscular injection, and within 15 min following intranasal spray. Maximal analgesia occurs 30–60 min after intravenous or intramuscular administration and within 1 h of nasal administration. The plasma half-life of butorphanol is about 3 h, and its analgesic effects after intravenous or intramuscular injection usually persist 3–4 h. Butorphanol nasal spray produces analgesia lasting 4–5 h and has been used for patients with headaches refractory to nonparenteral analgesics. The bioavailability of butorphanol nasal spray is 60–70%. Although this is not changed in patients with allergic rhinitis, the use of a nasal vasoconstrictor (oxymetazoline) slows the rate of absorption, resulting in a maximal plasma concentration about half that achieved without a vasoconstrictor.

The usual initial dose of injectable butorphanol is 1 mg every 3–4 h iv or 2 mg every 3–4 h im. In patients with hepatic or renal disease and in the elderly, the initial dose should generally be 0.5 mg iv or 1 mg im with the interval between doses up to 6 h or longer.

The recommended starting dose of butorphanol nasal spray is 1 mg (a single spray in one nostril). If adequate analgesia is not achieved within 60–90 min, an additional 1 mg spray may be administered in the opposite nostril. Alternatively, if the pain is quite severe and the patient will be able to remain recumbent in case drowsiness or dizziness occur, an initial dose of 2 mg (one spray in each nostril) may be administered. This regimen may be repeated every 3–4 h if needed. In elderly patients or patients with hepatic or renal disease, the initial dose should be 1 mg, followed by 1 mg in 90–120 min with subsequent doses administered at intervals of 6 h or more.

Each bottle of Stadol NS contains 2.5 mL of a 10-mg/mL solution of butorphanol tartrate. The bottle must be primed before use. Thereafter, each metered spray will deliver an average of 1.0 mg of butorphanol tartrate, and each bottle will provide an average of 14–15 doses. If not used for 48 h or longer, the bottle must be reprimed, which will decrease the total number of doses available.

Side effects of butorphanol include sedation, dizziness, sweating, nausea, and vomiting. Nasal butorphanol is associated with nasal congestion and insomnia. Butorphanol, like other mixed agonist–antagonist drugs with a high affinity for the κ-opioid receptor, may produce disturbing psychotomimetic effects in some individuals.

Dezocine

Dezocine (Dalgan) is a synthetic opioid agonist–antagonist available for parenteral administration. It possesses opioid agonist activity similar to morphine with greater opioid antagonist activity than pentazocine. Peak plasma concentrations occur between 10 and 90 min following a single injection. Plasma half-life ranges from about 1 to 7 (average 2.4) h.

The recommended intramuscular dose is 5–20 mg, adjusted according to factors such as the severity of pain and age. This dose may be repeated every 3–6 h as necessary, up to a probable upper limit of 120 mg/d. For intravenous administration, the usual dose is 2.5–10 mg every 2–4 h as needed. Dezocine is not recommended for subcutaneous administration due to the risk of subcutaneous inflammation and venous thrombosis following repeated injections. Dezocine is available in concentrations of 5, 10, and 15 mg/mL.

As with other agonist–antagonist opioids, this agent may induce withdrawal symptoms in patients physically dependent on narcotics. Dezocine and morphine produce a similar degree of respiratory depression, which is reversible with naloxone. Other side effects of dezocine include nausea, vomiting, sedation, dizziness, and injection-site reactions.

Nalbuphine

Nalbuphine (Nubain), chemically related to both oxymorphone and naloxone, is another synthetic drug with opioid agonist and antagonist activities. Nalbuphine is equianalgesic to morphine on a weight basis, but its analgesic effects are related to binding at κ-opioid receptors. Nalbuphine is a more potent antagonist at μ-receptors than pentazocine.

Onset of analgesia occurs within 15 min following subcutaneous or intramuscular administration and within 2–3 min following intravenous injection. The plasma half-life of nalbuphine is 5 h, with analgesic activity lasting 3–6 h. Since nalbuphine is metabolized by the liver and excreted by the kidneys, caution must be exercised in the administration of this agent to patients with impaired renal or hepatic function.

The usual adult dose is 10 mg/70 kg of body wt administered parenterally every 3–6 h for treatment of moderate to severe pain; the dose may be increased to 20 mg if necessary. Nalbuphine is available in concentrations of 10 and 20 mg/mL.

Side effects include sedation, sweating, nausea, vomiting, dizziness, dry mouth, and headache. CNS and cardiovascular effects occur less frequently. Nalbuphine causes respiratory depression approximately equal to morphine. However, in contrast to morphine, respiratory depression is not significantly greater with doses higher than the usual therapeutic dose. Nalbuphine may precipitate drug withdrawal in patients receiving morphine or other opioids.

Tolerance, Physical Dependence, and Addiction

Tolerance and physical dependence are normal physiological adaptations to repeated use of drugs from many categories. Tolerance, the most common response to repetitive use of a drug, may be defined as the reduction in response to a drug after repeated administration (Table 12). Thus, a higher dose is required to produce the same effect that was previously obtained at a lower dose. Tolerance develops at different rates to the analgesic, respiratory depressant, and emetic effects of opioids and slowly, if at all, to constipation (16).

Crosstolerance refers to the fact that repeated use of drugs in a given category confers tolerance not only to the drug being used but also to other drugs in the same category. However, crosstolerance is incomplete, since tolerance develops independently at each receptor subtype (16).

Table 12
Definitions of Physiological and Psychological Responses to Opioids

Tolerance	Reduction in response to opioid after repeated dosing
Physical dependence	Pharmacologic property of opioid drugs characterized by abstinence syndrome on abruptly stopping drug or administering antagonist drug
Addiction (psychological dependence)	Behavioral pattern characterized by compulsive securing and use of drug

Physical dependence refers to the physiologic state that develops as a result of the adaptation produced by resetting homeostatic mechanisms in response to repeated drug use. A person in this adapted or physically dependent state requires continued administration of the drug to maintain normal function. Physical dependence is an expected result of long-term administration of opioids and does not imply addiction or psychological dependence.

The appearance of a withdrawal syndrome when a drug is discontinued or an opioid antagonist is administered provides the only evidence of physical dependence. Withdrawal symptoms are characteristic of a given category of drugs, and they tend to be opposite to the original effects produced by the drug *(18)*. The development of physical dependence is not a cause for concern as long as opioid antagonists (including partial agonist and mixed agonist–antagonist opioids) are avoided and the drug is tapered rather than abruptly discontinued when dosage reduction is indicated *(19)*.

In contrast to tolerance and physical dependence, addiction or psychological dependence is not a pharmacologic property of opioids. Addiction is a psychological and behavioral state characterized by drug craving, use of the drug for other than analgesic purposes, overwhelming involvement in obtaining and using the drug, continued use despite harm, and a high probability of relapse to drug use following withdrawal *(14)*.

Addiction appears to be rare in patients using opioids for treatment of pain, in contrast to persons engaged in illicit use of these agents *(10)*. Data in patients with cancer as well as nonmalignant pain suggest that most patients with stable chronic pain syndromes do not require increasing opioid doses to maintain adequate analgesia. Rather, the need for increased opioid doses may indicate progression of the underlying process. The Boston Collaborative Drug Surveillance project studied almost 12,000 patients who received an opioid agent for acute pain; only four cases of substantiated psychological dependence were identified in patients without a prior history of drug abuse *(20)*. This may reflect the fact that addiction is a function not only of the substance but also the substrate: addicts often demonstrate aberrant psychological behavior and may also have a genetic predisposition toward addiction. The potential risk of developing addiction does not justify withholding opioid therapy in patients with no history of substance abuse.

Patients with pain are sometimes deprived of adequate opioid medication because they show evidence of tolerance and exhibit withdrawal symptoms if the analgesic medication is abruptly stopped. Appropriate management requires that the dose of opioid be increased to the level necessary to provide adequate analgesia. Adjuvant analgesics, local anesthetics, and nonpharmacologic therapy provide additional therapeutic options in patients tolerant to opioids. Failure to differentiate physical from psychological dependence represents a major obstacle to optimal pain management.

Legal Considerations in Prescribing Opioids

Although one reason for undertreatment of patients with intractable pain may be confusion between normal biological effects of opioids and addiction, another is that some physicians fear legal sanctions if they are perceived as prescribing excessive opioids. Undercover agents impersonating patients seeking opioids do not diminish this concern. In California, the legislature has established public policy as supportive of the responsible practice of pain management. The Business and Professional Code (Section 2241.5) indicates that no physician shall be subject to disciplinary action by the Medical Board of California (MBC) for "prescribing or administering controlled substances in the course of treatment of a person for intractable pain *(21)*." "Intractable pain," as defined in this code, represents a pain state in which "the cause of the pain cannot be removed or otherwise treated and which, in the generally accepted course of medical practice, no relief or cure of the cause of the pain is possible or none has been found after reasonable efforts," including, but not limited to, evaluation by the attending physician and one or more physicians "specializing in the treatment of the area, system, or organ of the body perceived as the source of the pain *(21)*." The MBC has established guidelines to help physicians treat intractable pain within the boundaries of state and federal law (Table 13) *(22)*. Physicians in other states should acquaint themselves with applicable laws that may provide similar guidance and protection. Adherence to these laws should allay unnecessary concerns as physicians prescribe analgesics in appropriate doses for their patients (*see also* Chapter 15).

ADJUVANT ANALGESICS

Adjuvant analgesics may be defined as agents that alleviate pain, even though their primary use is for another indication. These medications include antidepressants, anticonvulsants, muscle relaxants, adrenergic agonists, sympatholytics, and neuroleptics (Table 14).

Antidepressants

Antidepressants are frequently used to treat chronic pain, especially neuropathic pain. Pain relief is often achieved at doses that are subtherapeutic for the treatment of depression. The analgesic effects of these agents may result from their ability to block reuptake at presynaptic nerve endings of neurotransmitters, such as serotonin and norepinephrine, which are involved in pain and depression. Some agents, including amitriptyline, have been reported to potentiate the effects of morphine.

Tricyclic antidepressants represent the antidepressant drugs used most commonly as adjuvant analgesics. Amitriptyline (Elavil) may be used to treat postherpetic neuralgia, diabetic neuropathy, arthritis, low back pain, myofascial pain, cancer pain, migraine and tension-type headaches, central pain, and psychogenic pain *(23)*. Nortriptyline (Pamelor), desipramine (Norpramin), doxepin (Sinequan), imipramine (Tofranil), clomipramine (Anafranil), maprotiline (Ludiomil), and trazodone (Desyrel) are among

Table 13
Requirements for Treating Intractable Pain in California[a]

1. History and physical examination	A thorough medical history and physical examination must be accomplished. Prescribing controlled substances for intractable pain in California also requires evaluation by one or more specialists.
2. Treatment plan, objectives	The treatment plan should state objectives by which treatment success can be evaluated, such as pain relief and/or improved physical and psychosocial function, and indicate if any further diagnostic evaluations or other treatments are planned. Several treatment modalities or a rehabilitation program may be necessary.
3. Informed consent	The physician should discuss the risks and benefits of the use of controlled substances with the patient or guardian.
4. Periodic review	The physician should periodically review the course of opioid treatment of the patient and any new information about the etiology of the pain. Continuation or modification of opioid therapy depends on the physician's evaluation of progress toward treatment objectives.
5. Consultation	The physician should be willing to refer the patient as necessary for additional evaluation and treatment to achieve treatment objectives. Physicians should give special attention to those pain patients who are at risk for misusing their medications. The management of pain in patients with a history of substance abuse requires extra care, monitoring, documentation and consultation with addiction specialists, and may entail the use of agreements between the provider and the patient to specify rules for medication use.
6. Records	The physician should keep accurate and complete records.
7. Compliance with controlled substance laws and regulations	To prescribe substances, the physician must be appropriately licensed in California and comply with federal and state regulations for issuing controlled substances prescriptions. *Important:* Documented adherence to these guidelines will substantially establish the physician's responsible treatment of patients with intractable pain and will serve to defend that treatment practice in the face of complaints that may be brought.

[a]From ref. 22.

Table 14
Adjuvant Analgesics and Anesthetics

Class	Drugs
Antidepressants	Amitriptyline
	Clomipramine
	Desipramine
	Doxepin
	Imipramine
	Maprotiline
	Nortriptyline
	Paroxetine
	Trazodone
Anticonvulsants	Carbamazepine
	Clonazepam
	Gabapentin
	Phenytoin
	Valproate
Muscle relaxants	Baclofen
	Carisoprodol
	Cyclobenzaprine
	Methocarbamol
Topical agents	Capsaicin
	EMLA
	Lidocaine gel
Oral local anesthetics	Mexiletine
Intravenous local anesthetics	Lidocaine
Adrenergic agonists	Clonidine
Sympatholytics	Phenoxybenzamine
	Prazosin
	Propranolol
Neuroleptics	Fluphenazine
	Haloperidol
	Methotrimeprazine
	Pimozide

the other antidepressants that have been used as adjuvant analgesics. Antidepressants for which studies have demonstrated benefit in specific painful conditions are indicated in Table 15, and analgesic doses of antidepressants are listed in Table 16 *(24)*.

Amitriptyline (Elavil), often chosen as the initial agent, should be started in a dose of 10–25 mg at night. Morning sedation, a common side effect, may be decreased by administering the medication 2–3 h before bedtime. Tolerance to sedation often develops within several weeks. For those few patients unable to tolerate this beginning dose, the tablets may be divided. The dose may be increased every 5–7 d until improvement

Table 15
**Antidepressants Demonstrated
to Provide Analgesia in Controlled Trials[a,b]**

Medication	Analgesic Indication
Amitriptyline (Elavil)	Migraine and other headaches
	Postherpetic neuralgia
	Diabetic neuropathy
	Arthritis
	Low back pain
	Fibromyalgia
	Central pain
	Psychogenic pain
Clomipramine (Anafranil)	Neuropathic pain
	Idiopathic pain
Desipramine (Norpramin)	Postherpetic neuralgia
Doxepin (Sinequan)	Coexistent pain and depression
	Headache
	Low back pain
Imipramine (Tofranil)	Headache
	Diabetic neuropathy
	Low back pain
	Arthritis
Maprotiline (Ludiomil)	Postherpetic neuralgia
	Idiopathic pain
Nortriptyline (Pamelor)	Diabetic neuropathy
Paroxetine (Paxil)	Diabetic neuropathy

[a]Use of antidepressants for conditions other than those indicated may be appropriate; see text.
[b]From ref. 24.

is noted or significant side effects develop. One study noted that, while amitriptyline in doses of 25 and 50 mg was effective in reducing pain, doses of 75 mg provided greater analgesia, even in the absence of mood improvement. However, the 75-mg dose was associated with a greater incidence of adverse effects, primarily dryness of the mouth and drowsiness (25). Some patients may need even higher doses if analgesia is inadequate and the side effects are tolerable.

For patients who experience problems with these side effects, nortriptyline (Pamelor), the active metabolite of amitriptyline, may be administered. Nortriptyline is the tricyclic antidepressant least likely to cause orthostatic hypotension and should be considered in patients prone to falling. Desipramine (Norpramin) represents another antidepressant that causes less orthostatic hypotension and less sedation than amitriptyline. In fact, increased presynaptic levels of norepinephrine may cause stimulatory effects, making desipramine more appropriate for morning administration. As with most tricyclic antidepressants, the starting analgesic dose for these medications is 10 or 25 mg. If this dose

Table 16
Analgesic Doses of Antidepressants

Generic Name	Brand Name	Dosage Strengths	Starting Dose	Usual Dose
Amitriptyline	Elavil	10, 25, 50, 75, 100, 150 mg	10–25 mg qd[a]	25–150 mg qd
Desipramine	Norpramin	10, 25, 50, 75, 100, 150 mg	10–25 mg qd	25–150 mg qd
Doxepin	Sinequan	10, 25, 50, 75, 100, 150 mg	10–25 mg qd	25–150 mg qd
Imipramine	Tofranil	10, 25, 50 mg	10–25 mg qd	25–150 mg qd
Nortriptyline	Pamelor	10, 25, 50, 75 mg	10–25 mg qd	25–100 mg qd
Trazodone	Desyrel	50, 100, 150, 300 mg	50–100 mg qd	100–300 mg qd

[a]qd, once daily.

causes intolerable side effects, a liquid preparation of nortriptyline (Pamelor solution, 2 mg/mL) may be prescribed, allowing titration to minuscule doses.

Although newer agents such as selective serotonin reuptake inhibitors (SSRIs) are associated with fewer adverse effects, they appear to be less effective in relieving pain in the absence of depression. However, paroxetine (Paxil) has been reported to be effective in the treatment of diabetic neuropathy and represents an agent that may be prescribed for patients unable to tolerate any tricyclic antidepressant.

In general, an effective dose of antidepressant medication must be administered for a period of 1–3 wk to achieve analgesic effects. If required for pain control, full-dose antidepressant therapy should be administered for 1–2 mo to assess the efficacy of these agents. In an individual patient, therapy with one agent may be more effective than another. Thus, sequential trials using various tricyclic antidepressant drugs may be necessary.

Patients experiencing pain often develop depression. The use of these medications in antidepressant doses should be considered in patients with symptoms of depression, which may include dysphoria, lethargy, agitation, and insomnia *(23)*. Selective serotonin reuptake inhibitors (SSRIs) have generally replaced tricyclic antidepressants for the treatment of depression. However, SSRIs may not be optimal agents for patients with pain, for whom tricyclic antidepressant agents may be more effective as analgesic adjuvants. In addition, SSRIs may worsen symptoms such as nausea, agitation, insomnia, headache, and anorexia. On the other hand, some patients may not tolerate sedation associated with daytime use of tricyclic antidepressants; these patients may benefit from bedtime dosing with a tricyclic antidepressant and daytime administration of a selective serotonin reuptake inhibitor. However, caution is required since SSRIs such as fluoxetine (Prozac), paroxetine (Paxil), and sertraline (Zoloft) can significantly increase tricyclic antidepressant serum levels.

Tricyclic antidepressants are metabolized in the liver by the cytochrome P-450 isoenzyme system and excreted by the kidneys. Some of these metabolites possess pharmacologic activity, thereby increasing the duration of action of the compound. Examples

Table 17
Comparison of Antidepressant Side Effects

Drug	Sedative Effect	Anticholinergic Effect	Orthostatic Hypotension	Cardiac Toxicity	Seizures
Amitriptyline	+++	+++	+++	+++	++
Desipramine	+	+	+	++	+
Doxepin	+++	++	+++	++	++
Imipramine	++	++	++	+++	++
Nortriptyline	+	+	+	++	+
Trazodone	+++	0	++	+	0

Table 18
Selected Adverse Reactions to Tricyclic Antidepressants

System	Reaction
Anticholinergic	Dry mouth, blurred vision, glaucoma, sinus tachycardia, urinary retention, constipation, paralytic ileus, hyperpyrexia, memory dysfunction
Cardiovascular	Hypotension, hypertension, arrhythmias, conduction abnormalities, myocardial infarction
Endocrine	Impotence, altered libido, gynecomastia, testicular swelling, altered glucose levels, hyponatremia from inappropriate ADH secretion (SIADH)
Gastrointestinal	Altered taste, anorexia, black tongue, parotid gland swelling, nausea, vomiting, dyspepsia, abdominal cramping, hepatitis
Hematologic	Thrombocytopenia, leukopenia, agranulocytosis
Neurologic	Numbness, paresthesias, neuropathy, tremor, extrapyramidal symptoms, ataxia, headache, nightmares, hallucinations, seizures, stroke
Other	Weight gain or loss, sweating, alopecia

are nortriptyline from amitriptyline, nordoxepin from doxepin, and desipramine from imipramine.

Tricyclic antidepressants cause various side effects related to their blocking histaminic, muscarinic, and adrenergic receptors (Tables 17 and 18). These symptoms include dry mouth, blurred vision, tachycardia, urinary retention, constipation, and orthostatic hypotension. Precipitation of acute angle-closure glaucoma may occur due to anticholinergic activity. Ophthalmologic evaluation should be obtained in patients with glaucoma. Agents with little anticholinergic effect, such as desipramine or nortriptyline, should be considered in patients with prostatic hypertrophy. Because antidepressant medications may impair mental function, patients should be cautioned regarding driving or using potentially hazardous equipment when taking these drugs. These drugs may also decrease seizure threshold. Cardiac toxicity may include conduction disturbances and arrhythmias; these effects are most pronounced with high doses of amitriptyline and

Table 19
Selected Drug Interactions with Antidepressants

Medication	Interaction	Recommendation
MAO Inhibitors	May cause hyperpyretic crisis, seizures, death	Avoid concurrent use
Quinidine	May increase serum levels of tricyclic antidepressants	Avoid concurrent use
Cimetidine (Tagamet)	May increase serum levels of tricyclic antidepressants	Use another H_2-antagonist or lower dose of tricyclic antidepressant
Alcohol and sedatives	May potentiate sedation	Avoid or decrease dose
Warfarin (Coumadin)	May potentiate anticoagulant effects	Monitor carefully and adjust warfarin dose to maintain desired INR
Sulfonylureas	May increase action of sulfonylureas	Monitor glucose carefully
Phenytoin (Dilantin)	May increase toxicity of phenytoin; phenytoin decreases serum level of desipramine	Monitor phenytoin and desipramine levels
Carbamazepine (Tegretol)	May increase serum levels of both carbamazepine and tricyclic antidepressants	Use cautiously, monitor carbamazepine and antidepressant levels
Disulfiram (Antabuse)	May cause delirium	Avoid concurrent use
Selective serotonin reuptake inhibitors	May increase serum levels of tricyclic antidepressants	Monitor clinical status and antidepressant level

imipramine but may occur with other tricyclic antidepressants and trazodone. Baseline electrocardiogram should be obtained in older patients, and the EKG should be monitored during dose escalation in patients with cardiac disease and the elderly. The finding of significant conduction disturbance or arrhythmia contraindicates the use of these agents. Monitoring serum drug levels, when available, may further reduce the risk of adverse cardiac effects. Trazodone may cause priapism in men, sometimes causing permanent loss of erectile function.

Drugs that inhibit the cytochrome P-450 system—including cimetidine (Tagamet), quinidine, and selective serotonin reuptake inhibitors (SSRIs)—may lead to increased serum levels of tricyclic antidepressants. On the other hand, tricyclic antidepressants may potentiate the effects of warfarin (Coumadin), sulfonylureas, and other drugs. Selected drug interactions are listed in Table 19.

Anticonvulsants

Anticonvulsants are generally considered to be first-line agents for the treatment of neuropathic pain with a predominantly paroxysmal or lancinating quality, such as trigeminal neuralgia (26). Some of these drugs may also be used for treatment of migraine headaches and other pain syndromes (Table 20) (27). The mechanisms by which

Table 20
Pain Relief from Anticonvulsants
as Demonstrated by Controlled Studies[a,b]

Painful Disorder	Anticonvulsant Treatment
Trigeminal neuralgia	Carbamazepine
Diabetic neuropathy	Carbamazepine
	Phenytoin
Postherpetic neuralgia[c]	Carbamazepine and clomipramine
Migraine prophylaxis[d]	Valproate
	Carbamazepine
Central pain[e]	Carbamazepine
TMJ syndrome	Clonazepam
Cancer pain	Phenytoin

[a]Data derived from ref. 27.
[b]These are agents shown in controlled studies to be effective in controlling pain; this listing does not imply that these anticonvulsants are not used for other painful conditions or that other anticonvulsants may not be effective for treating the listed conditions.
[c]See Chapter 13 for current recommendations on treating postherpetic neuralgia.
[d]Other agents would generally be used initially.
[e]Amitriptyline was more effective than carbamazepine.

anticonvulsants relieve pain may be related to stabilizing neuronal membranes (phenytoin), altering sodium channel activity (carbamazepine), and modulating γ-aminobutyric acid activity (clonazepam and valproate) (23).

Doses of these medications are generally the same as used in treating seizures (Table 21). In general, therapy with an anticonvulsant medication should be initiated at the lowest possible dosage and then gradually increased every 3–7 d as tolerated until adequate analgesia is achieved. However, phenytoin can be started at the usual maintenance dose of 100 mg three times daily. Serum levels are available for these agents and should be used to monitor therapy. If significant pain relief is not attained following an adequate dose of one drug for 2–3 wk, another anticonvulsant may be tried.

Physicians prescribing these agents should have some familiarity with their side effects (Table 22). Drug interactions have been described among anticonvulsants such as carbamazepine, phenytoin, valproate, and other medications (Table 23). We recommend that potential drug interactions be analyzed before prescribing these agents. This may be readily accomplished with software available from *The Medical Letter* (Adverse Drug Interactions) or *Physicians' Desk Reference* (Drug Interactions and Side Effects).

Carbamazepine (Tegretol) is considered the drug of choice for lancinating pain and is useful for treating postherpetic neuralgia, diabetic neuropathy, and trigeminal neuralgia. Benefit has also been reported in the treatment of glossopharyngeal neuralgia, tabetic pain, postsympathectomy pain, pain in multiple sclerosis, and cancer pain. The usual starting dose is 100 mg twice daily with gradual increases over 3–4 wk up to a maximum dose of 1200 mg/d. Periodic attempts to reduce the dose to the minimum effective level are recommended.

Table 21
Analgesic Doses of Anticonvulsants

Generic Name	Brand Name	Dosage Strengths	Initial Dose	Maintenance Dose	Therapeutic Level,[a] μg/mL
Carbamazepine	Tegretol	100 mg chewable, 200 mg	100 mg po bid	200 mg po bid-qid; maximal daily dose is 1200 mg	4–12
Clonazepam	Klonopin	0.5, 1, 2 mg	0.5 mg po hs	0.5–1.0 mg po tid	0.013–0.072
Gabapentin	Neurontin	100, 300, 400 mg	100 mg po tid	300–600 mg po tid	Unknown
Phenytoin	Dilantin Infatabs	50 mg	100 mg po tid	100 mg po tid	10–20
	Dilantin Kapseals	30, 100 mg	300 mg po qd	300 mg po qd	10–20
Valproic acid	Depakene	250 mg	250 mg po qd	250–500 mg po bid-tid	50–100
Divalproex sodium	Depakote	125, 250, 500 mg	250 mg po qd	50–100 mg po bid-tid	50–100

[a]These represent therapeutic serum levels for treatment of epilepsy, which may be used as guidelines for analgesia.

Table 22
Selected Adverse Reactions and Recommendations for Anticonvulsants

Anticonvulsant	Reaction	Special Recommendations
Carbamazepine	Sedation Dizziness Diplopia Dry mouth Nausea, vomiting Leukopenia Thrombocytopenia Agranulocytosis Aplastic anemia Hepatotoxicity Congestive heart failure Hyponatremia Stevens-Johnson syndrome Teratogenicity	Monitor CBC before therapy, after 2–3 wk, then 2–3 mo Obtain baseline liver enzymes and creatinine Monitor serum drug level Use caution with tricyclic antidepressants
Clonazepam	Sedation Dizziness Ataxia Nausea Leukopenia Thrombocytopenia Withdrawal if abruptly stopped	Monitor serum drug level
Gabapentin	Somnolence Fatigue Dizziness Nystagmus Ataxia Nausea, vomiting Weight gain	
Phenytoin	Acne Hirsutism Coarse facies Sedation Confusion Dizziness Diplopia Nystagmus Ataxia Gingival hyperplasia Nausea, vomiting Megaloblastic anemia (folate, vitamin B_{12} deficiency) Leukopenia Thrombocytopenia Pancytopenia Agranulocytosis Hypocalcemia Hepatotoxicity	Discontinue drug if rash develops (may herald exfoliative dermatitis) Monitor CBC and liver enzymes Monitor serum drug level

(continued)

Table 22 *(continued)*

Anticonvulsant	Reaction	Special Recommendations
	Hypersensitivity reaction	
	Drug-induced lupus	
	Pseudolymphoma	
	Stevens-Johnson syndrome	
	Teratogenicity	
Valproic acid,	Sedation	Monitor CBC, liver enzymes
divalproex sodium	Encephalopathy	Check serum NH_3 if
	Dizziness	encephalopathy
	Ataxia	Monitor serum drug level
	Tremor	
	Alopecia	
	Nausea, vomiting	
	Dyspepsia	
	Thrombocytopenia	
	Acute pancreatitis	
	Hepatotoxicity (may be fatal)	
	Hyponatremia	
	Peripheral edema	
	Weight gain	
	Stevens-Johnson syndrome	
	Teratogenicity	

Approximately 20% of patients will develop leukopenia or thrombocytopenia; agranulocytosis and aplastic anemia are rare events *(26)*. Other reactions include sedation, dizziness, hepatotoxicity, and hyponatremia. Carbamazepine may inhibit the metabolism of tricyclic antidepressants, and tricyclic antidepressants may decrease the metabolism of carbamazepine, resulting in elevated levels of both drugs. Consequently, this combination of drugs should be used cautiously with monitoring of serum drug levels. Carbamazepine is seldom used in cancer patients due to concerns about bone marrow reserve following chemotherapy. Baseline laboratory studies should include complete blood count, liver enzymes, and creatinine. This drug should be discontinued if the leukocyte count is less than 4000 or decreases by 3000 or more, or if the absolute neutrophil count is less than 1500 *(26)*.

Phenytoin (Dilantin) is appropriate for treatment of postherpetic neuralgia, diabetic neuropathy, tabetic pain, posttraumatic neuralgia, trigeminal neuralgia, glossopharyngeal neuralgia, thalamic pain, postsympathectomy pain, and central pain. Extended-release phenytoin capsules (Dilantin Kapseals) permit once-daily dosing. Phenytoin may cause confusion, dizziness, ataxia, gingival hyperplasia, pseudolymphoma, hepatotoxicity, and a hypersensitivity syndrome. The development of a maculopapular rash may represent the harbinger of Stevens-Johnson syndrome and mandates that the drug be discontinued.

Valproate (Depakene, Depakote) represents an alternative agent for treatment of neuropathic pain states such as trigeminal neuralgia and postherpetic neuralgia in patients unable to tolerate or poorly responsive to carbamazepine and phenytoin. Depakene (valproic acid) and Depakote (valproic acid and sodium valproate in a 1:1 molar ratio),

Table 23
Selected Drug Interactions with Anticonvulsants

Anticonvulsant	Interacting Drug	Reaction
Carbamazepine	Doxycycline ((Vibramycin)	Decreased serum level of doxycycline
	Theophylline	Decreased serum levels of both carbamazepine and theophylline
	Tricyclic antidepressants	Increased serum levels of both carbamazepine and antidepressant
	Warfarin (Coumadin)	Decreased serum level of warfarin, which requires careful monitoring of INR
	Calcium-channel blockers	Increased serum carbamazepine level
	Cimetidine (Tagamet)	Increased serum carbamazepine level
	Erythromycin	Increased serum carbamazepine level
	Fluoxetine (Prozac)	Increased serum carbamazepine level
	Propoxyphene (Darvon)	Increased serum carbamazepine level
	Terfenadine (Seldane)	Increased serum carbamazepine level
Phenytoin	Corticosteroids	Decreased serum level of corticosteroid
	Doxycycline	Decreased serum level of doxycycline
	Meperidine (Demerol)	Increased metabolism to normeperidine, which may increase toxicity
	Oral contraceptives	Decreased efficacy of oral contraceptive
	Quinidine	Decreased serum level of quinidine
	Theophylline	Decreased serum level of theophylline
	Warfarin (Coumadin)	Decreased serum level of warfarin
	H_2-antagonists (Tagamet and others)	Increased serum level of phenytoin
	Salicylates	Increased serum level of phenytoin
	Sulfonamides	Increased serum level of phenytoin
Valproate	Cimetidine (Tagamet)	Increased serum level of valproate

a delayed-release preparation, both dissociate to the valproate ion in the gastrointestinal tract. This drug increases central levels of γ-aminobutyric acid (GABA), which may inhibit nociceptive pathways. Side effects include alopecia, sedation, dizziness, tremor, ataxia, nausea, vomiting, acute pancreatitis, and hepatic failure.

Clonazepam (Klonopin), an anticonvulsant agent with some properties characteristic of benzodiazepines, may also be useful for treating neuropathic pain, including trigeminal neuralgia and posttraumatic neuralgia. Although it is the most sedating of these agents, this property makes it appropriate for treating patients with pain associated with anxiety or insomnia. In addition, it is the most effective of the anticonvulsants in the treatment of myoclonic jerks associated with high-dose opioid therapy *(28)*. Side effects include dizziness, ataxia, leukopenia, and thrombocytopenia.

Gabapentin (Neurontin) represents a new anticonvulsant medication that is structurally related to the neurotransmitter GABA. Postherpetic neuralgia, reflex sympathetic dystrophy, phantom limb pain, and chronic diffuse and radicular pain have been reported to respond to gabapentin. An advantage of this agent is that it appears to have relatively few side effects, although it may cause dizziness, somnolence, and other evidence of CNS depression *(29)*. Its role in treating pain is promising but not yet well-defined.

Lamotrigine (Lamictal), another new anticonvulsant agent, may be useful for the management of headache and other pain syndromes. Additional data are necessary to determine its efficacy as an adjuvant analgesic.

Muscle Relaxants

Baclofen (Lioresal) is a GABA agonist with muscle relaxant and antispasmodic activity that has been demonstrated to decrease pain from trigeminal neuralgia in some patients. Baclofen is also used for treating lancinating or paroxysmal neuropathic pain of other types. Although baclofen may be categorized as a muscle relaxant, its efficacy as an adjuvant analgesic for treating neuropathic pain is not related to muscle relaxation. It may be used alone or in combination with other adjuvant analgesics.

The usual starting dose is 5 mg three times daily, with gradual increases in dose as needed up to 20 mg four times daily. Because it is primarily excreted unchanged through the kidneys, it should be used with caution in patients with decreased renal function. Side effects include sedation, confusion, dizziness, weakness, and nausea. Hallucinations and seizures may occur with abrupt drug withdrawal.

Cyclobenzaprine (Flexeril), a muscle relaxant structurally related to amitriptyline, may relieve pain associated with fibromyalgia and other myofascial pain syndromes. The most commonly reported side effects are drowsiness, dry mouth, and dizziness.

The usual initial dose is 10 mg or less at bedtime Although it may be prescribed up to 10 mg three to four times daily for severe myofascial pain, many patients experience intolerable sedation at these doses. According to the *Physicians' Drug Reference*, this medication should not be prescribed for more than 2–3 wk. However, cyclobenzaprine is commonly prescribed in low dose (10 mg or less at bedtime) for prolonged periods in patients with fibromyalgia without apparent toxicity.

Carisoprodol (Soma, Soma Compound) and methocarbamol (Robaxin) represent alternative muscle relaxants that may be used to treat myofascial pain in patients unable to tolerate or unresponsive to cyclobenzaprine. A metabolic product of carisoprodol is meprobamate, a sedative- hypnotic drug with potential for physical and psychological dependence. This raises concerns regarding long-term use of carisoprodol.

Alpha-2 Adrenergic Agonists

Clonidine (Catapres) exhibits analgesic effects for postherpetic neuralgia, diabetic neuropathy, migraine headaches, postoperative pain, and cancer pain. These effects are hypothesized to result from stimulation of dorsal horn adrenergic receptors that inhibit nociceptive impulses. Clonidine may be considered as an analgesic adjuvant for patients with pain unresponsive to NSAIDs, antidepressants, and anticonvulsants.

Therapy with clonidine may be initiated at a dose of 0.1 mg orally each day with subsequent increases until hypotension or other side effects develop. This medication is also available for transdermal administration (Catapres-TSS). Epidural clonidine may provide prolonged postoperative analgesia and has been reported to be as effective as epidural morphine in relieving low back pain from arachnoiditis *(30)*.

Common side effects of clonidine include sedation, hypotension, and dryness of the mouth. Particular caution must be exercised when prescribing this agent to the elderly or others predisposed to hypotension.

Sympatholytics

Sympatholytic agents may be utilized when treating patients with sympathetically maintained pain, especially if appropriate sympathetic nerve blocks are contraindicated or ineffective. Phenoxybenzamine (Dibenzyline), prazosin (Minipress), and propranolol (Inderal) have been reported to be effective in treating causalgia *(26)*. Orthostatic hypotension may limit the dose of these medications, especially in older patients.

Neuroleptics

The role of neuroleptic agents in the treatment of pain is limited. However, these drugs may be considered for patients with neuropathic pain refractory to other agents and for certain patients with cancer pain. Common side effects of neuroleptics include sedation, orthostatic hypotension, anticholinergic effects, and extrapyramidal reactions, including tardive movement disorders.

Methotrimeprazine (Levoprome) is a phenothiazine that has been demonstrated to possess analgesic effects. Use of this agent is limited by availability of only a parenteral formulation and side effects, including somnolence and orthostatic hypotension. Methotrimeprazine may be appropriate for patients with advanced cancer who are largely confined to bed, have other indications for a neuroleptic agent, and have continuous subcutaneous or intravenous access *(31)*.

Pimozide (Orap) has been reported to reduce symptoms of trigeminal neuralgia. One study found pimozide to be more effective than carbamazepine in such patients *(32)*. It may be considered for patients with refractory neuropathic pain characterized by lancinating or paroxysmal dysesthesia *(31)*. As with other neuroleptics, use of pimozide is limited by side effects, which include tremor and parkinsonian symptoms.

Fluphenazine (Prolixin), another phenothiazine, and haloperidol (Haldol) have been reported in various studies to decrease neuropathic pain and headaches. Addition of one of these agents to a tricyclic antidepressant or an anticonvulsant drug may provide enhanced analgesia in the treatment of neuropathic pain *(33)*.

TOPICAL AGENTS

Capsaicin (Zostrix, Capsin, Dolorac, and Others)

Topical administration of capsaicin, the active ingredient in hot chili pepper, stimulates the release of substance P, a chemomediator causing pain and inflammation, from the peripheral and central terminals of C fibers and Aδ fibers *(34)*. Prolonged application of capsaicin reversibly depletes substance P from these afferent neurons and prevents its reaccumulation. In addition, although capsaicin initially causes depolarization of nociceptive neurons, continued application leads to desensitization of these neurons, probably by inhibiting the specific calcium channels responsible for depolarization. Thus, noxious stimuli fail to release substance P and other neuropeptides. Either of these mechanisms may explain the analgesic and anti-inflammatory effects of capsaicin.

Benefit from topical administration of capsaicin has been described for treatment of various causes of chronic pain. The most extensive studies have documented decreased pain in patients with diabetic neuropathy and postherpetic neuralgia, but improvement has also been reported for patients with reflex sympathetic dystrophy, trigeminal neuralgia, cluster headache (100 µL of 10 mmol/L applied to the nasal mucosa), postmastectomy pain, fibromyalgia, osteoarthritis, and rheumatoid arthritis *(34)*. In general, the analgesic effects demonstrated in these studies required administration of capsaicin several times daily for a period of several weeks. Many patients failed to complete the trials due to the irritant effect of capsaicin, which causes a burning pain, especially during the initial applications. Capsaicin has also been used to treat pruritus, which is suppressed by blocking C fibers.

Capsaicin is available in strengths of 0.025, 0.075, and 0.25% for topical application to painful areas. The lower concentrations, available without prescription, should be applied three to four times daily; the highest concentration may be applied twice daily. Treatment should continue for at least 4–6 wk. A burning sensation is common at the site of application during the first few days of therapy; this may be transient or, if prolonged, may warrant preapplication of lidocaine 5% ointment. Contact with the eyes and broken or irritated skin should be avoided. Patients should avoid breathing the airborne material from the dried residue, which can cause irritation of the respiratory tract.

Local Anesthetics (EMLA)

EMLA cream is a eutectic mixture (the components are liquid at room temperature) of 2.5% lidocaine and 2.5% prilocaine which has been reported to relieve postherpetic neuralgia (*see* Chapter 13). By extension, this agent may also be utilized for treatment of other peripheral neuropathic pain, but data regarding efficacy are lacking.

Applied to intact skin under an occlusive dressing, EMLA provides topical analgesia for venous or arterial puncture, lumbar puncture, drug reservoir injections, and superficial skin surgery *(35)*. Dermal analgesia is achieved within 60 min of application, reaches a peak at 2–3 h, and persists for 1–2 h following removal. Transient, local blanching of the skin is common. EMLA cream is contraindicated in patients with methemoglobinemia and in infants receiving drugs associated with methemoglobinemia.

SYSTEMIC LOCAL ANESTHETICS
Oral Local Anesthetics

Mexiletine (Mexitil) is a local anesthetic and arrhythmic agent structurally similar to lidocaine but available for oral administration. Approved by the FDA for treatment of life-threatening ventricular arrhythmias, mexiletine has also been shown to be effective for treatment of diabetic neuropathy and other neuropathic pain syndromes. The analgesic use of mexiletine should generally be reserved for patients with continuous dysesthesia not controlled by antidepressants or patients with lancinating pain unresponsive to anticonvulsants *(26)*.

Therapy may be initiated at a dose of 150 mg once daily with gradual increases in dose up to 300 mg three times daily if needed. Adverse reactions include nausea, vomiting, dizziness, nervousness, tremor, incoordination, paresthesias, arrhythmias, hepatic disease, and blood dyscrasias. Patients should be monitored for cardiac toxicity with periodic electrocardiograms.

Intravenous Local Anesthetics

Although seldom used at this time, intravenous administration of lidocaine has been reported to provide analgesia in acute and chronic pain syndromes, including acute herpes zoster and postherpetic neuralgia. The duration of analgesia from intravenous infusion of lidocaine is relatively short, but this modality may be considered in occasional patients with refractory neuropathic pain despite treatment with an oral local anesthetic agent. This therapy is discussed further in Chapter 13.

NERVE BLOCKS

Although a detailed discussion of nerve blocks is beyond the scope of this chapter, health care providers should be aware of this therapeutic option, which may be performed by a variety of physicians, including anesthesiologists, neurosurgeons, neurologists, orthopedists, and radiologists. With current imaging techniques, virtually every nerve in the body is accessible for blockade.

Nerve blocks may be diagnostic, prognostic, or therapeutic (36). Diagnostic nerve blocks are used to determine the type of pain (such as somatic, visceral, or sympathetic) and its source. Thus, pain relief following infiltration of a sympathetic nerve with local anesthetic indicates that the pain is of sympathetic rather than somatic origin. Relief of abdominal pain following celiac plexus block identifies the pain as intraperitoneal rather than referred, and relief of pain following a peripheral nerve block excludes pain of central origin.

Prognostic nerve blocks temporarily produce the effects that occur after an irreversible procedure, such as neurolytic or surgical interruption of nerve pathways. This information is important to determine the location and assess the potential efficacy of an ablative procedure. However, pain relief after a prognostic nerve block does not guarantee satisfactory results from a neurolytic or surgical procedure; this may be related in part to the development of alternative pain pathways (36).

Therapeutic nerve blocks may provide analgesic benefit for a variety of acute and chronic pain conditions (37). Examples include treatment of an acute rib fracture or other thoracic pain with an intercostal nerve block and treatment of reflex sympathetic dystrophy or phantom limb pain with sympathetic nerve blocks. Cranial nerve blocks may be performed for intractable pain in the head and neck regions due to cancer or for cranial neuropathy, such as trigeminal neuralgia. Nerve roots may be blocked as they exit the intervertebral foramina at the cervical, thoracic, or lumbar level, depending on the location of the pain. Cervical nerve root blocks may be utilized for pain in the head, neck, and upper arm resulting from conditions such as whiplash. Blockade of the upper cervical nerve roots and greater and lesser occipital nerves may relieve occipital headache and neuralgia. Thoracic nerve root blocks may be indicated for pain following chest wall surgery, thoracic vertebral compression fracture, or acute herpes zoster or postherpetic neuralgia affecting thoracic dermatomes. Similarly, lumbar nerve root blocks may relieve pain from vertebral compression fracture, herpes zoster, or PHN affecting the lumbar area. Other regional pain syndromes may also be considered for nerve blocks. For example, shoulder pain may respond to blockade of the suprascapular nerve, and localized myofascial pain may improve following trigger-point injection with local anesthetic.

Nerve blocks may be performed using local anesthetics, in which case they are temporary and reversible, or neurolytics such as absolute alcohol or phenol, in which case they produce blockade that usually persists for months (but may last for years). Neurolytic blocks are often utilized for patients with intractable pain from cancer; they should be preceded by a prognostic nerve block using a local anesthetic.

EPIDURAL STEROIDS

Lumbar or caudal epidural injection of corticosteroids has been utilized for the treatment of various low back syndromes believed to be associated with inflammation or edema. These disorders include diskogenic disease and spinal stenosis.

The corticosteroid most often administered is methylprednisolone acetate in a dose of 80 mg per injection, but other preparations, such as triamcinolone, may be injected *(38)*. A local anesthetic, such as lidocaine, may be used as the diluent and often provides dramatic, albeit transient, pain relief. Some clinicians recommend epidural steroid administration for patients with low back pain associated with radicular symptoms following orthopedic or neurosurgical evaluation if symptoms fail to improve following conservative therapy for 2–6 wk *(39)*. Occasional patients will derive complete relief of pain following a single injection, whereas others may require two or three injections at intervals of at least 2 wk. Additional benefit from more than three injections is unlikely. Contraindications to this therapy include bleeding diathesis, local or systemic infection, and acute spinal cord compression *(38)*. Reported complications of this procedure include epidural abscess and bacterial meningitis.

Data concerning the efficacy of epidural corticosteroids show inconsistent results *(40)*. A recent review of controlled studies suggests that this treatment is probably efficacious for patients with lower extremity radicular pain syndromes at periods up to 3 mo *(38)*. Most studies have not demonstrated a long-term difference in outcome between patients who received epidural corticosteroids vs saline control. This may be related to the tendency for acute lumbar disk symptoms to improve even with conservative treatment. Factors reported to improve the response to epidural corticosteroids include acute pain, younger age, and no previous back surgery *(39)*.

Additional well-designed studies are needed to define further the role of epidural steroid injections. Based on the data presently available, epidural steroids seem appropriate for the treatment of low back pain with radicular symptoms in patients whose function is impared but who are not candidates for surgery by virtue of the lesion or other medical problems.

MARIJUANA

The use of marijuana (cannabis saliva) for medicinal purposes has recently become the focus of considerable attention and controversy. With few clinical trials assessing the therapeutic efficacy of marijuana, this debate relies heavily on anecdotes and emotional arguments.

Among the various compounds in marijuana, Δ-9-tetrahydrocannabinol (Δ-9-THC) accounts for most of the pharmacologic activity of smoked marijuana. Synthetic Δ-9-THC is available as dronabinol (Marinol) for oral administration. The Drug Enforcement Agency (DEA) categorizes marijuana as a Schedule I drug (no acceptable medical use with high potential for abuse) and dronabinol as a Schedule II drug (proven medical usefulness with high potential for abuse).

Tetrahydrocannabinols are highly lipid soluble and are readily absorbed from the lungs and gastrointestinal tract. Bioavailability of THC from smoking ranges from 15 to 20%, compared to about 6% following oral ingestion. Smoking marijuana produces an effect within minutes, whereas the maximal effect occurs 1–3 h after oral administration. Cannabinoid receptors are present in various regions of the brain, including the cerebral cortex, hippocampus, and cerebellum. An endogenous arachidonic acid derivative known as anandamide binds to these receptors, but the physiologic role of this ligand is unknown (41).

The pharmacologic effects of Δ-9-THC include changes in perception, motivation, cognitive function, learning, memory, judgment, and reaction time. Some individuals experience hallucinations, panic, or acute psychosis (18). Medicinal effects of marijuana have also been described. These include reduction of intraocular pressure, decreased muscle spasm in patients with spinal cord lesions or multiple sclerosis, anticonvulsant activity, appetite stimulation, antiemetic effects, and analgesia (41). Synthetic tetrahydrocannibol is approved by the FDA for the treatment of anorexia associated with weight loss in patients with AIDS and for nausea and vomiting associated with cancer chemotherapy in patients who have failed to respond adequately to conventional antiemetic treatments.

Purported advantages of marijuana over dronabinol and conventional medications include the ability to titrate the dose more precisely when the drug is delivered by inhalation rather than ingestion and the inability of some people with cancer to swallow medications. In addition, oral medications are unlikely to be effective in patients with vomiting. Opponents of the medical use of marijuana point to the effectiveness of conventional medications in the majority of patients. Moreover, smoking marijuana is associated with bronchopulmonary disease (including bacterial and fungal infections, squamous metaplasia, and probably cancer) and much higher levels of carboxyhemoglobin than tobacco cigarets (41). Both inhaled and ingested THC cause adverse CNS effects.

Recently, voters in California passed Proposition 215, which states that Californians have the right to obtain and use marijuana for medical purposes when recommended by a physician for treatment of seriously ill patients with cancer, anorexia, AIDS, chronic pain, spasticity, glaucoma, arthritis, migraine, or any other illness for which marijuana provides relief. Voters in Arizona passed a similar (though broader) measure known as Proposition 200. These propositions are in direct conflict with federal law, which prohibits possessing, dispensing, or distributing marijuana. Moreover, the federal government has indicated a willingness and intention to prosecute physicians who recommend or prescribe marijuana. A recent editorial in the *New England Journal of Medicine* characterized this federal policy as "misguided, heavy-handed, and inhumane (42)." Resolution of these contradictory laws will presumably require judicial intervention. In the meantime, the MBC recommends that physicians document responsible actions taken for their patients, consistent with the stated intent of the law *(43)*.

Within the context of pain treatment, a variety of other agents and techniques are available as outlined in this chapter. In general, these conventional therapies are effective and seem to represent safer alternatives to marijuana, whose side effects concern us. Consequently, we believe that marijuana has little, if any, use in the treatment of pain. Of interest is the ability to separate the analgesic effects of a synthetic cannabinoid from its mood altering effects in an animal model *(44)*. This suggests that it may be possible to synthesize cannabinoid drugs which possess analgesic properties without significant psychotropic effects. Such agents could prove useful in treating some patients with chronic pain.

SOMATOSENSORY STIMULATION

Acupuncture

Acupuncture, utilized as part of traditional Chinese medicine for thousands of years, is gaining acceptance in Western countries as an adjunct for the treatment of pain. The theory, according to Eastern medicine, is that stimulation of specific points along meridian channels, through which chi (or energy) flows, releases blocks in the meridians, thus balancing the opposing energy forces of yin and yang. The technique involves the insertion of fine needles into acupuncture points that are chosen based on the location of the pain. The needles remain in place for up to an hour, either rotated between the therapist's fingers or attached to an electrical current. Although the number of treatments may vary, acupuncture is usually administered two to three times per week for a period of at least 3–6 wk.

Acupuncture points, of which there are some 600, are reported to be areas with decreased electrical skin resistance that possess specific morphological characteristics. For example, a vasomotor-nerve bundle has been described as passing through the superficial fascia at 80% of acupuncture points. The acupuncture points on the extremities are described as lying on lines that generally follow major nerves and blood vessels, whereas on the face and head they lie near cranial nerves and blood vessels, and on the trunk they lie at segmental innervation levels where nerves and blood vessels penetrate muscle fascia *(45,46)*. The importance of these specific points is unresolved.

Theories to explain the mechanism of action of stimulation-induced analgesia according to Western notions of anatomy and physiology initially focused on selective stimulation of afferent fibers that may block the transmission of pain. One hypothesis, known as the gate control theory of pain, proposed that activation of large diameter Aβ peripheral afferent fibers, which transmit pressure and touch sensations, excites interneurons in the dorsal horn of the spinal cord, leading to presynaptic inhibition of pain transmission by the smaller C and Aδ fibers *(47)*.

Interest has also focused on endogenous chemical mediators of pain, such as endorphins and enkephalins, which bind to opiate receptors. Stimulation of the raphe magnus nucleus in the brainstem by endorphin or enkephalin activates descending neurons that terminate in the dorsal horn of the spinal cord and secrete serotonin. Serotonin in turn activates another set of neurons in the dorsal horn, causing them to release enkephalin, which is believed to inhibit C and Aδ pain fibers at their dorsal horn synapses with the spinothalamic and spinoreticular tracts.

Acupuncture is hypothesized to produce analgesia through several mechanisms. Activation of nerve fibers may trigger the release of enkephalin in the dorsal horn, causing presynaptic inhibition of afferent pain fibers and segmental analgesia, as proposed in the gate control theory. In addition, acupuncture is proposed to stimulate release of enkephalins in the midbrain, leading to activation of the raphe nucleus and the inhibitory serotonergic neurons described above, which could produce regional analgesia. A third potential mechanism involves release of β-endorphin from the hypothalamus and pituitary, the primary source of this mediator, which binds to opiate receptors and could induce generalized analgesia. Reports that β-endorphin and enkephalin levels in the cerebrospinal fluid increase following acupuncture and that the opioid antagonist naloxone may reverse acupuncture analgesia support the theory that endogenous opiate mechanisms are operative in this form of somatosensory-evoked analgesia *(48,49)*. Local physical changes, including muscle relaxation and vasodilatation, are also induced by the insertion of acupuncture needles and might provide benefit. Even fractals and chaos theory have been invoked to explain this modality *(45)*.

Although specific mechanisms involved in the induction of endogenous analgesia require clarification, it is apparent that acupuncture may modulate pain through various mechanisms at multiple levels. By employing both local and distant points, it is proposed that a combination of local and general analgesia can be produced *(45)*. Indeed, two patterns of analgesia have been described after acupuncture treatment of chronic back pain: a central-inhibitory pattern affecting the entire body and lasting only hours, and an origin-specific pattern affecting only the site of stimulation and lasting 10–14 d with cumulative effects at 4 mo *(50)*.

Regardless of mode of action, acupuncture is widely used to treat a variety of conditions, including headache, musculoskeletal pain, nausea and vomiting, and addiction. Other than anecdotal evidence, including reports of patients undergoing major surgery with no analgesia other than acupuncture, what is the evidence for the efficacy of this modality?

Various studies utilizing "placebo-controlled" conditions have examined the effects of acupuncture. In many of these studies, the acupuncture technique in the "real" acupuncture group was identical to that in the sham (placebo) group; the only difference was that needles were inserted into classical acupuncture points in the former and nonclassical points in the latter. Most studies analyzing the effect of acupuncture on the treatment of back pain have followed this protocol and have failed to show a significant difference between the study groups. However, such studies only reveal information about the most effective sites for needle insertion, not the effectiveness of acupuncture. In fact, an analgesic effect has been reported in 40–50% of patients receiving sham acupuncture, compared to 60% of patients receiving classical acupuncture *(51)*.

More reliable control techniques include "minimal" acupuncture (needles are inserted only 1–2 mm into nonclassical points and stimulated very lightly) and mock TENS (transcutaneous electrical nerve stimulators are used without current). A review of the literature for studies controlled in this manner revealed 10 reports describing the efficacy of acupuncture for treating chronic nonanginal pain, including facial pain, cervical pain, low back pain, osteoarthritis, migraine headache, and postherpetic neuralgia *(51)*. Among these studies, five showed significant benefit with acupuncture and three showed a tendency toward greater improvement with acupuncture than control. Benefit from acupuncture was reported in approximately 50–85% of patients with musculoskeletal pain (statistically significant difference in four of seven studies) and about 50% of patients with migraine headaches (statistically significant difference in one of two studies). A single study of postherpetic neuralgia showed very low response to either acupuncture or placebo. Several caveats should be noted regarding this analysis: the quality of these studies was not uniform, the duration of follow-up was generally short, the number of patients studied was often small, and even minimal acupuncture with slight penetration of the skin could possibly stimulate release of endorphins.

A recent study reported benefit from acupuncture for patients with tennis elbow pain lasting more than 2 mo *(49)*. Patients in the acupuncture group were treated at acupuncture points on the ipsilateral leg, whereas those in the control group were treated with placebo acupuncture on the back without penetration of the skin. After one treatment, 79% of the patients receiving traditional acupuncture noted pain relief of at least 50%, compared to 25% of patients in the placebo group. The average pain relief reported in the treatment group was 56%, compared to 15% in the placebo group. The average duration of analgesia after treatment was 20 h in the acupuncture group and 1.4 h in the placebo group. These differences reached statistical significance.

The effect of acupuncture mode has also been evaluated *(52)*. Patients with chronic nociceptive (neither neuropathic nor psychogenic) low back pain received manual stimulation, low-frequency electrical stimulation (2 Hz), or high-frequency electrical stimulation (80 Hz) of acupuncture needles, depending on their preference after a trial session with each one. Thereafter, they received up to 10 treatments using this preferred mode. After 6 wk, improvement was noted with each of these techniques. However, after 6 mo, significant improvement persisted only in those patients who had received low frequency stimulation.

These data support the efficacy of acupuncture in a proportion of patients with chronic musculoskeletal pain and possibly migraine headaches. Low-frequency electrical stimulation may represent the preferred mode for chronic musculoskeletal pain. We expect that, with greater appreciation of the methodological problems in earlier studies, properly designed trials will provide needed information concerning the role of acupuncture in treating a variety of disorders.

Transcutaneous Electrical Nerve Stimulation (TENS)

Transcutaneous electrical nerve stimulation (TENS) delivers low-voltage electrical impulses to the nervous system from surface electrodes placed over particular loci, often trigger points. The total electrical impulse delivered by the TENS unit is a function of the stimulator settings for amplitude, pulse width, and pulse rate. The amplitude varies from 0 to 60 mA on most TENS units; as the signal intensity increases, the reaction will range from paresthesias to muscle contraction. Pulse width refers to the duration of the pulse and usually ranges from 40–250 µs; longer pulse widths are associated with greater radiation and penetration of the signal. The pulse rate generally varies from 1 or 2 Hz to 100 Hz, adjusted to match the firing rate of the nerves being targeted. Generally, a biphasic (alternating) current is used.

High-frequency (conventional) TENS utilizes frequencies from 40 to 400 Hz with a pulse width of 20–250 μs. The amplitude should be adjusted to produce paresthesias without muscular contraction *(53)*. This mode stimulates large myelinated afferent fibers, which conduct rapidly and are postulated to inhibit nociceptive activity through the dorsal horn gating system (which may be modulated by descending serotonergic neurons). In addition, high-frequency stimulation (110 Hz) in combination with long pulse duration (200 μs) has been reported to inhibit peripheral sensory nerve conduction and decrease the threshold for mechanical pain *(54)*. Analgesia from this mode is characterized by rapid onset (usually within 20 min) and short duration of action (usually less than 1 h after cessation of stimulation).

Low-frequency TENS stimulates at a frequency of 1–5 Hz with a pulse width of 250–500 μs; the amplitude should be great enough to elicit strong, rhythmic muscular contraction *(53)*. These frequencies may activate smaller, slow conducting Aδ and C fibers, which are believed to stimulate the release of endorphins from the pituitary and to activate inhibitory descending serotonergic neurons. Reports that naloxone may inhibit analgesia induced by this mode are consistent with this hypothesis *(48)*. Analgesia produced by low-frequency TENS is associated with slow onset (usually more than 20 min) and prolonged benefit (up to 2–6 h after stimulation).

A burst or pulse train mode utilizes wide pulses delivered in bursts of 5–10 pulses at a rate of 1–2 bursts/s. This mode produces analgesia of onset and duration intermediate between high- and low-frequency TENS.

In addition, most TENS units feature a brief, intense mode, characterized by high-frequency bursts (up to 400 Hz) superimposed on low frequency TENS (1–5 Hz). This mode produces rapid analgesia of short duration. The high-frequency bursts are believed to stimulate large afferents and activate the segmental gating mechanism, whereas the low-frequency pulses are hypothesized to activate the endorphin system at the level of the pituitary.

Sites chosen for stimulation are anatomically and physiologically related to the involved area. These regions should be related segmentally to the source of pain and accessible to a TENS electrode. Most often, these sites are trigger-points, hypersensitive regions that elicit tenderness and referred pain when pressed. Stimulation at acupuncture points, superficial nerves, motor points (where nerves enter muscles), or distal sites may also provide benefit. Sequential stimulation of different sites is frequently recommended for patients who do not improve after the initial TENS treatment. Following instruction regarding stimulatory modes and placement of electrodes, the patient is able to apply the TENS unit on a regular basis without professional assistance. This represents an obvious advantage over acupuncture.

TENS is associated with few side effects, although allergic dermatitis and skin irritation have been described. It is recommended that the TENS unit not be placed over the eye, carotid sinus, trachea, larynx, or gravid uterus. TENS is not recommended for patients with cardiac pacemakers or a history of cardiac dysrhythmia.

Table 24
Pain Syndromes Treated with TENS

Musculoskeletal pain
Neurologic pain
Head and face pain
Abdominal and pelvic pain (including dysmenorrhea)
Cancer pain
Postoperative pain

Many acute and chronic pain syndromes have been reported to respond to transcutaneous electrical nerve stimulation (Table 24). However, well-controlled studies of efficacy in these conditions are few. As with acupuncture, one difficulty in conducting such studies is choosing an appropriate placebo. Most investigators have utilized sham TENS, in which electrodes are placed in the normal manner but no current is applied; some sham treatments include flashing lights, oscilloscope displays of waveforms, and sounds. Even in the absence of electrical current, the placebo patients usually receive a considerable amount of attention and sometimes other treatment (e.g., hot packs). In one study, 145 patients with chronic low back pain were assigned to one of four treatment groups: daily treatment with TENS, sham TENS, TENS plus a program of stretching exercises, or sham TENS plus exercises *(55)*. Improvement was progressive in all four study groups from wk 2 to wk 4. After 1 mo, about 45% of patients had improved with either TENS or sham TENS. Those patients who also performed exercises showed the most improvement within each group, but within 2 mo of the active intervention, most patients had discontinued the exercises and the initial improvement had disappeared. The authors concluded that TENS is no more effective than placebo in treating chronic low back pain and that TENS and exercise are no better than exercise alone. They noted that, for some persons with chronic pain, nociceptive stimulation may be minimal or nil, and learned pain behavior may be the major problem; TENS would not be expected to help these individuals. Another consideration is that TENS may not provide sufficient counterstimulation for some patients with low back pain but could be effective for other pain syndromes.

Given the widespread use of TENS for treating chronic back pain, other investigators also addressed the question of whether TENS provides only a placebo effect for this condition. One group divided 42 subjects with chronic low back pain into three treatment groups: TENS, sham TENS, or no treatment (control) *(56)*. Pain was quantitated using two visual analog scales: one to measure pain intensity and another to measure pain unpleasantness. These investigators found a significantly greater reduction in pain intensity immediately after treatment in the patients receiving TENS (43%) compared to sham TENS (17%). The pain unpleasantness rating decreased in both groups and showed a tendency toward greater reduction with TENS. Moreover, following repeated treatments, pain intensity and unpleasantness prior to each treatment session decreased over time for patients receiving TENS but not sham TENS, indicating cumulative benefit from TENS. Both TENS and sham TENS reduced pain intensity and unpleasantness at

3 and 6 mo following the 10-wk treatment period. Patients receiving TENS showed a tendency toward greater improvement at these intervals, though the difference did not reach statistical significance. Patients in the control group with neither TENS nor sham TENS showed a minor, nonstatistically significant tendency toward reduced pain intensity and unpleasantness over the same period. The authors acknowledged that the prolonged benefit noted with TENS may be related to increased physical activity as a consequence of reduced pain.

The efficacy of TENS in treating another painful condition, osteoarthritis, was recently evaluated (57). In this study, 36 patients with osteoarthritis of the knee participated in three treatment phases: TENS plus naproxen 500 mg twice daily; sham TENS plus naproxen 500 mg twice daily; or double placebo. No significant differences in pain measures were noted between these three groups. These data are difficult to interpret for several reasons: 10 subjects (28%) did not complete the study; the small number of patients may have precluded detecting a statistically significant difference (type II error); and the finding that placebo and 1000 mg naproxen daily provided equivalent benefit for osteoarthritis differs significantly from many drug trials and clinical experience.

Other investigators have described their experience with TENS in treating 193 patients with chronic pain of various etiologies (58). All patients utilized conventional TENS with an average stimulation frequency of 80 Hz and a mean pulse width of 140 μs. The results of treatment after 6 mo were retrospectively analyzed by an independent investigator. Decreased pain was reported in 69% of patients with musculoskeletal pain of mechanical or degenerative origin and 53% of those with peripheral nerve lesions. Only 24% of patients with pain of central origin, 9% of those with autonomic pain, and 9% of patients with pain related to psychological dysfunction noted benefit. This study suffers from the usual limitations of a retrospective uncontrolled trial but provides interesting preliminary data.

A reasonable synthesis of the available data is that TENS represents an appropriate modality for pain treatment in selected patients, particularly those with pain refractory to other therapy. TENS may be most effective when combined with other treatment, including exercise. The extent to which transcutaneous electrical nerve stimulation provides additional benefit over attention, physical therapy, and exercise in various conditions remains to be determined.

PHYSICAL THERAPY

Physical therapy is often utilized to reduce pain associated with disorders of the musculoskeletal system, such as muscle spasm, tendinitis, and arthritis. Heat, cold, manual therapies, and therapeutic exercises are commonly prescribed modalities and are discussed in this section.

Heat

The application of heat for muscle spasm often reduces spasm and associated pain. The responses that constitute the basis for the therapeutic use of heat include increased blood flow, muscle relaxation, decreased joint stiffness, and increased extensibility of collagen (59). Heat may also be applied as a counterirritant to decrease pain. Caution must be exercised when utilizing heat for patients with cardiovascular disease or sensory neuropathy.

Table 25
Therapeutic Heat Modalities[a]

Primary Mode of Heat Transfer	Modality	Depth
Conduction	Hot packs	Superficial
	Heating pads	Superficial
	Paraffin baths	Superficial
Convection	Hydrotherapy	Superficial
Conversion	Radiant heat (infrared)	Superficial
	Shortwaves	Deep
	Microwaves	Deep
	Ultrasound	Deep

[a]From ref. 59.

Heating may be vigorous, with elevation of tissue temperature near the tolerance level, or mild. Vigorous heating is utilized for treating joint contractures but may aggravate pain from acute arthritis. Moreover, use of vigorous heating for an acutely herniated intervertebral disk impinging upon a nerve root is contraindicated, as it may increase swelling and exacerbate the underlying condition.

Heating modalities may be divided into those that heat superficial tissues and those that heat deeper tissues (Table 25). Superficial heat may be administered using hot packs, heating pads, chemical packs, paraffin baths, or hot water in a tub or spa. Moist heat, which may be applied with a moist heating pad or hot, moist towels covered with plastic, appears to be more effective than dry heat. Deep heat is most often delivered using ultrasound, but diathermy (which employs short wave or microwave energy) is sometimes prescribed.

Hydrocollator and Related Packs

The most common commercially available packs are the Hydrocollator packs, which contain silicate gel in a cotton bag. They are heated in a water bath, where the gel absorbs hot water and attains a temperature of 160–175°F. Wrapped in towels to prevent excessive heating, the pack is applied to the affected region for 20–30 min. At home, moist heat can be delivered with hot, moist towels wrapped in plastic to retain heat. Also available for home use are gel packs that are heated in a microwave oven; these offer the advantages of greater convenience and more prolonged delivery of heat.

Electric Heating Pads

Transfer of heat to the body is more efficient with a moist heating pad than a regular (dry) heating pad. Heat output increases over time until a steady state is achieved. This may produce high temperatures, which are dangerous if the patient falls asleep on the pad, since the heat may produce analgesia that contributes to burns.

Paraffin Baths

Paraffin wax may be applied in layers to the hands, arms, or feet by repeatedly dipping the region into a thermostatically controlled container of melted paraffin wax. For therapeutic purposes, paraffin wax with a melting point of 125–130°F is used. An indication of the correct temperature (in addition to a thermometer) is the coexistence of liquid and solid paraffin in the container. This technique provides mild heating of the region and is utilized most often to decrease joint pain and stiffness and facilitate exercise in patients with rheumatoid arthritis. Vigorous heating can be achieved by immersing the extremity into the paraffin for 20–30 min (solid paraffin forms around the immersed region and protects it from excess heat).

Hydrotherapy

Whereas heat transfer with the above modalities occurs through conduction, hydrotherapy provides heat mainly through convection, since in most forms of hydrotherapy the water is agitated and warm water replaces the cooler water adjacent to the body. For total immersion, a whirlpool bath is generally used and temperatures usually do not exceed 105°F. For partial immersion, temperatures up to 115°F may be used.

Ultrasound

The penetration of ultrasonic energy into tissue depends on the absorption characteristics of the tissue and reflection at tissue interfaces. Ultrasound causes little temperature elevation in the superficial tissues but is the most effective deep heating modality. Biological interfaces such as myofascial boundaries in the musculature appear to be selectively heated by ultrasound. In addition, ultrasound can be used to decrease conduction velocity in peripheral nerves and to produce temporary nerve blocks. Nociceptive C fibers are reportedly the most sensitive to this modality.

The therapeutic ultrasound machine consists of a generator that produces an alternating current with a frequency of 0.8–1 MHz. This current is then converted by a transducer into acoustic vibrations with the same frequency. Therapeutic intensities range from 1 to 4 W/cm^2. Ultrasound is applied to tissues by moving the applicator head back and forth in an coupling medium that covers the skin. Treatment is usually administered to the target area for 7–10 min.

Ultrasound should not be applied to the eye, heart, areas of vascular insufficiency, pregnant uterus, or malignant tumors, and it should be used with caution over anesthetic areas. Interestingly, ultrasound can be used safely in the presence of surgical metallic implants. This is attributed to the high thermal conductivity of these implants, which results in more rapid heat dissipation than absorption. However, methyl methacrylate and high-density polyethylene, materials commonly used in total joint replacements, absorb more ultrasound than soft tissue. Since it is not known if this selective absorption could cause overheating or melting of the plastics, these materials should not be included in the ultrasound fields.

Cold (Cryotherapy)

Therapeutic application of cold may be utilized to treat conditions such as back pain and soft tissue injury associated with swelling. This modality may also be used to treat arthritis, but most patients prefer heat.

Cryotherapy is often employed to relieve muscle spasm associated with joint or skeletal disease or nerve root irritation. Muscle tone and spasticity seem to be reduced by the effect of cold on the muscle spindle *(59)*. In acute trauma such as sprains, cold application produces vasoconstriction, which reduces swelling and bleeding. Cold produces analgesic effects that may be related to impaired transmission by pain fibers, counterirritation, muscle relaxation, and decreased swelling. The duration of relief of pain and muscle spasm achieved with cold application is longer then with heat, but not all patients tolerate this modality. Cold should not be applied to tissues with compromised arterial blood flow and may not be appropriate for patients with Raynaud's phenomenon or other cold hypersensitivity.

Therapeutic cooling may be achieved by several methods, including immersion in ice water, application of cold packs, ice massage, or use of an evaporative coolant spray, such as fluoromethane. In addition to using commercially available cold packs, patients may improvise a cold pack by adding ice cubes to water in a plastic freezer bag. Ice massage is effective and easy to perform in the office or at home by applying an ice stick made by freezing water in a paper cup containing a tongue blade or similar handle. After peeling the paper cup from the ice, the ice stick is moved back and forth over the affected area for 10–12 min. If the patient is unable to tolerate this duration of treatment, a cold pack wrapped in a moist towel may be applied to the area for 10–15 min prior to the ice stick. Use of fluoromethane spray applied to the skin with a stroking motion has been advocated by some for treating fibromyalgia and trigger points.

Manual Therapies

Manual therapies include massage, traction, and joint mobilization. The primary goal of these techniques is to restore normal mobility to joints and tissues, thereby reducing abnormal forces and decreasing pain *(53)*.

Massage may be superficial or deep, applied to muscles, tendons, and fascia. For acute myofascial pain, deep but gentle massage may encourage elongation of the fibers and enhance blood flow *(53)*. In chronic stages, deep tissue massage may decrease scar tissue and increase mobility.

Manual traction is applied by a therapist to the involved area to distract joint surfaces. Applied to the spine, traction may relax the spinal muscles and separate the vertebral joint spaces, relieving compression on nerve roots or facet joints. Applied to an extremity, it may reduce resistance and improve range of motion of the joints and soft tissues.

Joint mobilization involves movement patterns that the patient is unable to produce independently but that are necessary for normal motion and function. These techniques include low-force rhythmic motions, sustained forces at the maximal range of passive joint motion, and short amplitude thrusts beyond the passive range (manipulation) *(53)*. Rhythmic mobilization techniques are used to elongate soft tissue structures when treating disorders such as adhesive capsulitis. Manipulation may be employed for treatment of neck and back pain, although its efficacy is controversial.

Therapeutic Exercises

Therapeutic exercises represent an integral part of the treatment program for most patients with musculoskeletal pain. They are utilized to increase flexibility, improve strength and endurance, and stabilize weak or lax joints.

Table 26
Walking: An Example of a Graduated Exercise Program
to Increase Speed and Endurance^{a,b}

1. Achieve activity level of walking 2000 ft (e.g., 10 laps of 200 ft each) without interruption. If necessary, this goal may be attained by increasing the distance walked by 200–400 ft each day.
2. Increase the distance walked to 2400 ft at previous pace or decrease time to walk 2000 ft by 30 s.
3. When this quota is reached, increase distance another 400 ft or decrease time another 30 s.
4. Continue reduction in time quotas until upper speed limit is reached, as determined by repeated time quota failures.
5. Increase time quota to level previously achieved and expand distance walked on successive days.
6. Provide positive reinforcement for achieving these goals by documenting increments in speed and distance on performance graphs.

[a]This program was designed for patients with distorted gait due to operant pain behavior, but the principles may be generalized and applied to other exercise programs.
[b]From ref. 61.

Patients with pain often decrease their level of physical activity due to concern that they may exacerbate pain or produce tissue damage. The consequences may include reduced flexibility, decreased muscle strength, muscle wasting, and overall deconditioning (60). Therapy to counter these effects should include exercises specific for the painful area in addition to general aerobic exercises. These exercises should optimize range of motion and muscle strength while demonstrating to the patient that exercises do not produce harm. Positive reinforcement is provided when patients reach established goals without displaying pain behavior. By improving physical condition and functional abilities, therapeutic exercises may provide pain relief and enhance the quality of life.

The exercises prescribed will depend on patient interest and the risk of exacerbating pain. Examples of appropriate exercises include rapid walking, running, aerobic dance, bicycling, swimming, rowing, and cross country skiing. This program should be graduated, starting with exercise to tolerance (as determined by pain, weakness, or fatigue), and increasing the level every few days. The goal should be to exercise for 15–60 min at least three times weekly. The patient should achieve either 60–65% of maximal aerobic capacity as determined by an exercise tolerance test or the training heart rate as calculated using the following formula: training heart rate = resting heart rate + 0.6 × (maximal heart rate – resting heart rate), with maximal heart rate obtained by subtracting the age of the patient from 220 (53). An example of an exercise program designed to shape rapid walking is summarized in Table 26 (61).

BEHAVIORAL THERAPY

Whereas traditional medical treatment approaches pain at the physicochemical level, behavioral therapy applies psychological principles to decrease pain. Behavioral approaches to the management of chronic pain incorporate several modalities, including operant conditioning, cognitive behavioral therapy, relaxation, and biofeedback.

Operant Behavioral Therapy

Operant behavioral therapy seeks to eliminate pain behaviors through negative reinforcement while increasing normal behaviors through positive reinforcement. The therapist ignores pain behaviors such as moaning or grimacing but provides attention and affection when the patient engages in healthy behaviors.

Cognitive Behavioral Therapy

Cognitive behavioral therapy assumes that our attitudes, beliefs, and expectations in certain situations determine our emotional and behavioral reactions to those situations *(62)*. Since cognitive factors affect the experience of pain, modifying these cognitions may alter the perception of pain. Patients learn to identify factors that exacerbate or improve their pain and are taught pain-control techniques such as relaxation, imagery, and self-coping statements. This approach can give the patient a feeling of control over pain, which may decrease feelings of anxiety, helplessness, and hopelessness. Cognitive behavioral approaches are reported to enhance tolerance to nociceptive stimuli and are used to treat various pain syndromes, including migraine and tension-type headaches, abdominal pain, and myofascial pain *(62)*.

Self-Management Approach

A self-management approach to behavioral therapy encourages the patient to assume most of the responsibility for these changes *(63)*. The physician or therapist provides information, support, and encouragement. This program involves relaxation, exercise, education, and occupation:

1. Deep relaxation is a key tool for pain reduction. This is an active process requiring daily practice. The therapist helps the patient find the most effective technique to achieve relaxation, be it muscle relaxation, gentle movement, breathing techniques, visualization, hypnosis, or meditation.
2. A graduated exercise program that incorporates stretching, aerobic, strengthening, and stabilizing exercises should be developed *(see above)*. Slow stretching of the entire body may reduce tension and provide a sense of well-being. Walking, swimming, and cycling are examples of appropriate aerobic exercise. The daily exercise routine should include strengthening and stabilizing exercises that may encompass not only areas of weakness but the entire body. Factors that discourage patients from exercising include the beliefs that exercise causes damage and that rest cures chronic pain. The therapist should assist the patient in creating a program that balances rest and movement.
3. Education may benefit both the physician and the patient. Whereas acute pain requires a search for the etiology, chronic pain may exist independently of the original stimulus. Pain is influenced by attention, anxiety, suggestion, prior conditioning, and other psychological factors. When negative thoughts and feelings evolve as a result of these factors (Table 27), the body may respond with

Table 27
A Sequence of Negative Thoughts and Feelings[a]

Thoughts	Feelings
The pain should be better now	Frustration
There must be something seriously wrong	Anxiety, fear
No one can diagnose what is wrong	Alarm
I will never get better	Depression
There is nothing anyone can do	Helplessness
I have to live with it	Hopelessness

[a]From ref. 63.

Table 28
Therapeutic Behavioral Modifications[a]

Behaviors to Increase	Behaviors to Decrease
Pleasurable activities	Searching for causes and cures
Meaningful activities	Focusing on pain
Relaxing	Resting
Pacing activities	Overdoing or underdoing
Movement for enjoyment, fitness, mobility	Avoidance of movement
Setting realistic goals	Panicking
Taking responsibility for treatment	Being helpless
Taking control of life	Being a victim

[a]From ref. 63.

increased muscle tension, postural changes, guarding, and restricted movement, leading to further pain and a vicious cycle of pain amplification. Whatever the cause of the pain, patients can learn techniques to make the pain more tolerable. Table 28 outlines therapeutic behavioral modifications. Developing a belief in reversibility creates opportunities for healing that are unavailable if the patient believes there is no hope for improvement (Table 29). An important part of the education process can be to dispel certain myths (Table 30).

4. Occupation can be an important tool in pain relief. Pain may be less significant when a person is occupied, especially if the occupation is satisfying and meaningful to the patient. Return to the work environment should be encouraged as soon as possible, even if the patient needs to begin with work restrictions and limited hours. Some employers do not accept this approach, and the patient may need to find a new occupation; this may also enhance the healing process by providing new opportunities and challenges.

Biofeedback

Biofeedback represents a form of behavioral therapy that utilizes instrumentation to provide information about otherwise nonconscious physiologic processes. Through

Table 29
A Comparison of Self-Defeating and Healing Thoughts[a]

Self-Defeating Thoughts	Healing Thoughts
I will never get better	I am learning to cope and heal myself
I am afraid of the pain	As I relax, the pain diminishes
I am afraid of the future	I am learning to live in the present
Nobody understands	I continue to heal myself whether or not they understand
There is nothing I can do	I am learning how I can help myself

[a]From ref. 63.

Table 30
Chronic Pain Myths[a]

You have to learn to live with it
Rest cures chronic pain
Let pain be your guide
Hurt is harm
Real pain is organic
Search long enough and you will find the cause and the cure
Abnormal imaging studies validate and explain the pain

[a]From ref. 63.

feedback from visual or auditory signals, the subject learns to control voluntarily a normally involuntary facet of physiology that may be linked to the pathogenesis of a given disease. This technique has been used to treat many pain syndromes as well as certain other disorders, such as Raynaud's phenomenon.

The most common use of biofeedback has been the treatment of headache or back pain using electromyographic (EMG) feedback from the affected region. In some headache studies, muscle tension levels did not correlate strongly with headache severity, and decreased muscle tension did not seem to decrease pain. This may reflect the involvement of factors other than muscle tension in the pathogenesis of these headaches rather than lack of efficacy of biofeedback. Other studies have reported that pseudobiofeedback is as effective as "real" biofeedback in the treatment of chronic pain, suggesting that benefit may be related to nonspecific factors such as the placebo effect (62).

A recent study analyzed the efficacy of biofeedback-assisted relaxation vs self-relaxation for treatment of migraine headache (64). Over an 8- to 12-wk period, the biofeedback group was trained to decrease forehead muscle tension using EMG biofeedback during four sessions and to increase finger temperature using thermal biofeedback during eight sessions. The authors reported that the biofeedback group had less headache pain and fewer medication requirements than the self-relaxation group upon evaluation 4–6 wk after treatment. Although the relaxation techniques varied somewhat between the groups and some differences did not achieve statistical significance, this study supports the benefit of biofeedback as an aid to relaxation.

The combination of biofeedback with operant behavioral therapy has been evaluated in an outpatient rehabilitation program treating patients with chronic pain and excess disability *(65)*. Patients were informed that the purpose of the treatment was neither to cure pain nor disease but rather to rehabilitate them to function as normally as possible. The program included 1 or 2 family sessions, 5–10 biofeedback sessions, and 15–20 sessions of physical and occupational therapy over a period of 5–6 wk.

The family sessions, which included a psychologist, the patient, and family members, utilized operant behavioral therapy techniques to reduce domestic and other reinforcements for disability and to increase reinforcements for activity. Biofeedback sessions offered muscle relaxation and stress management training, during which the therapists did not respond to or reinforce verbalizations of pain or other pain behaviors. The physical and occupational therapy program consisted of graduated, twice-daily exercises for strength, endurance, stretching, cardiovascular fitness, posture, body mechanics, and activities of daily living. Patients unable to perform exercise or activity at any level for three consecutive days were informed that they would be discharged from the program, since it would be unable to help them. At the conclusion of the program, participants were instructed to continue indefinitely a physical therapy exercise program at home for about 60 min each day. Outcomes were measured from patient responses to a questionnaire administered at intervals during a 2-yr period of evaluation.

The authors reported that pain reduction occurred within the first month of treatment and continued during the study period. Patients noted decreased disability with improvement in sitting, standing, walking, playing, family interactions, and sleeping. Of those patients answering the question as to whether the program helped them, virtually all described benefit after the first month, and 80–90% reported improvement at 6, 12, and 24 mo. No attempt was made to determine the relative contribution of each therapeutic modality to the improvement described. Although this study suffers from the absence of a control group, incomplete data collection, and reliance solely on patient self-assessment for all variables studied, it suggests that outpatient behavioral management of chronic pain is feasible in a cost-conscious society.

The difficulty in scientifically establishing the role of these behavioral techniques in the treatment of pain of various etiologies is illustrated by several additional studies. One study reported that among patients with chronic back pain or temporomandibular joint (TMJ) dysfunction, EMG biofeedback from the site of pain was more beneficial than cognitive behavioral therapy or conservative medical treatment *(66)*. Another concluded that, among patients with chronic low back pain, cognitive behavioral therapy and EMG biofeedback were equivalent but better than no intervention *(67)*. A third demonstrated no significant difference between treatment of chronic nonmalignant pain in a multidisciplinary pain clinic with outpatient cognitive behavioral therapy compared to supportive therapy with amitriptyline, although the authors noted a trend favoring the former *(68)*.

These data suggest that behavioral therapy provides benefit to some patients with chronic pain. Although the relative efficacy of cognitive behavioral therapy, operant conditioning, biofeedback, relaxation, and other behavioral techniques for treating pain remains to be established, some data suggest that a combination of these modalities may yield the greatest benefit. In most instances, these techniques will be provided in the setting of a multidisciplinary pain clinic.

PAIN CLINICS

The publication of *The Management of Pain* by Dr. John Bonica in 1953 marked the beginning of the systematic treatment of pain as an entity in itself. The recognition that a group of patients does not respond to conservative medical treatment combined with growing awareness of the role of psychosocial factors in the development and maintenance of chronic pain fostered an environment conducive to the emergence of multidisciplinary pain clinics *(69)*.

A comprehensive pain clinic may include staff from anesthesiology, neurology, psychiatry or psychology, physical and rehabilitation medicine, physical therapy, occupational therapy, nursing, nutrition, and pharmacy. Pain clinics may offer either inpatient or outpatient treatment, although outpatient therapy is considerably more likely in the current health care environment.

Pain clinic programs generally include a detailed evaluation during which the physical and psychological needs of the patient are incorporated into a treatment plan. In many instances, nerve blocks or trigger point injections will be utilized diagnostically or therapeutically. This may be of particular benefit to patients with regional pain. Psychological services may range from individual and group counseling to behavioral strategies, including coping techniques, relaxation training, biofeedback, and stress management. Treatment often includes physical therapy modalities such as hot or cold packs, ultrasound, or TENS to decrease pain as well as active physical therapy to increase muscle strength, flexibility, and endurance. An occupational therapist can analyze activities of daily living at home and other sites of work and suggest ways to pace these activities. Vocational services may be offered to help the patient return to productive activity. Educational services may include instruction on back care or other relevant topics. Attempts may be made to decrease drug dependence and abuse by gradual withdrawal of agents such as barbiturates, alcohol, benzodiazepines, and narcotics. However, some patients do require narcotics and may have been undertreated, whereas, for others, elimination of these drugs may actually decrease pain and promote other desirable goals, such as improved social interaction.

Diagnoses that may be appropriate for referral to a pain clinic include headache, chronic back pain and other myofascial pain syndromes, neuropathy, reflex sympathetic dystrophy, phantom limb pain, atypical facial pain, chest pain, abdominal pain, pelvic pain, cancer pain, and pain following surgery or trauma. Candidates for treatment at a pain clinic should be motivated individuals without major conscious secondary gain or malingering (Table 31). Patients involved in pain-related litigation may be advised to resolve the legal issues prior to enrollment.

The elimination of pain is an unrealistic objective for most patients with chronic pain syndrome, even though some patients will derive considerable benefit from local injections. The goal of the multidisciplinary pain clinic is to help the individual move from the illness role of "patient" to the wellness role of "person" by increasing activity level and vocational status and by reducing pain behaviors, life disruption, dependence on

Table 31
Criteria for Referral to Pain Clinic[a]

Adequate medical evaluation
Pain refractory to conventional therapy
Significant pain behavior and life disruption
Psychosocial difficulties
Medication dependence
Patient motivated to change

[a]From ref. *69.*

medication and the health care system, and secondary gain *(69).* To the extent that these objectives are fulfilled, pain clinics represent more cost-effective treatment than fragmented and prolonged medical care which fails to improve pain and function.

REFERENCES

1. Merskey H, Bogduk N, eds. Classification of Chronic Pain, 2nd ed. Seattle: IASP, 1994.
2. Rummans TA. Symposium on pain management. Introduction. Mayo Clin Proc 1994; 69: 373,374.
3. Cross SA. Symposium on pain management. Part I. Pathophysiology of pain. Mayo Clin Proc 1994; 69: 375–383.
4. Rains C, Bryson HM. Topical capsaicin: a review of its pharmacological properties and therapeutic potential in post-herpetic neuralgia, diabetic neuropathy and osteoarthritis. Drugs and Aging 1995; 7: 317–328.
5. Cancer Pain Guideline Panel. Management of cancer pain: adults. Am Family Physician 1994; 49: 1853–1868.
6. Hochberg MC, Altman RD, Brandt KD, et al. Guidelines for the medical management of osteoarthritis. Part I. Osteoarthritis of the hip. Arthritis Rheum 1995; 38: 1535–1540.
7. Hochberg MC, Altman RD, Brandt KD, et al. Guidelines for the medical management of osteoarthritis. Part II. Osteoarthritis of the knee. Arthritis Rheum 1995; 38: 1541–1546.
8. Taha AS, Hudson N, Hawkey CJ, et al. Famotidine for the prevention of gastric and duodenal ulcers caused by nonsteroidal antiinflammatory drugs. N Eng J Med 1996; 334: 1435–1439.
9. Insel PA. Analgesic-antipyretic and antiinflammatory agents and drugs employed in the treatment of gout. In: Hardman JG, Limbird LE, Molinoff PB, Ruddon RW, Gilman AG, eds. Goodman and Gilman's the Pharmacologic Basis of Therapeutics, 9th ed. New York: McGraw Hill, 1996: 617–656.
10. Tyler DC. Pharmacology of pain management. Ped Clin N Ann 1994; 41: 59–71.
11. Marshall KA. Managing cancer pain: basic principles and invasive treatments. Mayo Clin Proc 1996; 71: 472–477.
12. Lamer TJ. Symposium on pain management. Part II. Treatment of cancer-related pain: when orally administered medications fail. Mayo Clin Proc 1994; 69: 473–480.
13. Tutak U, Doleys DM. Intrathecal infusion systems for treatment of chronic low back and leg pain of noncancer origin. South Med J 1996; 89: 295–300.
14. Hammack JE, Loprinzi CL. Symposium on pain management. Part I. Use of orally administered opioids for cancer-related pain. Mayo Clin Proc 1994; 69: 384–390.
15. Reidenberg MM, Portenoy RK. The need for an open mind about the treatment of chronic nonmalignant pain. Clin Pharmacol Ther 1994; 55: 367–369.
16. Foley KM. Misconceptions and controversies regarding the use of opioids in cancer pain. Anti-Cancer Drugs 1995; 6: 4–13.
17. Tramadol—a new oral analgesic. Med Lett Drugs Ther 1995; 37: 59,60.
18. O'Brien CP. Drug addiction and drug abuse. In: Hardman JG, Limbird LE, Molinoff PB, Ruddon RW, Gilman AG, eds. Goodman and Gilman's The Pharmacologic Basis of Therapeutics, 9th ed. New York: McGraw Hill, 1996: 557–577.

19. Portenoy RK. Pharmacologic management of cancer pain. Sem Oncol 1995; 22: 112–120.
20. Porter J, Jick H. Addiction rare in patients treated with narcotics. N Eng J Med 1980; 302: 123.
21. Prescription or administration of controlled substances; intractable pain; application; denial, revocation, suspension of physician's and surgeon's license. California Business and Professions Code. 1994; section 2241.5.
22. Medical Board of California. Treatment of intractable pain: a guideline. Action Report 1996; 57: 1,6.
23. Rummans TA. Nonopioid agents for the treatment of acute and subacute pain. Mayo Clin Proc 1994; 69: 481–490.
24. Portenoy RK. Update on the pharmacotherapy of chronic pain. In: American Academy of Neurology Symposium on Pain, San Francisco, CA, 24 March 1996; 49–84.
25. McQuay HJ, Carroll D, Glynn CJ. Dose-response for analgesic effect of amitriptyline in chronic pain. Anaesthesia 1993; 48: 281–285.
26. Hegarty A, Portenoy RK. Pharmacotherapy of neuropathic pain. Sem Neurol 1994; 14: 213–224.
27. McQuay H, Carroll D, Jadad AR, Wiffen P, Moore A. Anticonvulsant drugs for management of pain: a systematic review. BMJ 1995; 311: 1047–1052.
28. Levy M. Pharmacologic management of cancer pain. Sem Oncol 1994; 21: 718–739.
29. Rosner H, Rubin L, Kestenbaum A. Gabapentin adjunctive therapy in neuropathic pain states. Clin J Pain 1996; 12: 56–58.
30. Glynn C, Dawson D, Sanders R. A double-blind comparison between epidural morphine and epidural clonidine in patients with chronic non-cancer pain. Pain 1988; 34: 123–128.
31. Portenoy RK, Kanner RM. Nonopioid and adjuvant analgesics. In: Portenoy RK, Kanner RM, eds. Pain Management: Theory and Practice. Philadelphia: FA Davis, 1996: 219–247.
32. Lechin F, van der Dijs B, Lechin ME, et al. Pimozide therapy for trigeminal neuralgia. Arch Neurol 1989; 46: 960–963.
33. Gomez-Perez FJ, Rull JA, Dies H, et al. Nortriptyline and fluphenazine in the symptomatic treatment of diabetic neuropathy: a double-blind cross-over study. Pain 1985; 23: 395–400.
34. Winter J, Bevan S, Campbell EA. Capsaicin and pain mechanisms. Br J Anaesthesia 1995; 75: 157–168.
35. Birmingham PK. Recent advances in acute pain management. Curr Probl Pediatr 1995; 25: 99–112.
36. Jain S. Nerve blocks. In: Warfield CA, ed. Principles and Practice of Pain Management. New York: McGraw-Hill, 1993: 379–400.
37. Katz N. Role of invasive procedures in chronic pain management. Sem Neurol 1994; 14: 225–236.
38. Spaccarelli, KC. Lumbar and caudal epidural corticosteroid injections. Mayo Clin Proc 1996; 71: 169–178.
39. Sandrock NJG, Warfield CA. Epidural steroids and facet injections. In: Warfield CA, ed. Principles and Practice of Pain Management. New York: McGraw-Hill, 1993: 401–412.
40. Koes BW, Scholten RJPM, Mens JMA, Bouter LM. Efficacy of epidural steroid injections for low-back pain and sciatica: a systematic review of randomized clinical trials. Pain 1995; 63: 279–288.
41. Doyle E, Spence M. Cannabis as a medicine? Br J Anaesth 1995; 74: 359–361 (editorial).
42. Kassirer J. Federal foolishness and marijuana. N Eng J Med 1997; 336: 366,367 (editorial).
43. Medical Board of California. Physicians, proposition 215, and the Medical Board of California. Action Report. 1997; 60: 5.
44. Little PJ, Compton DR, Johnson MR, Melvin LS, Martin BR. Pharmacology and stereoselectivity of structurally novel cannabinoids in mice. J Pharmacol Exp Ther 1988; 247: 1046–1051.
45. Nissel H. Pain treatment by means of acupuncture. Acup Electrother Res Int J 1993; 18: 1–8.
46. McLean B, Fives EH. Stimulation-induced analgesia. In: Warfield CA, ed. Principles and Practice of Pain Management. New York: McGraw-Hill, 1993; 413–425.
47. Wall PD. The gate theory of pain mechanisms: a reexamination and restatement. Brain 1978; 101: 1–18.
48. Price DD, Mayer DJ. Evidence for endogenous opiate analgesic mechanisms triggered by somatosensory stimulation (including acupuncture) in humans. Pain Forum 1995; 4: 40–43.
49. Molsberger A, Hille E. The analgesic effect of acupuncture in chronic tennis elbow pain. Br J Rheum 1994; 33: 1162–1165.
50. Price DD, Rafii A, Watkins LR, Buckingham B. A psychophysical analysis of acupuncture analgesia. Pain 1984; 19: 27–42.
51. Lewith G, Vincent C. Evaluation of the clinical effects of acupuncture. Pain Forum 1995; 4: 29–39.

52. Thomas M, Lundberg T. Importance of modes of acupuncture in the treatment of chronic nociceptive low back pain. Acta Anesthesiol Scand 1994; 38: 63–69.

53. Bengston R. Physical measures for pain relief. In: Warfield CA, ed. Principles and Practice of Pain Management. New York: McGraw-Hill, 1993; 427–436.

54. Walsh DM, Foster NE, Baxter GD, Allen JM. Transcutaneous electric nerve stimulation: relevance of stimulation parameters to neurophysiological and hypoalgesic effects. Am J Phys Med Rehabil 1995; 74: 199–206.

55. Deyo RA, Walsh NE, Martin DC, Schoenfeld LS, Ramamurthy S. A controlled trial of transcutaneous electrical nerve stimulation (TENS) and exercise for chronic low back pain. N Eng J Med 1990; 322: 1627–1634.

56. Marchand S, Charest J, Li J, Chenard J-R, Lavignolle B, Laurencelle L. Is TENS purely a placebo effect? A controlled study on chronic low back pain. Pain 1993; 54: 99–106.

57. Lewis B, Lewis D, Cumming G. The comparative analgesic efficacy of transcutaneous electrical nerve stimulation and a nonsteroidal antiinflammatory drug for painful osteoarthritis. Br J Rheum 1994; 33: 455–460.

58. Meyler WJ, de Jongste MJL, Rolf CAM. Clinical evaluation of pain treatment with electrostimulation: a study on TENS in patients with different pain syndromes. Clin J Pain 1994; 10: 22–27.

59. Lehmann JF, De Lateur BJ. Diathermy and superficial heat, laser, and cold therapy. In: Kottke FJ, Lehmann JF, eds. Krusen's Handbook of Physical Medicine and Rehabilitation, 4th ed. Philadelphia: WB. Saunders, 1990; 283–367.

60. Grabois M, McCann MT, Schramm D, Straja A, Smith A. Chronic pain syndromes: evaluation and treatment. In: Braddom, RL, ed. Physical Medicine & Rehabilitation. Philadelphia: WB Saunders, 1996; 876–892.

61. Fordyce WE. Distorted gait—a problem of shaping. In: Fordyce WE. Behavioral Methods for Chronic Pain and Illness. Saint Louis: CV Mosby, 1976; 184–189.

62. Domar AD, Friedman R, Benson H. Behavioral therapy. In: Warfield CA, ed. Principles and Practice of Pain Management. New York: McGraw-Hill, 1993; 437–444.

63. McIndoe R. A behavioural approach to the management of chronic pain. Aust Fam Physician 1994; 23: 2284–2292.

64. McGrady A, Wauquier A, McNeil A, Gerard G. Effect of biofeedback-assisted relaxation on migraine headache and changes in cerebral blood flow velocity in the middle cerebral artery. Headache 1994; 34: 424–428.

65. Roberts AH, Sternbach RA, Polich J. Behavioral management of chronic pain and excess disability: long-term follow-up of an outpatient program. Clin J Pain 1993; 9: 41–48.

66. Flor H, Birbaumer N. Comparison of the efficacy of electromyographic biofeedback, cognitive-behavioral therapy, and conservative medical interventions in the treatment of chronic musculoskeletal pain. J Consulting Clinical Psychology 1993; 61: 653–658.

67. Newton-John TRO, Spence SH, Schotte D. Cognitive-behavioural therapy versus EMG biofeedback in the treatment of chronic low back pain. Behav Res Ther 1995; 33: 691–697.

68. Pilowsky I, Spence N, Rounsefell B, Forsten C, Soda J. One patient cognitive-behavioural therapy with amitriptyline for chronic non-malignant pain: a comparative study with 6-month follow-up. Pain 1995; 60: 49–54.

69. Aronoff GM. The role of pain clinics. In: Warfield CA, ed. Principles and Practice of Pain Management. New York: McGraw-Hill, 1993; 481–491.

15 Legal Issues in Pain Management: Walking the Tightrope Between Legal Restrictions and Medical Ethics

Charles Bond, JD
Susan L. Ballard, JD

Key Points

- Physicians have an ethical and legal duty to effectively diagnose and manage pain.

- Physicians must be aware of federal and state laws, which have an impact on prescribing controlled substances for management of pain; and they must keep these in mind when developing treatment plans.

- Systematic adherence to medically based, peer-reviewed and nationally recognized guidelines, documentation of a good faith prior examination and outlining parameters of treatment plans will assist physicians in defending themselves against enforcement agency actions related to the prescribing of controlled substances.

- Physicians should become aware of cost issues and reimbursement biases for certain treatment approaches.

- The legality of physician-assisted suicide is in a state of flux, and susceptible to change in the next few years.

INTRODUCTION

A Canadian farmer took action: No longer able to tolerate helplessly watching his daughter exist—afflicted with cerebral palsy, a permanently dislocated hip, constant pain, and inability to walk, sleep, or eat by herself—he placed her in the cab of his pick-up truck and ran a hose from the gas pipe into the cab in order to end her life of pain. A Canadian jury heard testimony on this "mercy killing" in 1994 and found the father guilty of second-degree murder, which carries a minimum prison term of life with no possibility of parole for 10 yr. The Canadian Supreme Court ruled in February 1997 that Mr. Latmer would have a new trial.

This heart-wrenching scene may become only too common. In larger terms, that Canadian jury may as well have indicted the medical profession as a whole for its failure to effectively manage pain. How is it, in a world that has made amazing advances in medical technology to the extent of prolonging life, that the medical profession has not proved itself equally capable or willing to control pain? A 1995 editorial in *JAMA (1)* queried rhetorically, "When Will Adequate Pain Treatment Be the Norm?" According to a recent survey of oncologists, only 11% of the respondents believed they received good or excellent training in pain management during medical school, and only 27% though they had such training during residency *(2)*.

The challenge of effectively managing pain is not unique to American medicine: The World Health Organization (WHO) has recognized cancer pain, in particular, to be a problem of international scope and has urged that every nation considering legislation on euthanasia give a high priority to establishing a cancer pain relief policy *(3)*. In addition, the WHO published an analgesic ladder for pain treatment *(4)*. As a further indication of the international aspects of the problem, a recent feature story in a leading French periodical queried whether there should be a law against suffering in order to encourage physicians to consecrate more effort to alleviating that pervasive medical problem *(5)*.

It may be that inadequate pain management is less a function of insufficient knowledge than concern about legal controls governing the prescription of opiates, and public attitudes, as well as patient fears, regarding potential addiction to this method of pain control. This article will (1) provide a framework for reference on federal and state controls on drug prescribing; (2) review in depth California's approach to regulating prescription of controlled substances and exceptions for intractable pain as an example of one state's approach; (3) review the impact of "alternative medicine" to narcotics-based treatment and associated economic reimbursement issues; and (4) review the current debate on physician-assisted suicide and the status of that concept within the medical and legal field.

LEGAL RESTRICTIONS ON PRESCRIBING AND DISPENSING CONTROLLED SUBSTANCES

Physicians have traditionally treated pain through a narcotics-based approach. While most physicians recognize an ethical duty to manage pain and relieve a patient's suffering, some may feel constrained by legal limitations on prescribing controlled substances. This section will review the basic framework of federal and state regulation of the prescription of controlled substances as they relate to physician management of pain.

Federal Laws and the Jurisdiction of the Drug Enforcement Agency

Partially as a result of the American "war on drugs," several statutory and regulatory schemes are in place to control the availability of drugs, and particularly opiates, which are often used for cancer patients and patients with other types of chronic pain. The principal laws that govern the prescribing of controlled substances are the federal Controlled Substances Act (CSA) *(6)* and the Federal Food, Drug and Cosmetic Act (FFDCSA) *(7)*, which the Drug Enforcement Agency (DEA) and the Food and Drug Administration (FDA), respectively, enforce.

Physicians must become aware of the federal and state regulations concerning prescribing pain medication outlined below, since there are significant legal consequences associated with the unauthorized prescription of controlled substances. Under federal law, "a prescription for a controlled substance, to be effective, must be issued for a legitimate medical purpose by an individual practitioner acting in the usual course of his or her professional practice" (21 Code of Federal Regulations (CFR) Section 1306.4.). Any person who knowingly or intentionally issues a prescription, while not acting in the usual course of his or her professional practice or for a nonlegitimate medical purpose, is subject to prosecution under Title 21 of the United States Code Section 841 *(8)*. In addition, violation of laws governing the prescribing of controlled substances is likely to lead to a loss of a physician's DEA registration and prescribing privileges. Such convictions may also result in exclusion of the provider from the Medicare and Medicaid programs.

Most state drug laws are patterned after the model Uniform Controlled Substances Act (UCSA), developed by the National Conference of Commissioners on the Uniform State Laws (NCCUSL) *(9)*. The NCCUSL provides model laws for states in order to establish a consistent policy framework among the states and between the states and federal government. The UCSA, like the Federal CSA, was approved in 1970 and promulgated to the states for adoption. The law was subsequently amended in 1990 and 1994. (*See* Table 1 for a summary of state laws corresponding to that model federal law.)

The Prefatory Note to the 1990 Uniform Controlled Substances Act indicates that the drug abuse problem in the United States had reached epidemic proportions and manifested itself in every segment of society and every region of the United States. The Note further states that the primary purpose of the Uniform Act is to coordinate the codified system of drug control initiated by the 1970 Uniform Controlled Substances Act. The 1990 revision was intended to update and improve existing state laws and ensure legislative and administrative flexibility to enable the states to cope with both present and future drug problems. Of particular interest to physicians, the Prefatory Note observes:

> Because of the emphasis on controlling drug use, members of the medical profession may hesitate to prescribe narcotic drugs where use of such drugs is warranted. This Act addresses this concern. Legitimate use of controlled substances is essential for public health and safety, and the availability of these substances must be assured. At the same time, the illegitimate manufacture, distribution and possession of controlled substances must be curtailed and eliminated *(10)*.

The federal Controlled Substances Act and the variations adopted by individual states apply to all practitioners prescribing controlled substances in the course of professional practice or research *(11)*. The Act defines five categories of controlled substances (Class I-Class V), which range from those substances with high potential for abuse and no accepted medical use in the United States (Schedule I) to substances with a low potential for abuse and a currently accepted medical use in the United States (Schedule V) *(12)*.

Table 1
Uniform Controlled Substances Act
(Table of Jurisdictions Wherein Either the 1970, 1990, or 1994 Versions of the Act or a Combination Thereof Has Been Adopted[a])

Jurisdiction	Laws	Effective Date	Statutory Citation
Alabama	1971, no. 140	9-16-1971[c]	Code 1975 §§ 20-2-1 to 20-2-190
Alaska	1982, c. 45	1-1-1983	AS 11.71.010 to 11.71.900, 17.30.010 to 17.30.900
Arizona	1979, c. 103	7-1-1980	A.R.S. §§ 36-2501 to 36-2553
Arkansas[b]	1971, no. 590	4-7-1971	A.C.A. §§ 5-64-101 to 5-64-608
California	1972, c. 1407	3-7-1973	West's Ann. Cal. Health & Safety Code §§ 11000 to 11651
Colorado	1981, pp. 707 to 728		West's C.R.S.A. §§ 18-18-101 to 18-18-605
Connecticut	1967, no. 555	6-21-1967	C.G.S.A. §§ 21a-240 to 21a-308
Delaware	1972, c. 424	6-13-1972[c]	16 Del.C. §§ 4701 to 4796
District of Columbia	1981, D.C.Law 4-29		D.C.Code 1981, §§ 33-501 to 33-573
Florida	1973, c. 331	7-1-1973	West's F.S.A. §§ 893.01 to 893.165
Georgia	1974, p. 221	7-1-1974	O.C.G.A. §§ 16-13-20 to 16-13-56
Hawaii	1972, c. 10	1-1-1973	HRS §§ 329-1 to 329-58
Idaho	1971, c. 215	5-1-1971	I.C. §§ 37-2701 to 37-2751
Illinois	1971, P.A. 77-757	8-16-1971	S.H.A. 750 ILCS 35/1 to 35/26
Indiana	1976, P.L. 148	7-1-1977	I.C. 35-48-1-1 to 35-48-4-15
Iowa	1971, c. 148	7-1-1971	I.C.A. §§ 124.101 to 124.602
Kansas	1972, c. 234	7-1-1972	K.S.A. 65-4101 to 65-4141
Kentucky	1972, c. 226	7-1-1972	KRS 218A.010 to 218A.993
Louisiana	1972, no. 634	7-26-1972	LSA-R.S. 40:961 to 40:995
Maine	1975, c. 499	5-1-1976	17-A M. R.S. A §§ 1101 to 1116
	1941, c. 251	4-16-1941	22 M.R.S.A §§ 2383, 2383-A, 2383-B
Maryland	1970, c. 403	7-1-1970	Code 1957, an. 27, §§ 276 to 303
Massachusetts	1971, c. 1071	7-1-1972	M.G.L.A. c. 94C, §§ 1 to 48
Michigan	1978, no. 368	9-30-1978	M.C.L.A. §§ 333.7101 to 333.7545
Minnesota	1971, c. 937	6-18-1971	M.S.A. §§ 152.01 to 152.20
Mississippi	1971, c. 521	4-16-1971	Code 1972, §§ 141-29-101 to 41-29-185
Missouri	1971, H.B. No. 69	9-28-1971	V.A.M.S. §§ 1195.010 to 195.320
Montana	1973, c. 412	7-1-1973	MCA 50-32-101 to 50-32-405
Nebraska	1971, LB 326	5-26-1971	R.R.S. 1943 § 28-401 et seq.

Jurisdiction	Laws	Effective date	Code citation
Nevada	1971, c. 667	1-1-1972	N.R.S., 453.011 et seq.
New Jersey	1970, c. 226	1-17-1971	N.J.S.A. 2C:35-1 to 2C:35-23, 2C:36-1 to 2C36-9, 24:21-1 to 24:21-53
New Mexico	1972, c. 84	4-1-1973	NMSA 1978, §§ 30-31-1 to 30-31-41
New York	1972, c. 878	1-1-1972	McKinneys Public Health Law §§ 3300 to 3396
North Carolina	1971, c. 919	7-1-1971	G.S. §§ 90-86 to 90-113.8
North Dakota	1971, c. 919	7-1-1976	NDCC 19-03.1-01 to 19-03.1-43
Ohio	1975, p. 269	9-1-1971	R.C. §§ 3719.01 to 3719.99
Oklahoma	1971, c. 119	7-1-1978	63 Okl.St.Ann.§§ 2-101 to 2-610
Oregon	1977, c. 745	6-14-1972	ORS 475.005 to 475.295, 475.940 to 475.999
Pennsylvania	1972, no. 64	180 d after 6-23-1971	35.P.S. §§ 780-101 to 780-144
Puerto Rico	1971, no. 4		24 L.P.R.A. §§ 2101 to 2607
Rhode Island	1974, c. 183	7-1-1974	Gen. Laws 1956, §§ 21-28-1.01 to 21-28-6.02
South Carolina	1971, p. 800	6-17-1971	Code 1976, §§ 44-53-110 to 44-53-590
South Dakota	1970, c. 229	2-13-1970	SDCL 34-20B-1 to 34-20B-114
Tennessee	1971, c. 163	7-1-1971	West's Tenn. Code §§ 39-6-401 to 39-6-419, 53-11-30-1 to 53-11-414
Texas	1973, c. 429	8-27-1973	V.T.C.A Health & Safety Code, §§ 481.001 to 842.005
Utah	1971, c. 145	1-1-1972	U.C.A. 1953, 58-37-1 to 58-37-21
Virgin Islands	1971, no. 2961	30 d foll. 3-23-1971	19 V.I.C. §§ 591 to 631
Virginia	1970, c. 650	4-5-1970[c]	Code 1950, § 54.1-3400 et seq.
Washington	1971, c. 308	5-21-1971	West's RCWA §§ 69.50.101 to 69.50.609
West Virginia	1971, c. 54	6-10-1971	Code, 60A-I-101 to 60A-6-605
Wisconsin	1971 c. 219	10-1-1972	W.S.A. 161.001 to 161.62
Wyoming	1971, c. 246	3-4-1971	W.S. 1977, §§ 35-7-1001 to 35-7-1057

[a]The 1970 and 1990 versions of the Uniform Controlled Substances Act, while different, are similar in many of their provisions. The acts of the adopting jurisdictions will, therefore, generally contain many provisions common to both versions. Thus it is often difficult to say with certitude that a jurisdiction has adopted one version of the act rather than the other. For that reason, all jurisdictions adopting the Uniform Controlled Substances Act will be carried in the same table found at the beginning of each of the versions of the act.

[b]Note that Arkansas has adopted and retains the major provisions of both the Uniform Narcotic Drug Act and the Uniform Controlled Substances Act. (See General Statutory Note, infra.)

[c]Date of approval.

The CSA's reporting system provides for registration, record keeping, and reporting, which enable enforcement agencies to identify the manufacturer, distributor, physician, or pharmacist who diverts controlled substances to illicit uses. Violation of any of these provisions can result in a variety of penalties. It is generally recognized that the states, not the Federal Government, regulate the practices of medicine and pharmacy and that federal law generally refers to state law in areas that do not directly conflict with it *(13)*.

State Regulation of Controlled Substances—Overview

State regulation of medical practices involving the prescription of opiates is often complex, but generally involves at least three major sets of laws: (1) Controlled Substances, (2) Medical Practice, and (3) Pharmacy Practice. The relevant administrative agencies controlling these matters may have rules that may be more restrictive than federal or state law, and state agencies with authority to enforce law or rules generally have their own philosophy and set of priorities. Numerous local enforcement agencies and prosecutors also have the authority to enforce state-controlled substance laws.

In general, state laws recognize the ability of the physician to prescribe controlled substances in good faith and in the course of professional practice. These laws recognize that some drugs have "currently accepted medical uses" for purposes of placement in the proper schedule. State laws, however, often lack the federal law provisions that contain affirmative language recognizing the essential value of controlled substances or the importance of ensuring drug availability. In addition, not all state laws contain provisions recognizing the opioid treatment of intractable pain (discussed later in the California Intractable Pain Act Section). Physicians should contact their state licensing boards for statutes and regulations governing prescription of controlled substances in their particular state *(14)*.

At least 10 states, including California, have also adopted a multiple-copy prescription program *(15)*. The programs differ by state. All permit the states to monitor physician prescription of Schedule II controlled substances to patients. These laws protect the confidentiality of the information but also allow the information to be shared with local, state, and federal law enforcement agencies. Under this system, prescriptions for Schedule II Substances must be written in triplicate, with copies distributed in accordance with applicable law *(16)*.

CALIFORNIA: A CASE STUDY OF ONE STATE'S FRAMEWORK FOR REGULATING PRESCRIPTION OF CONTROLLED SUBSTANCES, AND ITS IMPACT ON PAIN MANAGEMENT

Ethical and Legal Duty to Treat Pain

The duty to treat pain from a medical ethics standpoint derives from the commitment of the physician to refrain from harming the patient, enhancing the patient's welfare while weighing and balancing the possible benefits against the possible harms in order to maximize the benefits and minimize the risks of harm,

The legal duty to treat pain stems from a health care provider's potential liability to patients for inadequate pain management, which could be translated into damages for physical pain and suffering and emotional distress. Failure to adequately treat pain may also subject a physician to professional discipline if it is determined to be representative of unprofessional conduct or gross negligence (Business and Professions Code Section 2234).

General Authority of Physicians and Surgeons under California Law

Physicians and surgeons may use drugs and devices on humans, as provided for by Section 2051 of the California Business and Professions Code. The primary limitations on this practice include prohibitions against: (1) prescribing without a good faith exam; (2) excessive prescribing; and (3) prescribing controlled substances to an addict. Investigating complaints about physicians relating to these three areas of medical practice represents one of the highest enforcement priorities of the Medical Board of California (MBC). This section will review the prohibitions and published policy of the MBC concerning these activities.

Prohibitions Against Prescribing Medication Without a Good Faith Exam

The necessity for physicians to perform a good faith examination prior to issuing a prescription cannot be overemphasized. *See* the California Business and Professions Code Section 2242, which prohibits prescribing dangerous substances (defined in Business and Professions Code section 4211 as any drug unsafe for self-medication and which can only be dispensed pursuant to a prescription) without an underlying medical condition. The impetus for enforcement on this front stems from concern of maintaining a patient's addiction, and/or providing drugs to be diverted for sale and distribution on the street. The MBC has also addressed this issue as follows in its Guidelines for Expert Reviewers:

> It is unprofessional conduct to prescribe, dispense, or furnish dangerous drugs (prescription medications including controlled substances) without a "good faith prior examination and medical indication therefor." This covers the situation [in which] a physician simply prescribes a medication, usually a controlled substance, without any underlying pathology indicating a need for that medication. This also covers the situation [in which] a physician, knowing that a patient is addicted to a dangerous drugs, continues to prescribe that drug. Needless to say, there are many instances [in which] prescribing without medical indication and excessive prescribing overlap. In addition, there are instances in which excessive prescribing of drugs or prescribing drugs without medical indication also constitutes an extreme departure, repeated departures, or lack of knowledge or skill, depending [on] the evidence presented *(17)*.

If the physician errs on the side of not treating such pain, he or she risks liability for professional negligence and pain and suffering experienced by the patient. So how can physicians best proceed on this issue? Perhaps some of the best advice is that physicians must respect the basic requirements for appropriate patient management: perform a good faith exam before prescribing medication, discuss the source and intensity of the pain, and clearly document any changes in the progression of the pain (particularly those that warrant increased dosages). One of the risks physicians in California face with the current medical board is that of physician reviewers merely looking at the numbers—the dosage and frequency of prescription—without reviewing the patient's underlying pain symptoms and history. Should this happen, a physician must be able to justify the course of treatment through the documentation described above. It would also be useful to reference medically sound and recognized pain treatment guidelines that are compatible with the treatment pursued. Two potential sources for this are the Agency for Health Care Policy and Research (AHCPR) guidelines on Acute Pain Management and on Management of Cancer Pain *(18)*.

The ability to refer to national peer-reviewed treatment guidelines that are medically sound and widely accepted will be of increasing importance for physicians. For example, a Florida court recently found it inappropriate for a medical board committee to negate a hearing officer's finding that a physician's treatment plan wars consistent with the standard of care and with the AHCPR guidelines *(19)*. The committee chose instead to rely on a pure analysis of the pharmaceutical records despite the fact that the medical reviewers themselves indicated they could not evaluate the appropriateness of the treatment without reviewing the patient's medical reports. One can only hope that other state licensing boards for health professionals will appreciate the need for reviewing patient records. In anticipation of this enlightenment, it will be important for physicians to maintain records that clearly support pain management decisions.

Prohibitions Against Excessive Prescribing

Despite the ethical and legal obligations that compel physicians to effectively manage their patients' pain, state regulation of prescribing and discipline of physicians, often based on review of numbers only, can present significant obstacles to this endeavor. This potential impediment to adequate pain management is grounded in the prohibition against excessive prescribing and administration of drugs found in Business and Professions Code Section 725.

The parameters of MBC enforcement action against excessive prescribing can probably best be appreciated by reference to the MBC Guidelines for Expert Reviewers:

> Excessive prescribing often involves controlled substances, but not always. Generally, the assessment as to whether prescribing for a particular patient was excessive has to do with the nature of the medical complaint and the amount and frequency of the prescription of drugs. This can be a single drug, a class of drugs (such as opiates or amphetamines), or a pattern of prescribing large amounts of drugs without justification. An action under this section can also be sustained if the drug itself is not being given in excessive amounts, by ordinary standards, but is being knowingly given in excessive amounts for a given patient's condition. For instance, repeatedly prescribing a drug in the same amounts for a patient who has repeatedly attempted suicide on that drug constitutes excessive prescribing *(20)*.

To date, only one California court has interpreted Section 725 of the Business and Professions Code. In the underlying case, the physician's conduct resulted in the death of the patient, and the court of appeal upheld the discipline imposed by the MBC, because it found that the unrefuted and uncontradicted expert testimony in the case established that the physician repeatedly prescribed lethal dosages of drugs to his patient: Therefore, the court found, the physician's conduct was an "extreme departure from the community standard of practice" *(21)*.

Pain Management and Addiction

Potential disciplinary action for unprofessional conduct on the basis of prescribing to an addict or habitué, which is prohibited under Section 2241 of the Business and Professions Code, represents a further concern physicians face in prescribing controlled substances for pain. This is an infraction on which the MBC has also focused particular attention during the last few years. It is generally unlawful for a physician to prescribe controlled substances to an addict, but there are some exceptions in which the physician is also trained in addiction management.

Identifying who is an addict, however, may be a daunting task. Even California case law recognizes the difficulties in making this determination as demonstrated in *People v. Shade* (1994) 32 Cal.Rptr. 2nd 59, a case in which the court demonstrates through its review of the meaning of "addict" that the case law and statutory definitions of addict are neither well-established nor static. Since the definition of an addict or habitué is murky at best, physicians should attempt to protect themselves against possible discipline under this statute by always performing a good faith exam and conducting a thorough history of the patient.

Physicians face the additional concern of public reproof for turning patients "into addicts" by prescribing opiates for pain. One must question, however, the accuracy of this perception. Some studies indicate that addiction to narcotics is less frequent than one might think in patients who use them for pain control *(22)*. It is true that a patient can develop tolerance to opiates and require increased dosages in order to achieve the same relief; however, if this is turning a patient into an addict, then a further balancing of interests must be undertaken. What are the costs to society and the benefits to the individual, particularly in terms of quality of life, with respect to not providing such pain control where it is warranted? Studies of cancer patients have demonstrated that uncontrolled pain can lead, among other things, to decreased functional capacity, severe depression, lack of social functioning *(23)*. On the other hand, one must also evaluate whether the side effects of narcotic-based pain control (dizziness, loss of memory, and so on) will negate any quality of life achieved by reduced pain. Certainly this is a difficult question, and a fine line must be observed by physicians in determining appropriate management, and providing, to the extent possible, a pain-free life.

California Intractable Pain Act

The exception to scrutiny of prescribing methods on which physicians should be able to rely is found in Business and Professions Code Section 2241.5, the Intractable Pain Act, which provides that a physician and surgeon may prescribe or administer controlled substances to a person in the course of treatment of that person for a diagnosed condition causing intractable pain. The provision defines "intractable pain" as "a pain state in which the cause of the pain cannot be removed or otherwise treated" and for which "in the generally accepted course of medical practice no relief or cure of the cause of the pain is possible or none has been found after reasonable efforts." "Reasonable efforts" are not limited to, but must include "evaluation by the attending physicians and surgeon and one or more physicians and surgeons specializing in the treatment of the area, system, or organ of the body perceived as the source of the pain" (Business and Professions Code Section 2241.5[b]). It should be noted, however, that the Intractable Pain Act does not apply to anyone being treated by the physician for chemical dependency because of the use of drugs or controlled substances, and it does not authorize a physician to prescribe or administer a controlled substance to a patient the physician knows to be using the drugs or substances for nontherapeutic purposes. Furthermore, that statute does not limit the Medical Board's authority to deny, revoke, or suspend the license of a physician who does any of the following:

1. Prescribes or administers a controlled substance (or treatment) that is non-therapeutic either in its nature or in the manner the controlled substance (or treatment) is administered or prescribed.
2. Prescribes or administers a controlled substance (or treatment) that is for a nontherapeutic purpose in a nontherapeutic manner.
3. Fails to keep complete and accurate records of purchases and disposal of controlled substances that are listed in the California Controlled Substance Act or in the Federal Comprehensive Drug Abuse Prevention and Control Act of 1970. These records must include date of purchase, date and record of the sale or disposal of the drugs by the physician, name and address of the person receiving the drugs, and reason for either the disposal or dispensing of those drugs. Such records must also comply with all state record keeping requirements for controlled substances.
4. Writes false or fictitious prescriptions for controlled substances.
5. Prescribes, administers, or dispenses controlled substances in a manner not consistent with public health and welfare.
6. Otherwise prescribes, administers, or dispenses in violation of Chapters 4 or 5 of the Uniform Controlled Substances Act (found in Health and Safety Code section 11150 and 11210 and following) or provisions in the Business and Professions code dealing with the Healing Arts.

Finally, the statute does nothing to diminish the ability of a governing body of a hospital from taking disciplinary actions against a physician or surgeon under professional peer review procedures.

It appears that the MBC has recognized that insufficient treatment of intractable pain can be an even more significant problem than overtreatment, and that the tendency to undertreat can be explained by fear that a complaint for over prescribing may put place a physician's license in jeopardy. Such concern persists, the MBC acknowledges, despite guidelines released in 1994 by the MBC to complement the California Intractable Pain Act, which established California public policy as supportive of the responsible practice of pain management. The MBC republished those guidelines in April 1996 and emphasized that, as with any medical treatment, treatment of chronic pain

Table 2
Guidelines for Treatment of Intractable Pain

1. History/physical exam and evaluation by one or more specialists if controlled substances are to be prescribed for intractable pain.
2. Development of a treatment plan that specifies objectives by which to measure treatment success, such as pain relief and/or improved physical and psychosocial functions.
3. Informed consent: The physician should discuss the risks and benefits of the use of controlled substances with the patient or guardian.
4. Periodic review of the course of opioid treatment of the patient should be undertaken by the physician and any new information about the etiology of the pain should be noted.
5. Consultation: The physician should be willing to refer the patient, as necessary, for additional evaluation and treatment to achieve treatment objectives. Special attention should be paid to pain patients at risk for abusing their medications. Pain management for patients with a history of substance abuse requires additional care, monitoring, documentation and consultations with addiction specialists, and may entail use of agreements between the provider and patient to specify rules for medication use.
6. Records: The physician should keep accurate and complete records, including the medical history and physical examination, other evaluations and consultation, treatment plan objectives, informed consent, treatments, medications, agreements with the patient, and periodic reviews.
7. Compliance with controlled substances laws and regulations: The physician must be appropriately licensed in California and comply with federal and state regulations for issuing controlled substances prescriptions.

must be consistent with established medical standards that serve the patient's total well-being *(24)*.

A framework for such pain management treatment, according to the MBC, would involve at least seven elements. These are outlined in the Summary of Guidelines shown in Table 2. According to the MBC publication containing these guidelines, documented adherence to these guidelines will "substantially establish the physician's responsible treatment of patients with intractable pain and will serve to defend that treatment practice in the face of complaints that may be brought" *(25)*.

COST AND REIMBURSEMENT ISSUES

Costs Associated with "Traditional" Medicine

The encouraging aspect associated with the clinical guidelines for the treatment of Acute and Chronic Pain and Cancer related pain released by the AHCPR and the emergence of intractable pain statutes is that attention is finally being placed on a significant medical and societal problem. The magnitude of the problem varies according to each study on the subject, but some estimates indicate that of the 526,000 Americans estimated to have died from cancer in 1993, as many as 70% of them died in unrelieved pain *(26)*.

Many observers and clinicians hope that the increased attention on pain management will translate positively into effective relief for the estimated 23 million Americans undergoing surgery each year and the over 1.2 million Americans annually diagnosed with cancer *(27)*. Current pain management techniques range from orally administered opiates to patient controlled analgesics (PCAs) to epidural injections and spinal pump implants. The costs, both economic and to the patient's overall well-being, can range from minimal to several thousand dollars per month. In addition, many methods involve associated personnel costs in the form of home nursing visits, for which private insurers may only pay 80% of the costs. These additional costs should be taken into consideration by physicians when designing a pain control approach.

Physicians should also take into consideration certain treatment reimbursement biases. For example, Medicare does not reimburse for outpatient oral analgesics but will reimburse for pain management in an inpatient facility. This results in a situation in which a person may well have reimbursement for a $4000 patient-controlled analgesia morphine system, but no coverage for $100 for oral morphine solutions *(28)*.

Costs Associated with "Alternative" Medicine

During the past 30 yr, there has been an increased interest in holistic medicine and focus on mind/body techniques to address some medical conditions *(29)*. A National Institutes of Health Technology Assessment Panel performed an extensive review of literature and survey results from expert panels regarding the effectiveness of behavioral and relaxation approaches in the treatment of pain and insomnia *(30)*. The panel concluded that there exist a number of well-defined behavioral and relaxation interventions that are effective in treating chronic pain and insomnia. According to the panel, there is strong evidence for using relaxation techniques in reducing chronic pain in a variety of medical conditions and for using hypnosis in alleviating pain associated with cancer *(31)*. The summary of conclusions indicated that, although scientific literature demonstrates the effectiveness of these techniques, there is a need for thoughtful interpretation of the findings and prompt translation of the conclusions into health care delivery programs *(32)*. The panel further recognized that specific structural, bureaucratic, financial, and attitudinal barriers have impeded integration of these techniques; all those obstacles are potentially surmountable with education and additional research as patients move from being passive participants in their treatment to becoming responsible, active partners in their rehabilitation *(33)*.

The AHCPR Guidelines on the Management of Pain Cancer endorse mind/body approaches such as those reviewed in the NIH study and promoted at alternative medicine centers *(34)*. In fact, many of the financial barriers that existed, including insurance coverage, are starting to show evidence of dissipation. Although previously difficult to imagine, some large insurance companies have started reimbursing for acupuncture, herbal medicine, and programs focusing on exercise, meditation, and diet *(35)*. Part of the appeal of such techniques to third-party payors may be reduced professional service fees. While alternative approaches can produce significant health benefits, physicians should be careful to distinguish between choices based on cost-effectiveness and insist on to what is effective and medically appropriate.

PHYSICIAN-ASSISTED SUICIDE

For some, physician-assisted suicide might be considered the ultimate admission of failure to manage pain. Others might argue that the availability of this mechanism represents a constitutional right for a terminally ill person to choose to end his or her often painful suffering. The contours of this debate are still forming, and one can expect its parameters to take on new dimensions in the next few years as courts attempt to grapple with this ethical and medical debate.

Legal Status of Concept

Case Law

Some studies indicate that the prospect of interminable unrelieved pain may prompt patients to request assistance from their physicians to end their pain through assisted suicide *(36)*. A 1996 federal appellate decision involving a Washington state statute prohibiting assistance to a person contemplating suicide eloquently addressed the legal, moral, and ethical debate behind the response of physicians to such patient requests *(37)*. Three physicians brought this case on behalf of three terminally ill patients who requested assistance in ending their pain. The physicians sought clarification of the law, since, when applied to its logical conclusion, the statute would criminalize such action by physicians. In its decision, the Ninth Circuit Court of Appeals found that an individual has a constitutionally protected liberty interest in choosing the time and place of one's death (Id at 1509).

At almost the same time that the decision in *Compassion in Dying* was published, the Second Circuit Federal Appeals Court in New York considered a similar scenario and found a prohibition against assisted suicide to be unconstitutional as applied to a physician who prescribes lethal drugs for a competent, terminally ill patient *(39)*. Unlike the Ninth Circuit, the Second Circuit did not find a substantive due process liberty interest in physician-assisted suicide. The court in *Quill* instead focused on an equal protection argument. It noted that a terminally ill person who refuses treatment is "similarly situated" to a terminally ill person who asks for a prescription of lethal drugs. It then found that criminalizing physician-assisted suicide would discriminate against terminally ill persons who are dependent on life-sustaining treatment and therefore do not have the choice of refusing treatment in order to hasten death. The US Supreme Court heard appeals on both of these cases in 1997, and reversed both federal appeals courts decisions. The Court observed that its decision should permit the earnest and profound debate about the morality, legality, and practicality of physician-assisted suicide in which our society is engaged to continue (*Vacco v. Quill* [1997] US No. 95-1858, and *Washington v. Glucksberg* [1997] US No. 96-110).

Statutes and Legislative Initiatives Concerning Physician-Assisted Suicide

Assistance (including assistance by a physician) in a suicide is criminal by statute in 35 states, criminal by common law in 8 other states and the District of Columbia, and its status is uncertain in 6 other states (Iowa, North Carolina, Ohio, Utah, Virginia, and Wyoming). In August 1996, the governor of Rhode Island signed legislation making it a felony for an individual or licensed health care professional to provide assistance or the means for another to commit suicide. The new law provides a limited exception for licensed health care professionals who administer, prescribe, or dispense medications or procedures to relieve another person's pain or discomfort, even if that medication or procedure may hasten the individual's death. The exception is only applicable as long as these medications or procedures are not knowingly administered to cause death. While state and federal courts struggle with interpreting case law and precedent on physician-assisted suicide, pending US Supreme Court review of the two federal appellate cases discussed above, one might expect more state legislatures to enact clarifying statutes on this issue.

In fact, the theme of physician-assisted suicide is not a new one: It has been an issue since the Hippocratic Oath—which technically prohibits such an action. But Greek literature was full of examples of physicians prescribing and administering drugs to hasten the death of those in pain.

Various states have recently considered the issue of physician-assisted suicide, particularly in the form of legislative initiatives. California voters narrowly rejected a legislative initiative (Proposition 161) in 1992 that would have created a mechanism allowing physician-assisted suicide in certain cases. By contrast, Oregon passed a statute in 1993 that would allow a terminally ill patient, once he or she has complied with several requirements, to request assistance from a physician to end his or her own life. To pursue this option, the patient must be diagnosed as terminally ill (i.e., less than 6 mo to live) by two independent physicians, make both oral and written requests (with specified waiting times between each request), and the physician must completely document the management of the case, the informed consent of the patient, and the absence of coercion. This initiative has not yet been implemented due to a successful court challenge by pro-life and disability activists who maintain that the initiative violates the Equal Protection clause of the 14th Amendment because it provides insufficient safeguards to protect the life and interests of those who may erroneously make a lethal medication request. The ruling, which has delayed implementation of the measure, is under appeal to the Ninth Circuit federal appeals court and may be reversed under the reasoning of *Compassion in Dying v. the State of Washington*, discussed above.

Physician Attitudes Regarding Physician-Assisted Suicide

The medical profession appears to be almost as divided as the general population on the issue of legalizing physician-assisted suicide. *The New England Journal of Medicine* conducted a survey of over one thousand physicians in Michigan and summarized the results as follows: 56% of the physicians responding favored legalization of physician-assisted suicide over an explicit ban, 37% favored an explicit ban, and 8% were uncertain *(40)*. The survey concluded that most physicians in Michigan prefer either the legalization of physician-assisted suicide or no ban at all; fewer than one-fifth prefer a complete ban on the practice. This survey has an additional interest since it was conducted in the state where Dr. Jack Kevorkian, has made his mark in this very debate. As of September 1996, Dr. Kevorkian had assisted in 41 suicides since 1990 and had been tried and acquitted three times. On July 25, 1996, Dr. Kevorkian filed a request with the US Supreme Court, asking the court to decide whether assisted suicide is a right guaranteed by the Constitution.

CONCLUSION

Physicians face a formidable challenge on the threshold of the 21st century. Advances in medical science and technology allow the medical profession to prolong life in many cases in which it was previously impossible to do so. As evidence of the profession's success in this area, life expectancies continue to increase for both men and women in industrialized countries. Having realized these advances, the medical profession must now devote equal attention to assuring that a prolonged life is worth living. In many case, making life worthwhile will require effective pain management for an individual patient.

In negotiating the course between ethical duties and legal restrictions on pain management, physicians must be aware of the federal and state bases for enforcement of laws concerning the prescribing of controlled substances, become knowledgeable about cost issues and alternative medicine, and balance all of these elements while formulating an effective pain management program.

REFERENCES

1. Stratton Hill, Jr. When will adequate pain treatment be the norm? JAMA 1995; 274:23: 1881,1882. (The author argues that both health care professionals and patients need education on effective means for treating chronic pain, which currently is woefully inadequate.)
2. Van Roenn JH et al. Physicians' attitudes and practice in cancer pain management. A survey from the Eastern Cooperative Oncology Group. Ann Intern Med 1993; 119: 121–126.
3. Foley K. The relationship of pain and symptom management to patient requests for physician-assisted suicide. J Pain Symp Mgmt 1991; 6: 5: 289–297.
4. *See* ref *1.*
5. *La Douleur.* L'Express, 23 mai 1996.
6. 21 United States Code (USC) Section 801 and following.
7. 21 USC Section 301 and following.
8. (Federal penalties under section 841 are based on the schedule classification of the involved controlled substance. Penalties for convictions involving a Schedule II controlled substance include imprisonment for as long as 20 yr plus a possible fine of up to $1 million. If a death or serious bodily injury results from the use of that Schedule II substance, imprisonment is mandated for not less than 20 yr plus the same possible fine. Punishment for convictions involving other controlled substances are as follows: Schedule III, imprisonment for not more that 5 yr and/or fine not to exceed $250,000; Schedule IV, imprisonment for not more that 3 yr and/or fine of not more than $250,000; Schedule V, imprisonment for not more than 1 yr and/or not to exceed $100,000. Fines and prison terms are generally greater for repeat offenses.)
9. Controlled Substances Act. Public Law 91-513, 84 Stat. 1242.
10. Prefatory Note for Uniform Controlled Substances Act. 1990; p. 4. (Additional information on federal restrictions concerning prescriptions for controlled substances can be found in "Physician's Manual: An Information Outline of the Controlled Substances Act of 1970" published by the US Department of Justice, Drug Enforcement Agency and periodically updated.)
11. (Section 101[19] of the that Act defines a practitioner as a physician, dentist, veterinarian, scientific investigator, pharmacist, pharmacy, or person licensed, registered or otherwise permitted to distribute, dispense, conduct research with respect to, administer, or use in teaching or chemical analysis, a controlled substance in the course of professional practice or research.)
12. (Physicians should consult their own state's medical practice acts and controlled substance schedules, since states have the option to vary which substances are in a particular schedule, and the requirements relating to substances varies according to its schedule. For example, Schedule II substances require a written prescription from the practitioner and cannot be refilled. Substances in Schedules III and IV require a written or oral prescription, must not be filled or refilled more than 6 mo after its date, or be refilled more than five times unless renewed by the practitioner. The variation in Schedule classification can also have an impact on the triplicate prescription requirements in place is some states, including California.)
13. *See* Section 202 of the 1962 Amendments to the Federal Food, Drug and Cosmetic Act. Public Law 87-871, 76 Stat. 780.

14. (California did enact, in 1990, special provisions concerning the treatment of intractable pain [California Business & Professions Code Section 2241.5]. In addition, the 1994 amendment to the Uniform Controlled Substances Act references that California statute and incorporates similar language in the model law. *See* Section 308(a),(f),(g) of the Uniform Controlled Substances Act.)

15. (These states include: New York, California, Hawaii, Illinois, Idaho, Rhode Island, Texas, Washington, Michigan, and Indiana. The requirements for California can be found in Health & Safety Code Section 11164; inpatient prescriptions are exempted from the triplicate form requirements. *See* Health and Safety Code Section 11159.)

16. (In California, for example, the original and duplicate of the prescription are submitted to the pharmacy when the prescription is filled. The pharmacy retains the duplicate and endorses and signs the original and submits it to the Department of Justice at the end of the month in which the prescription was filled. *See* California Health and Safety Code Section 11164.)

17. Medical Board of California, Division of Medical Quality. Guidelines for Expert Reviewers, June 1995; 14.

18. AHCPR. Acute Pain Management: Operative or Medical Procedures and Trauma, Publication 92-0032 (1992); and AHCPR Clinical Practice Guideline no. 9: Management of Cancer Pain, Publication 94-0592 (1994).

19. *Hoover v. Agency for Health Care Administration.* Florida District Court App. No. 95-3037, 6/26/96.

20. Medical Board of California, Division of Medical Quality. Guidelines for Expert Reviewers, June 1995; 14.

21. *Glover v. Board of Medical Quality Assurance.* (1991) 231 Cal.App.3d 203, 207,208.

22. Porter J, Jick H. Addiction rare in patients treated with narcotics. N Engl J Med, 1980; 302:123.

23. AHCPR Clinical Practice Guideline no. 9: Management of Cancer Pain, Publication 94-0592, 1994; 10–12.

24. Treatment of Intractable Pain: A Guideline, Action Report—Medical Board of California, April 1996; 57.

25. *See* ref. *24.*

26. Ferrell B. The cost of pain management. J Pain Symp Mgmt May 1994; 9, 4: 223.

27. Estimates are for 1993. *See* ref. *26.*

28. AHCPR Guidelines, Management of Cancer Pain. p. 19.

29. (The increased number of books on this subject written by physicians interested in integrating eastern and western medicine, such as those by Jon Kabat-Zinn, MD and Deepak Chopra, MD, illustrate the growing interest in this focus.)

30. Integration of behavioral and relaxation approaches into the treatment of chronic pain and insomnia. JAMA 1996; 276: 4: 313–318.

31. Cognitive behavioral techniques and biofeedback appeared to be moderately effective in relieving chronic pain. *See* ref. *30.*

32. *See* ref. *30.*

33. *See* ref. *30.*

34. AHCPR Clinical Practice Guideline no. 9: Management of Cancer Pain, 241–245.

35. Moultan K. Modern Healthcare (May 1996) 26:19:54.

36. Foley K. The relationship of pain and symptom management to patient requests for physician-assisted suicide. J Pain Symp Mgmt 1991; 6: 5: 289–297.

37. *Compassion in Dying v. State of Washington* 79 Fed.3d 790 (9th Circuit, 1996).

38. (Quite uncharacteristically for a Supreme Court justice, Anthony Scalia has already clearly stated his view against physician-assisted suicide. The Recorder [San Francisco] October 19, 1996; p. 2. It is expected that the US solicitor general will file a brief opposing physician-assisted suicide.)

39. *Quill v. Vaccaro* 80 F.3d 716 (Second Circuit, 1996).

40. Bachman J et al. Attitudes of Michigan physicians and the public towards legalizing physician-assisted suicide and voluntary euthanasia. N Engl J Med 1996; 334: 5: 303–309.

INDEX

ABOUT THE EDITORS

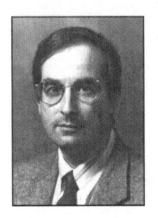

Dr. M. Eric Gershwin is the holder of the Jack and Donald Chia Endowed Chair of Medicine at the University of California at Davis School of Medicine. He graduated summa cum laude from Syracuse University with a major in zoology and received his medical degree from the Stanford University School of Medicine. Dr. Gershwin received his training in internal medicine at Tufts University and in immunology at the National Institutes of Health. He is a former Guggenheim fellow and has been chief of the Division of Allergy, Rheumatology and Clinical Immunology at the University of California since 1982. Dr. Gershwin has authored 15 books and more than 400 experimental research papers. He has received numerous honors and has lectured at more than 100 universities throughout the world.

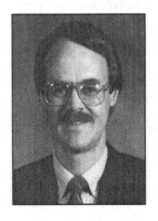

Dr. Maurice E. Hamilton is clinical professor at the University of California at Davis School of Medicine. After graduating magna cum laude from Carleton College with a major in physics, he performed graduate studies in biophysics at Stanford University. He received his medical degree from the University of California at San Diego. Dr. Hamilton was an NIH fellow in rheumatology at the University of Virginia and received his allergy training at the University of California at Davis. He was formerly on the faculty of SUNY Health Sciences Center and chief of the Division of Rheumatology at the VA Medical Center in Brooklyn. He is a fellow of the American College of Physicians, the American College of Rheumatology, and the American College of Allergy, Asthma and Immunology.